MW00527777

The Root of Chinese
Qìgōng

The Root of Chinese

Qìgōng

Secrets
for Health,
Longevity, and
Enlightenment

Dr. Yáng, Jwìng-Mǐng

YMAA Publication Center
Wolfeboro, NH USA

YMAA Publication Center
  PO Box 480
  Wolfeboro, NH, 03894
  1-800-669-8892 www.ymaa.com info@ymaa.com

Third Edition Copyright ©1989, 1997, 2022

ISBN 9781594399107 (print) • ISBN 9781594399114 (ebook) •
ISBN 9781594399121 (hardcover)

This book set in EB Garamond and Avenir.
All rights reserved including the right of reproduction in whole or in part in any form.
Copyright © 2022 by Yáng, Jwìng-Mǐng
Copyedit by Doran Hunter
Cover design by Axie Breen
Photos by YMAA Publication Center unless otherwise noted.

20220906

Publisher's Cataloging in Publication

Names: Yang, Jwing-Ming, 1946- author.

Title: The root of Chinese qìgōng = [Qi gong zhi ben] : secrets for health, longevity, & enlightenment / Dr. Yáng, Jwìng-Mǐng.

Other titles: Qi gong zhi ben.

Description: Third edition. | Wolfeboro, NH : YMAA Publication Center, [2022] | Revision of the 1997 edition. | Text in English, with some Chinese characters included. | Includes bibliographical references, translation and glossary of Chinese terms, and index.

Identifiers: ISBN: 9781594399107 (softcover) | 9781594399114 (ebook) | 978194399121 (hardcover) | LCCN: 2022936180

Subjects: LCSH: Qi gong. | Qi gong--Therapeutic use. | Qi (Chinese philosophy) | Mind and body. | Well-being. | Meditation. | Spiritual care (Medical care) | Spirituality. | Medicine, Chinese. | Holistic medicine. | BISAC: BODY, MIND & SPIRIT / Healing / Energy (Qigong, Reiki, Polarity) | BISAC: HEALTH & FITNESS / Tai Chi. | BODY, MIND & SPIRIT / Healing / Energy (Qigong, Reiki, Polarity) | PHILOSOPHY / Mind & Body. | SPORTS & RECREATION / Martial Arts / General.

Classification: LCC: RA781.8 .Y364 2022 | DDC: 613.7/1489--dc23

The authors and publisher of this material are NOT RESPONSIBLE in any manner whatsoever for any injury which may occur through reading or following the instructions in this manual.

The activities, physical or otherwise, described in this material may be too strenuous or dangerous for some people, and the reader(s) should consult a physician before engaging in them.

Neither the authors nor the publisher assumes any responsibility for the use or misuse of information contained in this book.

Figures 3-1, 3-2, 4-9, 4-10, 4-11, 6-1, 6-2, 6-3, 6-4, 9-6, 10-1, and 11-9 are used by permission from the LifeART Collection of Images © 1989-1997 by Techpool Studios, Cleveland, OH.

Printed in Canada.

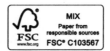

To My Brother Dr. Tim Chùn-Chíeh Yáng
楊俊杰醫師

Contents

Introduction

Qìgōng (氣功) is the science of cultivating the body's internal energy, which is called Qì (氣) in Chinese. The Chinese have been researching Qì for the last four thousand years and have found Qìgōng to be an effective way to improve health and to cure many illnesses. Most important of all, however, they have found that it can help them to achieve both mental and spiritual peace.

Until recently, Qìgōng training was usually kept secret, especially within martial arts systems or religions such as Buddhism and Daoism. Only acupuncture and some health-related Qìgōng exercises were available to the general public. During the last forty years, these secrets have become available to the general public through publications and open teaching. Medical professionals have finally been able to test Qìgōng more widely and scientifically, and they have found that it can help or cure a number of diseases that Western medicine has difficulty treating, including some forms of cancer. Many of my students and readers report that after practicing Qìgōng, they have changed from being weak to strong, from depressed to happy, and from sick to healthy.

Since Qìgōng can bring so many benefits, I feel that it is my responsibility to collect the available published documents and compile them, filter them, understand them, and introduce them to those who cannot read them in their original Chinese. It is, however, impossible for one person alone to experience and understand the fruit of four thousand years of Qìgōng research. I hope that other Qìgōng experts will share this responsibility and publish the information that they have been taught, as well as what they have learned through research and experimentation.

Even though Qìgōng has been researched in China for four thousand years, there are still many questions which can only be answered through recourse to today's technology and interdisciplinary knowledge. Contemporary, enthusiastic minds will have plenty of opportunity to research and promote the art. This is not a job that can be done through one individual's effort. It requires a group of experts, including Western-style doctors, Qìgōng experts, acupuncturists, and equipment-design specialists to sit down and work together and exchange their research results. A formal organization with adequate financial support will be needed. If this research is properly conducted, it should succeed not only in providing validation of Qìgōng for the Western mind, but it may also come up with the most efficient methods of practice. I feel certain that Qìgōng will become very popular in a short time and bring many people a healthier and happier life. This is a new field for Western science, and it will need a lot of support to catch up to the research that has already been done in China. I hope sincerely that Qìgōng science will soon become one of the major research fields in colleges and universities in this country.

Foreword

Thomas G. Gutheil, M.D.

First Edition

When Nixon opened China to the West in the 1970s, great interest was kindled in the possibilities of Americans learning many previously hidden secrets of the "inscrutable" Orient. One of the realms of exploration most eagerly awaited, particularly by Western physicians, was the science of Oriental healing: exotic practices such as acupuncture, Shiatsu massage, Tàijíquán, and the curious and puzzling notion of Qì, or vital energy. Popular magazines at the time featured arresting photographs of men and women lying calmly on operating tables, nearly disemboweled during major surgery, yet apparently requiring no more anesthesia than a few gleaming needles thrust into the skin of their foreheads.

Since these earliest dramatic harbingers, serious investigation of phenomena based on Chinese conceptualizations have both waxed and waned. Interest in Tàijíquán, for example—a form of exercise, health maintenance, and combat—has risen steadily, especially in the western United States, stimulated in part by the fact that a large part of the Chinese citizenry practices this exercise daily to apparently good effect, and in part by the fact that Tàijíquán masters, who regularly win mixed martial arts tournaments, seem to become better with age, rather than slower and weaker as do aging practitioners of other martial forms such as Gōngfū.

In contrast, after a spate of studies and articles attempting to define the physiologic bases for the generally unchallenged efficacy of acupuncture, interest in this area has waned markedly. Most early investigators tended toward the beliefs either that some form of suggestibility was involved, like that of hypnosis, another time-honored and effective anesthetic; or else that some known neural mechanism was being employed, such as "gating," where stimulation of some nerves with acupuncture needles functionally blocked impulses (presumably pain impulses) in others.

At the present time in the public mind a mixed feeling, an ambivalence, seems to hold sway, between forces of acceptance and of resistance toward these oriental concepts. To place the value of the present book in some perspective, therefore, it will be useful to understand these opposing forces.

The current forces tending toward acceptance of Chinese healing theory and practice draw from multiple origins. The first is the upsurge of interest in physical fitness. A few years ago the "high energy, high effort" fitness wave swept over the country; thousands of formerly sedentary individuals ran, jogged, danced, pumped and stretched in search of greater health and strength or, at least, an improved silhouette. Then, as many would-be athletes nursed injured or over-strained muscles, bones and joints, interest in "low-impact" exercise surfaced. Ironically, Qìgōng practices were already providing this valuable type of conditioning centuries ago. Thus, the Westerner familiar with low-impact aerobics can readily understand the value of Qìgōng forms.

A second force tending toward acceptance is the average person's awareness of the link between mind and body; the concept of psychosomatic illness—mental conditions causing physical illnesses—is familiar from the popular press, from the revelations of celebrities and from everyone's personal experience of tension headaches, stress ulcers, and the like. In a comparable fashion, some recent investigations by Herbert Benson, M.D. and others on the beneficial physical effects of mental calmness (as in the "relaxation response") have given solid support to the power of mental states to heal or harm. Thus the emphasis in Qìgōng practice on mental conditioning as a prerequisite and companion to physical improvement is not so foreign a notion at all.

On the other side of the ledger, certain factors tend to elicit resistance to these Eastern teachings and disbelief in both their relevance to modern persons and their scientific validity. One such factor is the radical interweaving in Qìgōng of what purports to be an essentially physiologic theory with philosophy and even religion or cosmology. Westerners used to partaking of their philosophy and science at separate tables may be alienated by their frank combination in Qìgōng principles.

A second factor is the absence at the present time of a "hard-science" physiology for Qì, its vessels and its actions. Some provocative preliminary findings have emerged correlating alterations in electric impedance in the skin at those points thought to be significant as acupuncture meridians and points; yet, alas, careful and replicable research with impeccable methodology has largely been lacking in this area. Instead, dubiously convincing, largely anecdotal material dominates the written works on the subject.

Another factor causing resistance is the tendency of writers in this field, following very ancient traditions and philosophical themes, to use the names of familiar body organs to describe conditions of the body related to Qì for which no other terminology exists. The Western reader becomes lost in the question of whether such phrases as "weakness of the liver" are meant to be metaphoric (that is, meaning, more literally, "a certain condition of bodily energy, otherwise indescribable, which affects those body sites which historical tradition has identified with the liver"); or whether the reader should, indeed, look to the condition of the actual liver to find some form of pathology, for which no clear picture comes to mind, since the liver performs so many different functions that "weakness" conveys nothing meaningful.

Finally, many Westerners appear to be put off by the inherently poetic and metaphoric terminology common in Chinese nomenclature for, say, types of Qì and physical exercise techniques. To pick one example, a particular stance in Shàolín style Gōngfū is called "Golden Rooster Stands on One Leg"; such flowery language can have a jarring effect on the Westerner who is accustomed to such mundane descriptions as "side deltoid stretch."

For the Westerner who can bridge the gap between Western and Oriental conceptualizations, this book (and, indeed, the planned series) offers an exceptionally valuable resource in summarizing in a clear and straightforward way the historical development of this ancient field of learning. Through his exhaustive efforts to bring together ancient and more recent

Chinese texts in this book, Dr. Yáng has performed essential services in two ways. First, by tracing the history and evolution of these concepts, the reader can gain a sense of the development of ideas whose roots reach back over the centuries—ideas which are desperately in need of just such cross-cultural illumination as this book provides. Second, Dr. Yáng is issuing a challenge to others to bring the focus of careful research to this area to provide a durable empirical basis for both theory and practice of these sciences and arts. For both of these important steps, clearly, the time has come.

Thomas G. Gutheil, M.D.
Associate Professor of Psychiatry
Harvard Medical School

Foreword

Irwin H. Rosenberg, M.D.

Second Edition

As much of the world undergoes fundamental re-evaluation of methods and goals of health care in the face of the growing wave of older citizens, there has never been such openness to expanding our concepts of treatment and health promotion. The wisdom and experience of Eastern healing traditions, accumulated and enriched over millennia, is brilliantly presented in this text on Qìgōng. These Eastern healing traditions have added to the growing recognition that proper exercise is essential to health maintenance and amelioration of disease, and have expanded the scope and definition of healing. Perhaps, most importantly in the West, we are learning humility about the limits as well as the genius of Western scientifically-based medical techniques in relation to Eastern practices and learning.

Dr. Yáng, Jwìng-Mǐng is a rare teacher/treasure who bridges the gap between Western science and the highest traditions of Eastern healing. This book on Qìgōng—literally the study, research, and practices related to Qì the energy circulating in our bodies and in the universe—is an accessible expression of the Chinese approach to the fusion of concepts of body and mind. The book is also a practical guide to the devoted trainee or practitioner of Qìgōng and Tàijíquán.

The Root of Chinese Qìgōng is an archive which will help preserve as well as expand the use of time-honored healing traditions. In both the West and East, we are in Dr. Yáng's debt for this definitive guide to better health and well-being.

Irwin H. Rosenberg, M.D.
Professor of Medicine and Nutrition
Director of The Human Nutrition Research
Center on Aging, Tufts University

Foreword

Daniel Reid

Second Edition

Qìgōng is an ancient art and science of health care and energy management that has been practiced continuously in China for at least 5,000 years. Formerly reserved exclusively for members of the imperial family and aristocracy as a secret practice for preserving health and prolonging life, and for the most advanced adepts of Daoist and Buddhist sects as a means of attaining spiritual immortality, Qìgōng has in recent years become available to the general public as a simple but profoundly effective method of self health care. While Western medical science continues to question the very existence of Qì (energy) as a factor in human health, millions of people throughout the world have already begun to experience the power of Qìgōng both for curing disease and for preventing it, as well as for enhancing overall vitality, achieving emotional and mental equilibrium, and cultivating spiritual awareness.

Modern physics has already established the fact that all matter in the universe, from atoms and molecules to planets and stars, ultimately consists of nothing more or less than energy vibrating at various frequencies and in particular patterns of relationship. That energy, which is the fundamental "stuff" of the universe is what the Chinese refer to as "Qì." Qìgōng therefore is a system whereby each and every individual may learn to work with the energies of the body, the planet, and the cosmos itself, in order to achieve the optimum state of balance and harmony upon which health and longevity depend.

The Root of Chinese Qìgōng is one of the first books to explore the nature of Qì and explain the ancient practice of Qìgōng in the light of modern science while still remaining faithful to the original Daoist principles that gave birth to this profound system of health care and spiritual cultivation. Indeed, the author has clearly demonstrated that Qìgōng is based entirely on scientific principles of energy that were known to the ancient Daoist masters who developed it long before Einstein first informed Western science that energy and matter are relative and transmutable elements.

Dr. Yáng, Jwìng-Mǐng is uniquely qualified to explore the topic of Qìgōng in terms of Western thought. Backed by over thirty years of personal experience as both a practitioner and teacher of Qìgōng, trained in classical forms by traditional masters in Táiwān, and the founder of a school in America that transmits this ancient practice to contemporary Western students, Dr. Yáng has gained full command of both the classical Daoist principles and the modern science concepts required to elucidate this traditional Chinese practice in a way that is meaningful to contemporary readers without a prior background in Chinese studies. What distinguishes *The Root of Chinese Qìgōng* from so many other books that have appeared in recent years on the same subject is the scientific validity he bestows on the principles of Qìgōng practice, the simplicity and clarity of language used to present the traditional ideas involved, and the concurrent adherence to the original spirit, or "root" of Qìgōng in ancient China.

The West has long given lip service to the idea of imposing "mind over matter" but has never developed an effective method whereby this goal may be accomplished. That's because Western thought divided body and mind into two mutually exclusive realms. Matters of the body were approached either chemically or mechanically, while the mind became the domain of religion and later psychology. Traditional Eastern thought has always cited a third, pivotal element in the human system, and that element is energy, known as prana in ancient India, and Qì in China. Qì is the bridge that links body and mind into an integrated and functional system, and it is the medium through which the mind may gain command over the body. The method whereby the medium of energy may be utilized to gain control over the body is Qìgōng, or "energy-work."

According to the Daoist tradition of China, the Three Treasures of life are essence (the essential secretions of the body), energy (the vital energies that animate the body and may be controlled by proper breathing), and spirit (awareness, intent, and the various facilities of the mind). When these three aspects of existence are brought into balance and harmony, the health of the entire organism is protected and life prolonged. Qìgōng is the fulcrum of balance between the body and mind, with energy serving as the common force upon which both depend. Energy is also the medium through which the powers of nature and the cosmos enter and influence the human system, and Qìgōng provides a way whereby the practitioner may synchronize his or her system in order to harness those powers to promote human health and support human life.

For those who are interested in learning the basic concepts and practical applications of Qìgōng as a means of cultivating health and longevity, *The Root of Chinese Qìgōng* provides an excellent and comprehensive overview on the subject, a view that will no doubt awaken the reader's mind to the importance of energy as the most fundamental fact of life.

Daniel Reid
Author of *The Complete Book of
Chinese Health & Healing,
The Tao of Health, Sex, and Longevity,*
and *Chinese Herbal Medicine*

Preface

First Edition, as published 1989

Since my first Qìgōng book *Chì Kūng: Health and Martial Arts* appeared, I have received many compliments and thank-you's, as well as numerous questions, and many valuable suggestions from doctors, readers with medical problems, and the general public. This has led me to believe that my introductory book has opened the door to Qìgōng for many people and has brought health benefits to more than a few. This response has encouraged me to continue my research and publishing. However, most of my Qìgōng experience and knowledge was obtained through my Tàijíquán and Shàolín practice, and was therefore limited to a few Daoist and Buddhist Qìgōng exercises, as well as some of the common Qìgōng exercises which are popular in China. Because of this limitation in my Qìgōng knowledge, I have spent a lot of time analyzing, researching, pondering, and experimenting with many other Qìgōng styles about which I have read in my collection of Qìgōng documents. This research has greatly increased my knowledge.

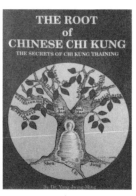

First edition, as published in 1989.

In August of 1986 I had a chance to go back to Táiwān to visit my family. This visit also gave me the opportunity to see what Qìgōng documents had been published since I left Táiwān in 1974. To my surprise, there are a great many new publications available. I was so happy to learn that many documents had been published which described training techniques heretofore kept secret. With my brother's encouragement and financial support, I was able to purchase all of the expensive documents which I found worthwhile. Once I returned to the United States, I started to read and study them, and to experiment with some of the methods. These documents made me realize how limited my knowledge was, and opened up a whole new field of Qìgōng study for me.

In my excitement and enthusiasm I decided to compile them, filter out the parts which seemed questionable, and introduce the results to my readers. An unfortunate problem arose in that most of the documents explain what to do, but do not explain why, and some will even just tell the process without explaining how to do it. Despite the obstacles, I decided to try my best, through research and contemplation, to determine the secrets of the techniques.

After two years of research and experimentation, I feel that it will take at least five years and eight volumes of introductory books to initiate the reader into the broad field of Chinese Qìgōng. Although these eight volumes will be based on the documents available to me, they will not be direct translations of these documents, except for the ancient poetry or songs which are the root of the training. This approach is necessary simply because these documents do not have any systematic introduction or way of tying everything together. What I can do is read them and study them carefully. Then I can compile and organize the information, and discuss it carefully in the light of my own Qìgōng knowledge and experience.

This approach will allow me to cautiously bring long-concealed Qìgōng knowledge to the reader. The only thing lacking is the experience. Many of the methods require more than twenty years of training to complete, and I would have to spend more than three lifetimes studying the various methods before I could discuss them with authority. I realize that it is impossible for me alone to introduce the results of four thousand years of Qìgōng research with these eight books, but I would still like to share the knowledge which I have gained from these documents, and the conclusions which I have drawn from my training. Please take these books in the tentative spirit in which they are written, and not as a final authority or bible. I sincerely hope that many other Qìgōng experts will step forward and share the traditional teachings which were passed down to them, as well as the fruits of their experience.

At present, the following books are planned:

1. *The Root of Chinese Qìgōng—Secrets for Health, Longevity, and Enlightenment*
2. *Muscle/Tendon Changing and Marrow/Brain Washing Qìgōng—The Secret of Youth* (*Yìjīnjīng* and *Xǐsuǐjīng*, 易筋經、洗髓經) (published, new title: *Qìgōng—The Secret of Youth*, by YMAA Publication Center)
3. *Qìgōng Massage—Fundamental Techniques for Health and Relaxation* (Qìgōng Ànmó and Qìgōng Diǎnxuè, 氣功按摩、氣功點穴) (published by YMAA Publication Center)
4. *Qìgōng and Health—For Healing and Maintaining Health* (published by YMAA Publication Center)
5. *Qìgōng and Martial Arts—The Key to Advanced Martial Arts Skill* (Shàolín, Wǔdāng, Éméi, and others) (published, new title: *The Essence of Shàolín White Crane*, by YMAA Publication Center)
6. *Buddhist Qìgōng—Chǎn, the Root of Zěn* (禪)
7. *Daoist Qìgōng* (*Dāndǐng Dàogōng*, 丹鼎道功)
8. *Tibetan Qìgōng* (*Mìzàng Shéngōng*, 密藏神功)

In this first volume we will discuss the roots of Chinese Qìgōng by dividing them into four parts. The first part will introduce the history of Qìgōng, the basic concepts and terminology commonly used in Qìgōng society and documents, the different Qìgōng categories, and the relationship between Qì and the human body, and fundamental Qìgōng training theory and principles. This first part will give you a general concept of what Qìgōng is and the various subjects that it includes. The second part will discuss the general keys to Qìgōng training and give you the foundation of knowledge necessary for successful practice. This part serves as a map of the what and the how of Qìgōng training, so that you can choose your goal and the best way to get there. The third part will review the Qì circulatory system in your body, which includes the twelve primary Qì channels and the eight extraordinary Qì vessels. This part will give you a better understanding of how Qì circulates in your body.

Finally, the fourth part of the book will list some of the many questions about Qìgōng that remain unanswered.

The second volume in this series will cover Yìjīn and Xǐsuǐ Qìgōng (易筋經、洗髓經氣功), which are translated as "Muscle/Tendon Changing" and "Marrow/Brain Washing Qìgōng." Marrow/Brain Washing is deep, and difficult to understand. It has been found in documents detailing both Buddhist and Daoist Qìgōng and meditation training, and it has been known in China since the Liáng dynasty (梁朝), more than fourteen hundred years ago. Because, however, the training usually involves stimulation of the sexual organs, it has traditionally been passed down only to a few trusted students.

In addition to the eight in-depth books, YMAA is also introducing a series of instructional books and videotapes on specific Qìgōng exercise sets. This series is designed for people who want to learn exercises that they can do on their own to improve or maintain their health. These books and videos will be easy to understand both in theory and in practice. The first book and tape are on the Eight Pieces of Brocade (Bāduànjǐn, 八段錦), one of China's most popular Qìgōng sets.

Preface

Second Edition, as published 1997

Since 1989, when this book was first introduced to the public, more than thirty thousand copies have been sold. This is better than I originally expected. The reason for this is simply because the subject of Qìgōng was still very new to Western readers, even though it has been studied and practiced in China, Japan, and India for many thousands of years. Therefore, the market is very small and restricted to those already interested in Chinese culture. In addition, this book is considered to be an in-depth theoretical treatise on Qìgōng. It is like a piece of classical music, instead of rock music, which can be understood and accepted easily by the general society.

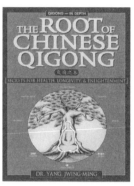

Second edition, as published in 1997.

Qìgōng today, like Tàijíquán in the early 1980s, is being understood and welcomed in the West. I believe that there are a few reasons for this. First, since President Nixon visited mainland China in 1973 and opened the gates to the nation, there has been more and more culture exchange between China and the West. The Western world has a better understanding of Chinese culture. This has agitated and stimulated many Westerners to take an interest in Chinese culture, study it, and accept it. Second, Chinese acupuncture and Qìgōng healing techniques have been widely accepted. Alternative medicine, as it was originally called, is now considered to be "complementary medicine." Finally, the general public is more open minded, and the bondage of tradition, especially religious tradition, has been reduced to its lowest point ever. This open-minded attitude has generated great interest in foreign cultures.

Since 1989, I have written and published ten more books and fifteen videotapes to introduce Chinese culture to the Western society. YOAA, Inc. (Yáng's Oriental Arts Association, Inc.) was established to expedite this cultural exchange. YMAA Publication Center is the division that handles the publications. In addition, YMAA has also established more than thirty schools and three publication centers in Europe to translate these books into non-English languages. Currently, many YMAA books have been translated into French, Italian, Spanish, Polish, Hungarian, Bulgarian, Russian, and Czech.

In 1989 when this book was written, I had a dream of introducing in-depth Qìgōng books to the West. The books I wanted to write include:

1. *The Root of Chinese Qìgōng—Secrets for Health, Longevity, and Enlightenment*
2. *Qìgōng—The Secret of Youth (Dámó's Muscle/Tendon Changing and Marrow/Brain Washing Classics) (Yìjīnjīng and Xǐsuǐjīng, 易筋經、洗髓經)*
3. *Qìgōng Massage—Fundamental Techniques for Health and Relaxation (Qìgōng Ànmó and Qìgōng Diǎnxuè, 氣功按摩、氣功點穴)*
4. *Qìgōng for Health & Martial Arts: Exercises and Meditation*

5. *Qìgōng and Martial Arts—The Key to Advanced Martial Arts Skill* (Shàolín, Wǔdāng, Éméi, and others) (new title: *The Essence of Shàolín White Crane*, by YMAA Publication Center)
6. *Buddhist Qìgōng—Chǎn, the Root of Zěn* (禪)
7. *Daoist Qìgōng* (Dāndǐng Dàogōng, 丹鼎道功)
8. *Tibetan Qìgōng* (Mìzàng Shéngōng, 密藏神功)

This is the first of those books. The second, *Muscle/Tendon Changing and Marrow/ Brain Washing Chì Kūng* (new title: *Qìgōng—The Secret of Youth*), was also published in 1989. The first half of the *Chinese Qìgōng Massage, General Massage* was published in 1992. The second half, about Tuīná, Diǎnxuè, and Qì massage, is still being written. *Qìgōng and Health* has not yet been started. *Qìgōng and Martial Arts* has been written under the title *The Essence of Shàolín White Crane*, which was published in 1996. *Buddhist Qìgōng* and *Tibetan Qìgōng* have not yet been started. Currently, I am working on *Daoist Qìgōng*, which will be published as two new titles: *Small Circulation Meditation* and *Grand Circulation and Enlightenment Meditation*. I plan to complete these two volumes by 1999. The writing process is slow and time consuming. This is especially significant since almost all of the Qìgōng documents were released to the general public in the last ten years, both in China and Táiwān. This has provided me with ten-fold the amount of information. Naturally, this has also offered me a greater chance to make the future books more complete and in-depth.

There is another reason for the slow progress. The market for the in-depth books, especially those that relate to inner Qìgōng feelings and spiritual cultivation, is very limited. In order to prevent any financial difficulty in the publication business, I have also put a lot of time and effort into writing other smaller introductory books for Qìgōng healing and martial arts. As I pointed out in the original preface, the translation and interpretation of the Qìgōng from Chinese to English is not easy. We will need an organization that has strong financial support and many Qìgōng experts to do the job. I will just try my best to contribute what I can. I sincerely hope that the government, universities, or private organizations will sponsor this project to expedite this Qìgōng cultural exchange.

In this new edition, some new concepts have been added and some old concepts have been deleted. Not only that, for those readers who understand, the Chinese characters are immediately included in the text when the Chinese is mentioned. In addition, when this book was written, the Chinese romanization system called Pinyin was not yet popular. Therefore, an older system was used. However, Pinyin is now widely used in the West in both scholastic and lay societies, so this book follows the Pinyin romanization system. In addition, new typesetting has been done to make this book easier to read. Finally, the glossary and translation of Chinese terms have been combined, and an index has been added.

Dr. Yáng, Jwìng-Mǐng
Boston, January 15, 1997

Publisher's Note on the 3rd Edition

This 3rd edition includes pinyin with tonal marks, a new Chinese character font (Biau-Kai), and selected illustration enhancements.

An important contribution to this new edition is the use of tonal marks on the pinyin. Pinyin is the current standard for Romanizing Chinese characters so they can be read by non-Chinese speaking readers. By adding tonal marks to the Romanized Chinese words (pinyin), we can have a guide for properly pronouncing these words.

Before we can begin learning how to pronounce pinyin words, we must recognize some common differences in how some letters sound.[1]

ü Start pronouncing "ee" in English and then round your lips to pronounce "oo".
q Pronounced like "ch" in chin.
x Pronounced like a blend of "she" and "he".
z Pronounced like "ds" in kids.
c Pronounced like "ts" in bats.
zh Pronounced like "ger" in germ.
ch Pronounced like "chur" in church.
sh Pronounced like "sur" in sure.
er Pronounced like "ar" in are.
i When i follows z, c, s, it sounds like "zz": zzz, czz, szz.
   When i follows zh, ch, sh, r, it sounds like "rr": zhrr, chrr, shrr, rrr.

There are primarily four tonal categories written in pinyin.[2]
   1. mā 媽 (mom). Begins high and stays high.
   2. má 麻 (hemp). Begins at mid-range and ends high.
   3. mǎ 馬 (horse). Begins mid-range, dips low, ends mid-range.
   4. mà 罵 (scold). Begins high and ends low.

There are many websites offering guides for the pronunciation of Chinese words and how to interpret and pronounce pinyin words with the tonal marks. We encourage readers to explore these valuable online tools. Some are provided below for your reference.

https://dictionary.hantrainerpro.com/
https://en.wikipedia.org/wiki/Pinyin
https://ymaa.com/publishing/spoken-chinese-glossary

---

1.   https://www.mandarintutor.com/resources/pinyinintro
2.   https://www.duchinese.net/blog/learn-to-read-chinese-tones/

PART ONE

General Introduction

CHAPTER 1

Introduction

1-1. PRELUDE (XÙYÁN, 序言)

In their seven thousand years of history, the Chinese people have experienced all possible human suffering and pain. Chinese culture is like a very old man who has seen and experienced all of the pain of human life. Yet through his experience, he has also accumulated a great store of knowledge. Chinese culture, as reflected in its literature and painting, ranks among the greatest achievements of the human spirit. It reflects humankind's joy and grief, pleasure and suffering, peace and strife, vitality, sickness, and death.

Within this complex cultural and historical background, the Chinese people have long sought ways of living healthy and happy lives. However, as they looked for ways to better themselves and seek spiritual fulfillment, they have also tended to believe that everything that happens is due to destiny and that it is prearranged by heaven. Despite this fatalistic belief, they have still looked for ways to resist the apparent inevitability of sickness and death.

The Chinese have devoted a large part of their intellectual effort to self-study and self-cultivation in the hope of understanding the meaning of their lives. This inward-feeling and looking, this spiritual searching, has become one of the major roots of Chinese religion and medical science. Qì, the energy within the human body, was studied very carefully. As people perceived the link between the Qì in the human body and the Qì in nature, they began to hope that this Qì was the means whereby man could escape from the trap of sickness and death. Over the years, many different sectors of Chinese society have studied and researched Qì.

Of all the researchers, the scholars and the doctors have had the longest history, and they have brought the understanding of Qì to a very deep level. It was they who learned the methods of maintaining health and curing sickness. Chinese medical science has developed out of the Qì research of the physicians.

When Indian Buddhism was imported into China, it profoundly influenced Chinese culture. Naturally, Chinese Qìgōng was also affected by the Buddhist meditative practices. The Daoist religion (Dàojiào, 道教) was created out of a mixture of traditional scholarly Daoism (Dàoxué, 道學) and Buddhism (Fóxué, 佛學). Since that time, Buddhist and Daoist Qìgōng have been considered among the greatest achievements of Chinese culture.

Daoism and Buddhism have not only brought the Chinese people a peaceful, spiritual mind which may untie the mystery of human life and destiny, they have also created a hope that the development of Qìgōng may give people a healthy and happy life while they are alive and an eternal spiritual life after death. When viewed from this historical background, it is not hard to understand why a major part of Chinese culture in the last two thousand years, other than warfare and possibly medical science, were based on the religions of Daoism and Buddhism, and spiritual science.

The emphasis on the spiritual life, rather than the material, is one of the major differences between Eastern and the Western cultures. An example of this is in the maintenance of health, where the West emphasizes the physical body more, while the East tends to also treat the person's spiritual and mental health.

Most Westerners believe that if you strengthen your physical body, you also improve your health. They emphasize the exercising and training of the physical body, but they ignore the balancing of the body's internal energy (Qì), which is also related to the emotions and the cultivation of spiritual calmness. Daoists call this "Cóngwài Jiàngōng" (從外健功) (building the strength externally) or "Yuǎnxīn Zhī Wàigōng Yùndòng" (遠心之外功運動) (distant mind's external exercises, meaning "external exercises without mental concentration or attention").

People who exercise a lot and whose bodies are externally strong are not necessarily healthier or happier than the average person. In order to have true good health you must have a healthy body, a healthy mind, and also smooth and balanced Qì circulation. According to Chinese medicine, many illnesses are caused by imbalances in your mind. For example, worry and nervousness can upset your stomach or harm your spleen.[1] Fear or fright can hinder the normal functioning of your kidneys and bladder. This is because your internal energy (Qì circulation) is closely related to your mind. In order to be truly healthy, you must have both a healthy physical body and a calm and healthy mind. True good health is both external and internal.

When someone gets involved in body building, he will emphasize building strong muscles. According to acupuncture and Qìgōng theory, he will also energize his body, stimulate his mind, and increase the level of the Qì circulation. If he trains properly, he will naturally gain physical health. However, if he exercises too much, he will over-energize his body and over-excite his mind and Qì. This will make his physical body too Yáng (positive). According to Chinese philosophy, too much of something is excessive Yáng (陽) and too little is excessive Yīn (陰), and neither extreme is desirable. When your body is too Yáng or too Yīn, your internal organs will tend to weaken and to degenerate sooner than they ordinarily would. A person who seems to be externally strong and healthy may be weak internally.

---

1. When Chinese medicine refers to an organ, such as the spleen, kidney, or bladder, they are not necessarily referring to the physical organ, but rather to a system of functions which are related to the organ.

In addition, when a body builder gets older, his over-stressed muscle fibers may lose their elasticity and degenerate faster than those of the average person. This causes the Qì to stagnate in the Qì channels. This phenomenon is well known among older practitioners of external martial arts, where it is called Sàngōng (散功), meaning "energy dispersion." The proper amount of exercise will generate only enough Qì to stimulate the organs and help them function normally and healthily. Overdoing exercise is like getting too much sunshine, which we now know will cause your skin cells to degenerate faster than the lack of sun.

Qìgōng practitioners believe that in order to gain real health you must not only do external exercises but must also "Cóngnèi Zhújī" (從內築基) ("build the foundation internally"), or do "Xiàngxīn Zhī Nèigōng Yùndòng" (向心之內功運動) (literally "toward the mind's internal exercise," meaning internal exercise with mental concentration). Strengthening yourself internally and externally at the same time is called "Xìngmìng Shuāngxiū" (性命雙修). Xìng means natural characteristics, personality, temperament, or disposition. It is shown internally. Mìng is life and refers to the life or death of the physical body. Shuāngxiū means dual cultivation. The expression therefore means that if you desire to gain real health, you must cultivate your character internally and strengthen your body both internally and externally. The internal side is approached through meditation and Qìgōng exercises.

Many people believe that Qìgōng is a product only of China, India, or other Oriental countries. As a matter of fact, internal energy cultivation has also been common in the Western world, usually within the context of religion. Many people have been able to find their internal foundation and strength through meditation or praying in their church, temple, or mosque. Through their devotions and the practice of prayer, they are able to build up their concentration, confidence, and will, all of which are prerequisites to internal strength. The practice of such disciplines allows the energy in the body to become balanced, bringing health and strength to some, and even, in some cases, seemingly supernatural powers. Jesus is credited with many miracles, but he told his disciples, "He that believeth on me, the works that I do, shall he do also, and greater works than these shall he do" (John 14:12). All of the major Western religions have had branches or sects that used practices similar to the Oriental Qìgōng disciplines.

However, there have also been people without any particular religious belief who have meditated by themselves and, through the buildup and circulation of Qì, developed psychic or healing abilities. Unfortunately, in earlier times such people were often killed as witches or heretics, so people who found they had such powers tended to view themselves as freaks or worse, and hid their powers. These negative attitudes only kept people from researching and understanding such abilities.

Many people in China and India have developed amazing powers through their meditation training. Fortunately, these powers were understood as being a result of Qìgōng, and so people were encouraged to train and research the subject. Although Qìgōng is becoming a more acceptable subject in the West, the Chinese and Indians are still way ahead in this internal mental and physical science.

Since 1973, acupuncture has been widely accepted by the American people, and even by many in the medical establishment. More and more people are becoming familiar with the concept of Qì. Qì-related arts such as Tàijíquán and Qìgōng exercises are getting much more attention than ever before. Many people are learning that the study of Qì can be very beneficial, and I feel certain that in the next twenty years Qìgōng will become one of the hottest fields of research.

1-2. General Definition of Qì and Qìgōng (Qì Yǔ Qìgōng De Yībān Dìngyì, 氣與氣功的一般定義)

Before we define Qì and Qìgōng, you should understand that so far, there is no one scientific definition of Qì that is accepted generally by Qìgōng practitioners and Chinese medical society. The way people define Qì varies depending upon their individual background and experience. Some people think Qì is an electric energy, others believe that it is a magnetic energy, and many others believe that Qì is heat or some other type of energy. However, anyone who has carefully researched the historical background of Qì would not define it by any one of these narrow definitions.

It is the same with Qìgōng. Qìgōng is often narrowly thought of as only exercises or meditations that can be used to improve one's health or to cure sickness. In fact, however, the range of Qìgōng and the scope of its research is much wider. You should understand this point so you will be able to view Qì and Qìgōng in an accurate and open way.

In this section we will discuss the general definition of Qì and Qìgōng. Specific terms concerning Qì and Qìgōng that are directly related to the human body will be discussed later in a separate section.

General Definition of Qì (Qì Zhī Yībān Dìngyì, 氣之一般定義)

Qì is the energy or natural force that fills the universe. Heaven (the sky or universe) has Heaven Qì (Tiānqì, 天氣), which is made up of the forces that the heavenly bodies exert on the earth, such as sunshine, moonlight, and the moon's effect on the tides. In ancient times, the Chinese believed that it was Heaven Qì that controlled the weather, climate, and natural disasters. In China, the weather is still referred to as Tiānqì (Heaven Qì). Every energy field strives to stay in balance, so whenever the Heaven Qì loses its balance, it tries to rebalance itself. Then the wind must blow, rain must fall, even tornadoes or hurricanes must happen in order for the Heaven Qì to reach a new energy balance.

Under Heaven Qì, which is the most important of the three, is Earth Qì (Dìqì, 地氣). It is influenced and controlled by Heaven Qì. For example, too much rain will force a river to flood or change its path. Without rain, the plants will die. The Chinese believe that Earth Qì is made up of lines and patterns of energy, as well as the earth's magnetic field and the heat concealed underground. These energies must also balance, otherwise disasters such as earthquakes will occur. When the Qì of the earth is balanced, plants will grow and animals thrive.

Finally, within the Earth Qì, each individual person, animal, and plant has its own Qì field, which always seeks to be balanced. When any individual thing loses its Qì balance, it will sicken, die, and decompose. All natural things, including man, grow within and are influenced by the natural cycles of Heaven Qì and Earth Qì. Human Qì (Rénqì, 人氣) is usually considered a separate type of Qì, different from the Qì of the earth, and of plants and animals. The reason for this is simply that because we are human, we are particularly concerned with Human Qì, and have devoted a great deal of study to it.

Qì can be generally defined as any type of energy that is able to demonstrate power and strength. This energy can be electricity, magnetism, heat, or light. In China, electric power is called Diànqì (Electric Qì, 電氣), and heat is called Rèqì (Heat Qì, 熱氣). When a person is alive, his body's energy is called Rénqì (Human Qì, 人氣).

Qì is also commonly used to express the energy state of something, especially living things. As mentioned before, the weather is called Tiānqì (Heaven Qì) because it indicates the energy state of the heavens. When a thing is alive it has Huóqì" (Vital Qì, 活氣), and when it is dead it has Sǐqì (Dead Qì, 死氣) or "Guǐqì" (Ghost Qì, 鬼氣). When a person is righteous and has the spiritual strength to do good, he is said to have Zhèngqì (Normal Qì or Righteous Qì, 正氣). The spiritual state or morale of an army is called Qìshì (energy state, 氣勢).

You can see that the word Qì has a wider and more general definition than most people think. It does not refer only to the energy circulating in the human body. Furthermore, the word "Qì" can represent the energy itself, and it can also be used to express the manner or state of the energy. It is important to understand this when you practice Qìgōng, so that your mind is not channeled into a narrow understanding of Qì, which would limit your future understanding and development.

General Definition of Qìgōng (Qìgōng Zhī Yībān Dìngyì, 氣功之一般定義)

We have explained that Qì is energy, and that it is found in the heavens, in the earth, and in every living thing. In China, the word "Gōng" is often used instead of "Gōngfū," which means energy and time. Any study or training which requires a lot of energy and time to learn or to accomplish is "Gōngfū" (功夫). The term can be applied to any special skill or study as long as it requires time, energy, and patience. Therefore, the correct definition of Qìgōng is any training or study dealing with Qì which takes a long time and a lot of effort.

The Chinese have studied Qì for thousands of years. Some of the information on the patterns and cycles of nature has been recorded in books, one of which is the *Yìjīng* (*Book of Changes*, 易經) (1122 BCE). When the *Yìjīng* was introduced to the Chinese people, they believed that natural power included Tiān (Heaven, 天), Dì (Earth, 地), and Rén (Man, 人). These are called Sāncái (The Three Natural Powers, 三才) and are manifested by the three Qì's: Heaven Qì, Earth Qì, and Human Qì (Figure 1-1). These three facets of nature have their definite rules and cycles. The rules never change, and the cycles repeat periodically. The Chinese people used an understanding of these natural principles and the *Yìjīng* to calculate the changes of Natural Qì. This calculation is called Bāguà (the Eight Trigrams, 八卦). From the Eight Trigrams are derived the Sixty-Four Hexagrams. Therefore, the *Yìjīng* was probably the first book that taught the Chinese people about Qì and its variations in nature

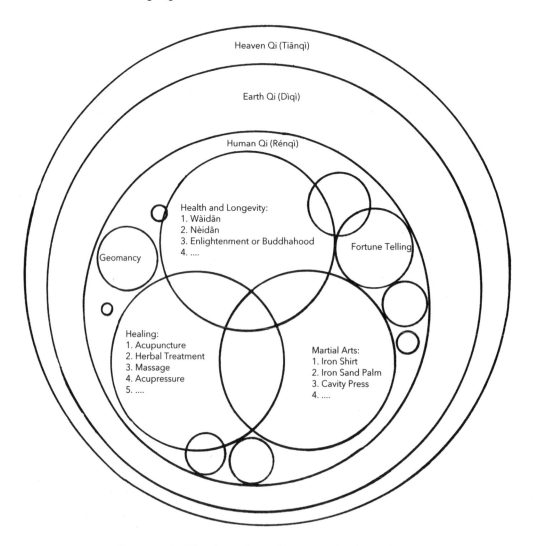

Figure 1-1. The three Qì's of Heaven, Earth, and Man

and man. The relationship of the Three Natural Powers and their Qì variations were later discussed extensively in the book *Qìhuàlùn* (*Theory of Qì's Variation*, 氣化論).

Understanding Heaven Qì is very difficult, however, and it was especially so in ancient times when the science was just developing. But since nature is always repeating itself, the experience accumulated over the years has made it possible to trace the natural patterns. Understanding the rules and cycles of "Tiānshí" (heavenly timing, 天時) will help you to understand natural changes of the seasons, climate, weather, rain, snow, drought, and all other natural occurrences. If you observe carefully, you will be able to see many of these routine patterns and cycles caused by the rebalancing of the Qì fields. Among the natural cycles are those of the day, the month, and the year, as well as cycles of twelve years and sixty years.

Earth Qì is a part of Heaven Qì. If you can understand the rules and the structure of the earth, you will be able to understand how mountains and rivers are formed, how plants grow, how rivers move, what part of the country is best for someone, where to build a house and which direction it should face so that it is a healthy place to live, and many other things related to the earth. In China today there are people, called "geomancy teachers" (Dìlǐshī, 地理師) or "wind water teachers" (Fēngshuǐshī, 風水師), who make their living this way. The term Fēngshuǐ (風水) is commonly used because the location and character of the wind and water in a landscape are the most important factors in evaluating a location. These experts use the accumulated body of geomantic knowledge and the *Yìjīng* to help people make important decisions such as where and how to build a house, where to bury their dead, and how to rearrange or redecorate homes and offices so that they are better places to live and work in. Many people even believe that setting up a store or business according to the guidance of Fēngshuǐ (風水) can make it more prosperous.

Among the three Qì's, Human Qì is probably the one studied most thoroughly. The study of Human Qì covers a large number of different subjects. The Chinese people believe that Human Qì is affected and controlled by Heaven Qì and Earth Qì, and that they in fact determine your destiny. Therefore, if you understand the relationship between nature and people, in addition to understanding human relations (Rénshì, 人事), you will be able to predict wars, the destiny of a country, or a person's desires and temperament and even his future. The people who practice this profession are called Suànmìngshī (calculate life teachers, 算命師).

However, the greatest achievement in the study of Human Qì is in regard to health and longevity. Since Qì is the source of life, if you understand how Qì functions and know how to regulate it correctly, you should be able to live a long and healthy life. Remember that you are part of nature, and you are channeled into the cycles of nature. If you go against this natural cycle, you may become sick, so it is in your best interests to follow the way of nature. This is the meaning of "Dào" (道), which can be translated as "The Natural Way."

Many different aspects of Human Qì have been researched, including acupuncture, acupressure, herbal treatment, meditation, and Qìgōng exercises. The use of acupuncture, acupressure, and herbal treatment to adjust Human Qì flow has become the root of Chinese medical science. Meditation and moving Qìgōng exercises are used widely by the Chinese people to improve their health or even to cure certain illnesses. Meditation and Qìgōng exercises serve an additional role in that Daoists and Buddhists use them in their spiritual pursuit of enlightenment.

You can see that the study of any of the aspects of Qì including Heaven Qì, Earth Qì, and Human Qì should be called "Qìgōng." However, since the term is usually used today only in reference to the cultivation of Human Qì through meditation and exercises, we will only use it in this narrower sense to avoid confusion.

Before we finish this section, we would like to discuss one more thing. The word Nèigōng (內功) is often used, especially in Chinese martial society. "Nèi" means "internal" and "Gōng" means "Gōngfū." Nèigōng means "internal Gōngfū," as opposed to Wàigōng (外功), which means "external Gōngfū." Nèigōng is martial arts training, existing in all Chinese martial styles, which trains Qì internally and manifests it in external actions. Typical Chinese martial styles that focus on internal training first and then manifest it externally are "internal styles" (Nèijiā, 內家) such as Tàijíquán (太極拳), Liùhé Bāfǎ (六合八法), Bāguàzhang (八卦掌), and Xíngyìquán (形意拳). In contrast to internal styles, external styles (Wàijiā, 外家) emphasize developing the muscles' strength first and then applying it to the martial techniques. Then, they train Qì's strength internally so their martial power can be manifested to a higher level. Typical Wàigōng martial styles are: Praying Mantis (Tángláng, 螳螂), Tiger Claw (Hǔzhǎo, 虎爪), Eagle (Yīngzhǎo, 鷹爪), White Crane (Báihè, 白鶴), Dragon (Lóngxíng, 龍形), and so on. Many of the external styles originated in the Shàolín Temple.

1-3. ABOUT THIS BOOK (GUĀNYÚ ZHÈ BĚNSHŪ, 關於這本書)

I hope this book will lay down a theoretical foundation that interested Qìgōng practitioners can use in their training. Hopefully this book can explain to you the How, Why, and What of Qìgōng, and help you to avoid being confused and misled.

It is extremely difficult to write a book that covers more than four thousand years of study and research, especially since a large portion of the knowledge was kept secret until the last forty years. Even though the study of Qìgōng has reached very high, there are still many questions that must be answered through recourse to today's technology and interdisciplinary knowledge. Contemporary, enthusiastic minds will have plenty of opportunity to research and promote the art.

One of the major purposes of this book is to stimulate Western scholars and medical society to get involved with and study this newly revealed science. Hopefully other Qìgōng experts will be encouraged to share their knowledge with the public. I believe that in a short time Qìgōng will reach new and exciting heights in the Western world. This would be one of the greatest cross-cultural achievements since East and West opened their doors to each other.

Most available documents are not systematically organized and do not explain the subject very well. As I compile them and try to explain them in a logical and scientific way, I must use my own judgment, and I must explain them based on my personal Qìgōng background and my understanding of the documents. It is impossible for one person alone to do justice to this enormous field. You are encouraged to question everything stated in this text, and to always remember that many conclusions come from my own judgment. The main purpose of this book is to lead you to the path of study—it is not meant to be the final authority.

When you read this book, it is important that you keep your mind open and let go of your habitual ways of thinking. When we find ourselves in a new environment or start studying something new, it is human nature to view the new from the standpoint of what we have already learned. Unfortunately, this tends to make us conservative and narrow minded. This is commonly seen in tourists who visit another country but judge the local customs and behavior according to their own country's standards. This usually leads to a lot of confusion and misunderstanding. If, however, you try to understand other people according to their own culture and historical background, you will have a much better chance of understanding their behavior. Please do this when you start studying this science of Qìgōng. If you keep your mind open and try to understand it according to its historical background, you will find it a fascinating and challenging subject.

It is true that it is very hard to break from tradition. In many old cultures, tradition must be obeyed absolutely. If anyone is against the tradition, he is considered a traitor to the culture. However, the correct approach to research and study involves questioning tradition and proving its inaccuracies through the use of modern thought and technology. This is especially necessary in regard to ancient sciences that were developed before the last century. New study will allow us to prove and establish their accuracy. You should understand that this is not a form of betrayal. It is our responsibility to prove the truth and bring facts to light.

Many of the theories that have been passed down were based upon many years of experience. Regardless of how you modify a theory, the fact is, it is still the root of the entire science. Therefore, the correct approach to study and research involves respect and study of the past. From this respect and study, you will be able to find the root of the entire science. If you forget this root, which has been growing for thousands of years, you are studying only the branches and flowers.

You should judge this inner science of Qìgōng in a logical and scientific manner. Of course, the words "logic" and "scientific" are not absolute terms. They are relative to the science and understanding we possess. Remember, though, that although science has been developing for thousands of years, it was only in the last hundred years or so that it suddenly began to swell in the width and depth of its understanding. We can be sure, therefore, that our understanding today is still in its infancy. There are many facts and phenomena that cannot be explained by today's science. Therefore, when you read about this new inner science, be logical and scientific, yet don't reject explanations that lie outside of what you presently accept as true. What is accepted as true in a few years may be quite different from what we now accept.

All sciences were developed from daring assumptions that were then proven by careful experimentation. The results we get from our experiments allow us to modify our assumptions and to create new experiments that explore our new hypotheses. This process enables us to develop a complete theory and determine what next needs to be studied.

It is the same with Qìgōng practice. If you look and study carefully, you will see that, although many of the Qì-related theories were proven accurate and have been widely used in China, there are still many questions that still need to be answered.

During the course of study you must be patient and persevering. Strong will, patience, and perseverance are the three main components of success. This is especially true in Qìgōng training. Your will and wisdom must be able to dominate and conquer your emotional laziness. I believe that a person's success depends on his attitude toward life and his moral character, rather than his wisdom and intelligence. We've all known people who were wise, yet ended up losers. They may be smart, and they pick things up more quickly than other people, but they soon lose interest. If they don't persevere, they stop learning and growing, and they never achieve their goals. They never realize that success demands moral virtues, and not just wisdom. A person who is truly wise knows that he must develop the other requirements for success.

In addition, a person who is truly wise will know when to start and when to stop. Many opportunities to succeed are lost by people who are too proud of their intelligence. There is a Chinese story about a group of people who competed in a snake-drawing contest. One man completed his drawing of a snake faster than anybody else. He was very proud of himself, and he thought, "I'm so fast I could even draw four legs on the snake and still win!" So he drew the legs on, but when the judge chose the winner, it was somebody else. The man was very upset and asked the judge why he didn't win; after all, he had finished before everyone else. The judge said: "You were supposed to draw a snake. Since snakes don't have legs, what you drew was not a snake." So, as smart as the man was, he didn't have the sense to know when to stop.

A person who is really wise understands that real success depends not only on his wisdom but also on his moral character. Therefore, he will also cultivate his moral character and develop his good personality. Confucius said: "A man who is really wise knows what he knows and also knows what he does not know."[2] Too often, people who are smart become satisfied with their accomplishments and lose their humility. They feel that they know enough, and so they stop learning and growing. In the long run they will only lose. Remember the story of the tortoise and the hare. If the rabbit had not been so proud and satisfied, he would not have lost the race.

Once you understand what has been passed down to you, you should be creative. Naturally, this creativity must be under one condition: that you must understand the old way clearly and thoroughly. Only after you understand the old knowledge to a deep level will your mind be qualified to think, "What if...?" Then you will be able to come up with good ideas for further study and research. If all Qìgōng practitioners only practice the old ways and never search for new ones, the science of Qìgōng will stagnate at its current level. In that case, we will have lost the real meaning of and attitude toward learning.

This book is the most fundamental of the YMAA Qìgōng book series. It offers you the foundation of knowledge and training practices required to understand subsequent YMAA Qìgōng books. This book consists of four major parts. The first part will briefly summarize Qìgōng history, explain the necessary Qìgōng terminology, and discuss the major Qìgōng categories. The second part will discuss the theory and major keys to Qìgōng training. This will enable the Qìgōng beginner to enter the door to the Qìgōng garden and will offer the experienced practitioner a directory to the various types of Qìgōng. The third part will review the Qì channels and vessels to help you understand the Qì circulatory system in the human body. Finally, the fourth part will conclude the discussion in this book and list some of the many questions I have about Qìgōng.

---

2. 孔子曰：〝知之為知之，不知為不知，是智也。〞

CHAPTER 2
History of Qìgōng

The history of Chinese Qìgōng can be roughly divided into four periods. We know little about the first period, which is considered to have started when the *Yìjīng* (*Book of Changes*, 易經) was introduced sometime before 1122 BCE and to have extended until the Hàn dynasty (206 BCE, 漢) when Buddhism and its meditation methods were imported from India. This infusion brought Qìgōng practice and meditation into the second period, the religious Qìgōng era. This period lasted until the Liáng dynasty (502–557 CE, 梁), when it was discovered that Qìgōng could be used for martial purposes. This was the beginning of the third period, that of martial Qìgōng. Many different martial Qìgōng styles were created based on the theories and principles of Buddhist and Daoist Qìgōng. This period lasted until the overthrow of the Qīng dynasty (清) in 1911, when the new era started in which Chinese Qìgōng training is being mixed with Qìgōng practices from India, Japan, and many other countries.

2-1. BEFORE THE HÀN DYNASTY (BEFORE 206 BCE) (HÀNQIÁN, 漢前)

The *Yìjīng* (*Book of Changes,* 易經) (1122 BCE) was probably the first Chinese book related to Qì. It introduced the concept of the three natural energies or powers (Sāncái, 三才): Tiān (Heaven, 天), Dì (Earth, 地), and Rén (Man, 人). Studying the relationship of these three natural powers was the first step in the development of Qìgōng.

In 1766–1154 BCE (the Shāng dynasty, 商), the Chinese capital was in today's Ānyáng in Hénán province (河南、安陽). An archaeological dig there at a late Shāng dynasty burial ground called Yīnxū (殷墟) discovered more than 160,000 pieces of turtle shell and animal bone that were covered with written characters. This writing, called "Jiǎgǔwén" ("Oracle-Bone Scripture," 甲骨文), was the earliest evidence of the Chinese use of the written word. Most of the information recorded was of a religious nature. There was no mention of acupuncture or other medical knowledge, even though it was recorded in the *Nèijīng* (內經) that during the reign of the Yellow Emperor (2690–2590 BCE, 黃帝) Biānshí (stone probes, 砭石) were already being used to adjust people's Qì circulation. The archaeologists did, however, discover stones at the dig that they believed were Biānshí (Figure 2-1).

During the Zhōu dynasty (1122–934 BCE, 周), Lǎozi (老子; or Lǐěr, 李耳) mentioned certain breathing techniques in his classic *Dào Dé Jīng* (*Classic on the Virtue of the Dào,* 道德經). He stressed that the way to obtain health was to "concentrate on Qì and

13

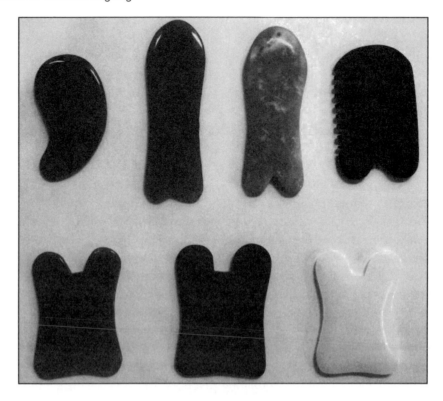

Figure 2-1. Acupuncture stone probes (Biānshí)

achieve softness" (Zhuānqì Zhìróu, 專氣致柔). Later, *Shǐjì* (*Historical Record*, 史記) also described more complete methods of breath training. About 300 BCE the Daoist philosopher Zhuāngzi (莊子) described the relationship between health and the breath in his book *Nánhuájīng* (南華經). It states: "The real person's (i.e., immortal's) breathing reaches down to their heels. The normal person's breathing in the throat."[1] This suggests that a breathing method for Qì circulation was already being used by some Daoists at that time.

During the Qín and Hàn dynasties (221 BCE–220 CE, 秦，漢), there are several medical references to Qìgōng in the literature, such as the *Nànjīng* (*Classic on Disorders*, 難經) by the famous physician Biǎnquè (扁鵲), which describes using breathing to increase Qì circulation. *Jīnguì Yàolüè* (*Prescriptions from the Golden Chamber*, 金匱要略) by Zhāng, Zhòng-Jīng (張仲景) discusses the use of breathing and acupuncture to maintain good Qì flow. *Zhōuyì Cāntóngqì* (a comparative study of the Zhōu (dynasty) *Book of Changes*, 周易 參同契) by Wèi, Bó-Yáng (魏伯陽) explains the relationship of human beings to nature's forces and Qì. It can be seen from this list that up to this time, almost all of the Qìgōng publications were written by scholars such as Lǎozi (老子) and Zhuāngzi (莊子), or physicians such as Biǎnquè (扁鵲) and Wèi, Bó-Yáng (魏伯陽).

1.　莊子曰：〝真人之息以踵，眾人之息以喉。〞

Let us conclude with a few important points about Qìgōng in this period:

1. Historical documents for this period are scarce today, and it is difficult to obtain detailed information, especially about Qìgōng training.
2. There were two major types of Qìgōng training. One type was used by the Confucian and Daoist scholars, who used it primarily to maintain their health. The other type of Qìgōng was for medical purposes, using needles or exercises to adjust the Qì or to cure illness.
3. There was almost no religious color to the training.
4. All of the training focused on following the natural way and improving and maintaining health. Actively countering the effects of nature was considered impossible.

2-2. FROM THE HÀN DYNASTY TO THE BEGINNING OF THE LIÁNG DYNASTY (206 BCE–502 CE) (HÀN ZHÌ LIÁNGCHŪ, 漢至梁初)

Because many Hàn emperors were intelligent and wise, the Hàn dynasty was a glorious and peaceful period. It was during the Eastern Hàn dynasty (ca. 58 CE, 東漢) that Buddhism was imported to China from India. The Hàn emperor became a sincere Buddhist; Buddhism soon spread and became very popular. Many Buddhist meditation and Qìgōng practices, which had been practiced in India for thousands of years, were absorbed into the Chinese culture. The Buddhist temples taught many Qìgōng practices, especially the still meditation of Chán (Rěn, 禪，忍), which marked a new era of Chinese Qìgōng. Much of the deeper Qìgōng theory and practices that had been developed in India were brought to China. Unfortunately, since the training was directed at attaining Buddhahood, the training practices and theory were recorded in the Buddhist bibles and kept secret. For hundreds of years the religious Qìgōng training was never taught to laymen. Only in the last century has it been available to the general populace.

Not long after Buddhism had been imported into China, a Daoist by the name of Zhāng, Dào-Líng (張道陵) combined the traditional Daoist principles with Buddhism and created a religion called "Dàojiào" (道教). Many of the meditation methods were a combination of the principles and training methods of both sources.

Since Tibet had developed its own branch of Buddhism with its own training system and methods of attaining Buddhahood, Tibetan Buddhists were also invited to China to preach. In time, their practices were also absorbed.

It was in this period that the traditional Chinese Qìgōng practitioners finally had a chance to compare their arts with the religious Qìgōng practices imported mainly from India. While the scholarly and medical Qìgōng had been concerned with maintaining and improving health, the newly imported religious Qìgōng was concerned with far more. Contemporary documents and Qìgōng styles show clearly that the religious practitioners trained their Qì to a much deeper level, working with many internal functions of the body, and strove to obtain control of their bodies, minds, and spirits with the goal of escaping from the cycle of reincarnation.

While the Qìgōng practices and meditations were being passed down secretly within the monasteries, traditional scholars and physicians continued their Qìgōng research. During the Jìn dynasty (晉) in the 3rd century CE, a famous physician named Huátuó (華陀) used acupuncture for anesthesia in surgery. The Daoist Jūnqiàn (君倩) used the movements of animals to create the Wǔqínxì (Five Animal Sports, 五禽戲), which taught people how to increase their Qì circulation through specific movements (some say that the Wǔqínxì was created by Huátuó). Also, in this period a physician named Gé, Hóng (葛洪) mentioned, in his book *Bàopǔzi* (抱朴子), using the mind to lead and increase Qì. Sometime in the period of 420 to 581 CE, Táo, Hóng-Jǐng (陶弘景) compiled the *Yǎngxìng Yánmìng Lù* (*Records of Cultivating Temperament and Extending Life*, 養性延命錄), which showed many Qìgōng techniques.

Characteristics of Qìgōng during this period were:

1. There were three schools of religious Qìgōng that influenced and dominated the Qìgōng practice in this period. These are Indian Buddhism, Tibetan Buddhism, and Daoism.
2. Almost all of the religious Qìgōng practices were kept secret within the monasteries.
3. Religious Qìgōng training worked to escape from the cycle of reincarnation.
4. Relatively speaking, religious Qìgōng theory is deeper than the theory of the non-religious Qìgōng, and the training is harder.
5. Qì circulation theory was better understood by this time, so the Qìgōng sets created in this period seem to be more efficient than the older sets.

2-3. FROM THE LIÁNG DYNASTY TO THE END OF THE QĪNG DYNASTY (502–1911 CE) (LIÁNG ZHÌ QĪNGMÒ, 梁至清末)

During the Liáng dynasty (502–557 CE, 梁), the emperor invited a Buddhist monk named Dámó (達摩), who was once an Indian prince, to preach Buddhism in China. The emperor decided he did not like Dámó's Buddhist theory, so the monk withdrew to the Shàolín Temple (少林寺). When Dámó arrived, he saw that the priests were weak and sickly, so he shut himself away to ponder the problem. He emerged after nine years of seclusion and wrote two classics: *Yìjīnjīng* (*Muscle/Tendon Changing Classic*, 易筋經) and *Xǐsuǐjīng* (*Marrow/Brain Washing Classic*, 洗髓經). *The Muscle/Tendon Changing Classic* taught the priests how to gain health and change their physical bodies from weak to strong. The *Marrow/Brain Washing Classic* taught the priests how to use Qì to clean the bone marrow and strengthen the blood and immune system, as well as how to energize the brain and attain enlightenment. Because the *Marrow/Brain Washing Classic* was harder to understand and practice, the training methods were passed down secretly to only a very few disciples in each generation.

After the priests practiced the Muscle/Tendon Changing exercises, they found that not only did they improve their health, but they also greatly increased their strength. When this training was integrated into the martial arts forms, it increased the effectiveness of their techniques. In addition to this martial Qìgōng training, the Shàolín priests also created five animal styles of Gōngfū that imitated the way different animals fight. The animals imitated were the tiger (Hǔxíng, 虎形), leopard (Bàoxíng, 豹形), dragon (Lóngxíng, 龍形), snake (Shéxíng, 蛇形), and crane (Hèxíng, 鶴形).

Outside of the monastery, the development of Qìgōng continued during the Suí and Táng dynasties (581–907 CE, 隋，唐). Cháo, Yuán-Fāng (巢元方) compiled the *Zhūbìng Yuánhòu Lùn* (*Thesis on the Origins and Symptoms of Various Diseases*, 諸病源候論), which is a veritable encyclopedia of Qìgōng methods, listing 260 different ways of increasing the Qì flow. The *Qiānjīnfāng* (*Thousand Gold Prescriptions*, 千金方) by Sūn, Sī-Miǎo (孫思邈) described the method of leading Qì, and also described the use of the Six Sounds. The Buddhists and Daoists had already been using the Six Sounds to regulate Qì in the internal organs for some time. Sūn, Sī-Miǎo also introduced a massage system called Lǎozi's Forty-Nine Massage Techniques. *Wàitái Mìyào* (*The Extra Important Secret*, 外台祕要) by Wáng, Táo (王燾) discussed the use of breathing and herbal therapies for disorders of Qì circulation.

During the Sòng, Jīn, and Yuán dynasties (960–1368 CE, 宋，金，元), *Yǎngshēngjué* (*Life Nourishing Secrets*, 養生訣) by Zhāng, Ān-Dào (張安道) discussed several Qìgōng practices. *Rúmén Shìshì* (*The Confucian Point of View*, 儒門視事) by Zhāng, Zi-Hé (張子和) describes the use of Qìgōng to cure external injuries such as cuts and sprains. *Lánshì Mìcáng* (*Secret Library of the Orchid Room*, 蘭室祕藏) by Lǐ, Guǒ (李果) describes using Qìgōng and herbal remedies for internal disorders. *Gézhì Yúlùn* (*A Further Thesis of Complete Study*, 格致餘論) by Zhū, Dān-Xī (朱丹溪) provided a theoretical explanation for the use of Qìgōng in curing disease.

During the Sòng dynasty (960–1279 CE, 宋), Zhāng, Sān-Fēng (張三豐) is believed to have created Tàijíquán (or Tài Chí Chuán, 太極拳). Tàijíquán followed a different approach in its use of Qìgōng than did Shàolín (少林). While Shàolín emphasized Wàidān (External Elixir, 外丹) Qìgōng exercises, Tàijíquán emphasized Nèidān (Internal Elixir, 內丹) Qìgōng training.

In 1026 CE the famous brass man of acupuncture was designed and built by Dr. Wáng, Wéi-Yī (王唯一). Before that time, the many publications that discussed acupuncture theory, principles, and treatment techniques disagreed with each other and left many points unclear. When Dr. Wáng built his brass man, he also wrote a book called *Tóngrén Yúxuè Zhēnjiǔ Tú* (*Illustration of the Brass Man Acupuncture and Moxibustion*, 銅人俞穴鍼灸圖). He explained the relationship of the twelve organs and the twelve Qì channels, clarified many of the points of confusion, and, for the first time, systematically organized acupuncture theory and principles.

In 1034 CE, Dr. Wáng used acupuncture to cure the emperor Rénzōng (仁宗). With the support of the emperor, acupuncture flourished. In order to encourage acupuncture medical research, the emperor built a temple to Biǎnquè, who wrote the *Nànjīng* and worshiped him as the ancestor of acupuncture. Acupuncture technology developed so much that even the Jīn (金) race in the distant north requested the brass man and other acupuncture technology as a condition for peace. Between 1102 to 1106 CE, Dr. Wáng dissected the bodies of prisoners and added more information to the *Nànjīng*. His work contributed greatly to the advancement of Qìgōng and Chinese medicine by giving a clear and systematic idea of the circulation of Qì in the human body.

Later, in the Southern Sòng dynasty (1127–1279 CE, 南宋), Marshal Yuè, Fēi (岳飛) was credited with creating several internal Qìgōng exercises and martial arts. It is said that he created Bāduànjǐn (the Eight Pieces of Brocade, 八段錦) to improve the health of his soldiers. He is also known as the creator of the internal martial style Xíngyìquán (形意拳). Eagle-style martial artists also claim that Yuè, Fēi was the creator of their style.

From then until the end of the Qīng dynasty (1911 CE, 清), many other Qìgōng styles were founded. The well-known ones include Hǔbùgōng (Tiger Step Gōng, 虎步功), Shíèrzhuāng (Twelve Postures, 十二庄) and Jiàohuāgōng (Beggar Gōng, 叫化功). Also in this period, many documents related to Qìgōng were published, such as *Bǎoshēn Mìyào* (*The Secret Important Document of Body Protection*, 保身秘要) by Cáo, Yuán-Bái (曹元白), which described moving and stationary Qìgōng practices; and *Yǎngshēng Fūyǔ* (*Brief Introduction to Nourishing the Body*, 養生膚語) by Chén, Jì-Rú (陳繼儒), about the three treasures: Jīng (essence, 精), Qì (internal energy, 氣), and Shén (spirit, 神). Also, *Yìfāng Jíjiě* (*The Total Introduction to Medical Prescriptions*, 醫方集解) by Wāng, Áng (汪昂) reviewed and summarized the previously published materials; and *Nèigōng Túshuō* (*Illustrated Explanation of Nèigōng*, 內功圖說) by Wáng, Zǔ-Yuán (王祖源) presented the Twelve Pieces of Brocade (Shíèr Duànjǐn, 十二段錦) and explained the idea of combining both moving and stationary Qìgōng.

In the late Míng dynasty (ca. 1640 CE, 明), a martial Qìgōng style, Huǒlónggōng (Fire Dragon Gōng, 火龍功), was created by the Tàiyáng martial stylists (太陽宗). The Well-known internal martial art style Bāguàzhang (Eight Trigrams Palm, 八卦掌) is believed to have been created by Dǒng, Hǎi-Chuān (董海川) late in the Qīng dynasty (1644–1911 CE, 清). This style is now gaining in popularity throughout the world.

During the Qīng dynasty, Tibetan meditation and martial techniques became widespread in China for the first time. This was due to the encouragement and interest of the Manchurian emperors in the royal palace, as well as others of high rank in society.

Characteristics of Qìgōng during this period were:

1. Qìgōng was adapted into the martial arts, and martial Qìgōng styles were created.
2. Qì circulation theory and acupuncture reached a peak. More documents were published about medical Qìgōng than the other categories of Qìgōng exercises.
3. Religious Qìgōng practice remained secret.
4. Qìgōng exercises had become more popular in Chinese society.

2-4. FROM THE END OF THE QĪNG DYNASTY TO THE PRESENT (QĪNGMÒ ZHÌJĪN, 清末至今)

Before 1911 CE, Chinese society was still very conservative and old-fashioned. Even though China had been expanding its contact with the outside world for the previous hundred years, the outside world had little influence beyond the coastal regions. With the overthrow of the Qīng dynasty in 1911 and the founding of the Chinese republic, the nation began changing as never before. Since this time, Qìgōng practice has entered a new era. Because of the ease of communication in the modern world, Western culture now has great influence on the Orient. Many Chinese have opened their minds and changed their traditional ideas, especially in Táiwān (台灣) and Hong Kong (Xiānggǎng, 香港). Various Qìgōng styles are now being taught openly, and many formerly secret documents have been published. Modern methods of communication have opened up Qìgōng to a much wider audience than ever before, and people now have the opportunity to study and understand many different styles. In addition, people are now able to compare Chinese Qìgōng to similar arts from other countries such as India, Japan, Korea, and the Middle East.

I believe that in the near future Qìgōng will be considered the most exciting and challenging field of research. It is an ancient science just waiting to be investigated with the help of the new technologies now being developed at an almost explosive rate. Anything we can do to speed up this research will greatly help humanity to understand and improve itself.

CHAPTER 3
Basic Concepts of Qìgōng

There are a number of special terms that are commonly used by Qìgōng practitioners and are found in the documents that have been passed down from generation to generation. Since most of these terms are key words that will help you to grasp the basic concepts of Qìgōng practice, it is important that you understand their real meaning. In this chapter we will discuss the major terms which are directly related to Qìgōng training. Other terms will be discussed in the appendix.

3-1. THE THREE TREASURES—JĪNG, QÌ, AND SHÉN (SĀNBĚN-JĪNG, QÌ, SHÉN, 三本-精、氣、神)

Understanding Jīng (essence, 精), Qì (internal energy, 氣), and Shén (spirit, 神) is one of the most important requirements for effective Qìgōng training. They are the root of your life and therefore also the root of Qìgōng practice. Jīng, Qì, and Shén are called "Sānbǎo" (三寶), which means "The Three Treasures," "Sānyuán" (三元), which means "The Three Origins," or "Sānběn" (三本), which means "The Three Foundations." In Qìgōng training, a practitioner learns how to "firm his Jīng" (Gùjīng, 固精; Gù means to firm, solidify, retain, and conserve) and how to convert it into Qì. This is called "Liànjīng Huàqì" (煉精化氣), which means "to refine the Jīng and convert it into Qì." Then he learns how to lead the Qì to the head to convert it into Shén (also called nourishing Shén). This is called "Liànqì Huàshén" (煉氣化神), which means "to refine the Qì and convert it into (nourish) the Shén." Finally, the practitioner learns to use his energized Shén to govern the emotional part of his personality. This is called "Liànshén Liǎoxìng" (煉神了性), or "to refine the Shén to end human (emotional) nature."

These conversion processes are what enable you to gain health and longevity. As a Qìgōng practitioner, you must pay a great deal of attention to these three elements during the course of your training. If you keep these three elements strong and healthy, you will live a long and healthy life. If you neglect or abuse them, you will be sick frequently and will age fast. Each one of these three elements or treasures has its own root. You must know the roots so that you can strengthen and protect your three treasures.

Jīng (精)

The Chinese word Jīng means a number of things depending on where, when, and how it is used. Jīng can be used as a verb, an adjective, or a noun. When it is used as a verb, it means "to refine." For example, to refine or purify a liquid to a high quality is called "Jīngliàn" (精煉). When it is used as an adjective, it is used to describe or signify something which is "refined," "polished," and "pure without mixture." For example, when a piece of art work is well done, people say "Jīngxì" (精細), which means "delicate and painstaking" (literally, "pure and fine"), or "Jīngliàng" (精良), which means "excellent quality" (literally "pure and good"). When Jīng is used to apply to personal wisdom or personality, it means "keen" and "sharp." For example, when someone is smart or wise, they are called "Jīngmíng" (精明), which means "keen and clever." When Jīng is applied to a thought, it means "profound" or "astute," and indicates that the idea or plan was well and carefully considered. When used as a noun for an object, Jīng means "the essence" or "the essentials." When it is used for the energy side of a being, it means "spirit" or "ghost." Since Chinese people believe that the male sperm or semen is the refined and the most essential product of a man, Jīng also means sperm or semen.

When Jīng is used as "essence," it exists in everything. Jīng may be considered the primal substance or original source from which a thing is made, and which exhibits the true nature of that thing. When Jīng is used in reference to animals or humans, it means the very original and essential source of life and growth. This Jīng is the origin of the Shén (spirit) that makes an animal different from a tree. In humans, Jīng is passed down from the parents. Sperm is called "Jīngzǐ" (精子), which means "the sons of essence." When this essence is mixed with the mother's Jīng (egg), a new life is generated which is, in certain fundamental respects, an intertwining of the Jīngs of both parents. The child is formed, the Qì circulates, and the Shén grows. The Jīng that has been carried over from the parents is called "Yuánjīng" (元精), which means "Original Essence."

Once you are born, Original Jīng is the fountainhead and root of your life. It is what enables you to grow stronger and bigger. After your birth you start to absorb the Jīng of food and air, converting these Jīngs into the Qì which supplies your body's needs. You should understand that when Jīng is mentioned in Qìgōng society, it refers usually to Yuánjīng (Original Jīng, 元精). Qìgōng practitioners believe that Original Jīng is the most important part of you, because it is the root of your body's Qì and Shén. The amount and quality of Original Jīng is different from person to person, and it is affected significantly by your parents' health and living habits while they were creating you. Generally speaking, it does not matter how much Original Jīng you have carried over from your parents. If you know how to conserve it, you will have more than enough for your lifetime. According to Chinese medicine, you probably cannot increase the amount of Jīng you have. It is believed, however, that Qìgōng training can improve its quality.

In Qìgōng training, knowing how to conserve and firm your Original Jīng is of primary importance. To conserve means to refrain from abusing your Original Jīng through overuse.

For example, if you overindulge in sexual activity, you will lose Original Jīng faster than other people and your body will degenerate faster. To firm your Jīng means to keep and protect it. For example, you should know how to keep your kidneys strong. Kidneys are thought of as the residence of Original Jīng. When your kidneys are strong, the Original Jīng will be kept firm and will not be lost without reason. The firming of your Original Jīng is called "Gùjīng" (固精), which is translated "to make solid, to firm the essence." Only after you know how to retain (meaning, to conserve and firm) your Original Jīng can you start seeking ways to improve its quality. Therefore, conserving and firming your Jīng is the first step in training. In order to know how to conserve and firm your Jīng, you must first know the root of your Jīng, where the Original Jīng resides and how Original Jīng is converted into Qì.

As mentioned, the root of your Original Jīng before your birth is in your parents. After birth, this Original Jīng stays in its residence, the kidneys, which are now also its root. When you keep this root strong, you will have plenty of Original Jīng to supply to your body.

If you look carefully at how you were formed, you can gain interesting insights into life. You started as one sperm which, because it managed to reach and penetrate the egg before any of the other millions of sperm could, was one of the strongest and luckiest sperm alive. Once this sperm entered the egg, one human cell formed and then started to divide, from one to two, and from two to four. Finally, the baby formed. All of the baby's health depended on the sperm and egg that were generated from the Jīng of the parents. As the baby was being formed it was immersed in liquid, and it received all of its nutrition and oxygen from the mother through the umbilical cord. Notice that the umbilical cord connects at the navel, which is very close to both the Dāntián (丹田) and your body's center of gravity. The umbilical cord is very long, and because it is hard for the mother alone to push the necessary supplies to the baby, the baby needs to help. The baby must draw the nutrients to itself with an in-and-out pumping motion of its abdomen.

Once you are born, you start taking in oxygen through your nose and food through your mouth. Since you no longer need the abdominal motion to pump in nutrients, it gradually stops, and, finally, you forget how to use it. In Qìgōng, the Lower Dāntián (Xià Dāntián, 下丹田) or abdomen is still considered the original Qì source because it is here that Qì is made from the Original Jīng that you inherited from your parents.

According to Chinese medical and Qìgōng society, the Original Jīng you obtained from your parents stays in your kidneys after your birth. This Original Jīng is the source of your life and growth. This Original Jīng is converted continuously into Qì, which moves into the Lower Dāntián and stays stored there in its residence for future use. The Dāntián is located on the Conception Vessel—one of the eight Qì "reservoirs" in the body which regulate the Qì flow in the other Qì channels (this will be discussed further in Part Three). Dāntiánqì is considered "Water Qì" (Shuǐqì, 水氣) and is able to cool down the "Fire Qì" (Huǒqì, 火氣) generated from the Jīng of food and air and that resides at the Middle Dāntián.

As you may realize from the above discussion, if you wish to stay strong and healthy, you must first conserve your Original Jīng. Remember that Original Jīng is like the principal in your savings account in that it is an original investment that will continue to return interest as long as it is conserved. Jīng can produce Qì, so if you handle this Jīng carefully, you will continue to have Jīng and Qì. However, if you abuse yourself with an unhealthy lifestyle, you may damage and reduce your Original Jīng.

In order to conserve your Jīng, you must first control your sexual activity. The gonads are called the "external kidneys" (Wàishèn, 外腎) in Chinese medical society. This is because Chinese doctors believe that sperm is a product of Original Jīng and the Jīng from food and air. The more ejaculations you have, the faster you will exhaust your Original Jīng, and the shorter your life will be.

Please understand that the Chinese doctors and Qìgōng practitioners are not saying that in order to conserve your Jīng, you must stop your sexual activity completely. As a matter of fact, they encourage the proper amount of sexual activity, believing that it will energize and activate the Jīng, which makes the Jīng-Qì conversion more efficient. Remember, Jīng is like fuel, and Qì is like the energy generated from this fuel. The more efficiently you can convert your fuel into energy, the less you will waste.

In addition, the proper amount of sexual activity will energize the Qì so that it nourishes the Shén (spirit). This will help you stay mentally balanced and raise your Shén. It is very important to keep your Shén raised, otherwise you will tend to get depressed and will be afraid to face life. It is very hard to define how much sex is the proper amount. It depends on the individual's age and state of health. According to Qìgōng, the Jīng that resides in the external kidneys (gonads) is the main source of the Qì that fills up the four major Qì vessels in the legs. These four Qì reservoirs (vessels) keep the legs strong and healthy. Therefore, if you feel that your legs are weak due to the amount of sexual activity, you have lost too much of your Jīng.

The second thing you must do in order to conserve your Original Jīng is to prevent your Original Qì from leaking out of your body. There are two acupuncture cavities called "Shènshū" (B-23, 腎俞) or "Jīngmén" (Essence Doors, 精門). These two cavities are the doors through which the kidneys communicate with the outside, and they are used to regulate the Qì production in the kidneys. When Qì is converted from Original Jīng, most of it moves forward to the Dāntián. However, some Qì is lost backward through the Kidney Doors. If you lose too much Qì, your Jīng will be depleted as you try to make up for the loss. In Qìgōng practice, one of the major training goals is to learn how to lead the converted Qì from the kidneys to the Dāntián more efficiently.

Qì (氣)

Since we have already discussed Qì at the beginning of this chapter in general terms, we will now discuss Qì in the human body and in Qìgōng training. Before we start, we would like to point out one important thing. At this time, there is no clear explanation of the relationship between all of the circulatory systems and the Qì circulatory system. The Western world knows of the blood system, nervous system, and lymphatic system. Now, there is the Qì circulation system from China. How are, for example, the Qì and the nervous system related? If the nervous system does not match the Qì system, where does the sensing energy in the nervous system come from? How is the lymphatic system related to the Qì system? All of these questions are still waiting for study by modern scientific methods and technology. Here, we can only offer you some theoretical assumptions based on the research conducted up to now.

Chinese medical society believes that the Qì and blood are closely related. Where Qì goes, blood follows. That is why "Qìxuě" (Qì Blood, 氣血) is commonly used in Chinese medical texts. It is believed that Qì provides the energy for the blood cells to keep them alive. As a matter of fact, it is believed that blood is able to store Qì, and that it helps to transport Air Qi especially to every cell of the body.

If you look carefully, you can see that the elements of your physical body such as the organs, nerves, blood, and even every tiny cell are all like separate machines, each with their own unique function. Just like electric motors, if there is no current in them, they are dead. If you compare the routes of the blood circulatory system, the nervous system, and the lymphatic system with the course of the Qì channels, you will see that there is a great deal of correspondence. This is simply because Qì is the energy needed to keep them all alive and functioning.

Now, let us look at your entire body. Your body is composed of two major parts. The first part is your physical body, and the second is the energy supply your body needs to function. Your body is like a factory. Inside your body are many organs, which correspond to the machines required to process the raw materials into the finished product. Some of the raw materials brought into a factory are used to create the energy with which other raw materials will be converted into finished goods. The raw materials for your body are food and air, and the finished product is life.

The Qì in your body is analogous to the electric current that the factory power plant obtains from coal or oil. The factory has many wires connecting the power plant to the machines and other wires connecting telephones, intercoms, and computers. There are also many conveyer belts, elevators, wagons, and trucks to move material from one place to another. It is no different in your body where there are systems of intestines, blood vessels, complex networks of nerves, and Qì channels to facilitate the supply of blood, sensory information, and energy to the entire body. However, unlike the digestive, circulatory, and central nervous systems—all of whose supportive vessels can be observed as material structures in the body—Qì channels are non-material and cannot be observed as physical objects. The circulatory, nervous, and Qì systems all possess similar configurations within the body and are distributed rather equally throughout the body.

In a factory, different machines require different levels of current. It is the same for your organs, which require different levels of Qì. If a machine is supplied with an improper level of power, it will not function normally and may even be damaged. In the same way, your organs, when the Qì level running to them is either too positive or too negative, will be damaged and will degenerate more rapidly. The ancient Chinese character for Qì (炁) was formed of two words. On the top is the word "nothing" (无) and at the bottom is the word "fire" (灬). This implies that Qì is "no fire." That means that when the organs are supplied with the proper amount of Qì, they will not be overheated and "on fire."

In order for a factory to function smoothly and productively, it will not only need high quality machines, but also a reliable power supply. The same goes for your body. The quality of your organs is largely dependent upon what you inherited from your parents. To maintain your organs in a healthy state and to ensure that they function well for a long time, you must have an appropriate Qì supply. If you don't have it, you will become sick.

Qì is affected by the quality of air you inhale, the kind of food you eat, your lifestyle, and even your emotional make-up and personality. The food and air are like the fuel or power supply, and their quality affects you. Your lifestyle is like the way you run the machine, and your personality is like the management of the factory.

The above discussion clarifies the role Qì plays in your body. However, it should be noted that the above metaphor is an oversimplification, and that the behavior and function of Qì is much more complex and difficult to handle than the power supply in a factory. You are neither a factory nor a robot; you are a human being with feelings and emotions. Unfortunately, your feelings have a major influence on your Qì circulation. For example, when you pinch yourself, the Qì in that area will be disturbed. This Qì disturbance will be sensed through the nervous system and interpreted by your brain as pain. No machine can do this. Moreover, after you have felt the pain, unlike a machine, you will react either as a result of instinct or conscious thought. Human feelings and thought affect Qì circulation in the body, whereas a machine cannot influence its power supply. In order to understand your Qì, you must use your feelings, rather than just the intellect, to sense its flow and make judgments about it.

Now a few words as to the source of Human Qì. As mentioned, Chinese doctors and Qìgōng practitioners believe that the body contains two general types of Qì. The first type is called "Pre-birth Qì" or "Original Qì" (Yuánqì, 元氣). Original Qì is also called "Xiāntiānqì" (先天氣) which, translated literally, means "Pre-heavenly Qì." Heaven here means the sky, so preheaven means before the baby sees the sky. In other words, before birth. Original Qì comes from converted Original Jīng which you received before your birth. This is why Original Qì is also called "Pre-birth Qì."

The second type is called "Post-birth Qì" or "Hòutiānqì" (後天氣), which means "Post-heaven Qì." This Qì is drawn from the Jīng (i.e., essence) of the food and air we take in. The residence of the Post-birth Qì is the Middle Dāntián (Zhōng Dāntián, 中丹田) (solar plexus). This Qì then circulates down and mixes with the Pre-birth or Dāntiánqì (Original Qì, 丹田氣). Together, they circulate down, passing into the Governing Vessel (Dūmài, 督脈), from where they are distributed to the entire body.

Pre-birth Qì is commonly called "Water Qì" (Shuǐqì, 水氣) because it is able to cool down the Post-birth Qì, which is called "Fire Qì" (Huǒqì, 火氣). Fire Qì usually brings the body to a positive (Yáng) state, which stimulates the emotions and scatters and confuses the mind. When the Water Qì cools your body down, the mind will become clear, neutral and centered. It is believed in Qìgōng society that Fire Qì supports the emotional part of the body, while Water Qì supports the wisdom part.

After the Fire Qì and Water Qì mix, this Qì will not only circulate to the Governing Vessel but will also supply the "Thrusting Vessel" (Chōngmài, 衝脈), which will lead the Qì directly up through the spinal cord to nourish the brain and energize the Shén and soul. As will be discussed later, energizing the brain and raising the Shén are very important in Qìgōng practice.

According to its function, Qì can be divided into two major categories. The first is called "Yíngqì" (Managing Qì, 營氣), because it manages or controls the functioning of the body. This includes the functioning of the brain and the organs, and even body movement. Yíngqì is again divided into two major types. The first type circulates in the channels and is responsible for the functioning of the organs. The circulation of Qì to the organs and the extremities continues automatically as long as you have enough Qì in your reservoirs and you maintain your body in good condition. The second type of Yíngqì is linked to your Yì (mind, intention, 意). When your Yì decides to do something, for example to lift a box, this type of Yíngqì will automatically flow to the muscles needed to do the job. This type of Qì is directed by your thoughts, and therefore is related closely to your feelings and emotions.

The second major category of Qì is "Wèiqì" (Guardian Qì, 衛氣). Wèiqì forms a shield on the surface of the body to protect you from negative outside influences. Wèiqì is also involved in the growth of hair, the repair of skin injuries, and many other functions on the surface of the skin. Wèiqì comes from the Qì channels and is led through the millions of tiny channels (Luò, 絡) to the surface of the skin. This Qì can even reach beyond the body. When your body is positive (Yáng, 陽), this Qì is strong, and your pores will be open. When your body is negative (Yīn, 陰), this Qì is weak, and your pores will close up more to prevent Qì from being lost.

In the summertime, your body is Yáng and your Qì is strong, so your Qì shield will be bigger and extend beyond your physical body; the pores will be wide open. In the wintertime, your body is relatively Yīn (negative), and you must conserve your Qì in order to stay warm and keep pathogens out. The Qì shield is smaller and doesn't extend out much beyond your skin.

Wèiqì functions automatically in response to changes in the environment, but it is also influenced significantly by your feelings and emotions. For example, when you feel happy or angry, the Qì shield will be more open than when you are sad.

In order to keep your body healthy and functioning properly, you must keep the Yíngqì functioning smoothly and, at the same time, keep the Wèiqì strong to protect you from negative outside influences such as the cold. Chinese doctors and Qìgōng practitioners believe that the key to doing this is through Shén (spirit, 神). Shén is considered to be the headquarters that directs and controls the Qì. Therefore, when you practice Qìgōng you must understand what your Shén is and know how to raise it. When people are ill and facing death, very often the ones with a strong Shén, which is indicative of a strong will to live, will survive. The people who are apathetic or depressed will generally not last long. A strong will to live raises the Shén, which energizes the body's Qì and keeps you alive and healthy.

In order to raise your Shén, you must first nourish your brain with Qì. This Qì energizes the brain so that you can concentrate more effectively. Your mind will then be steady, your will strong, and your Shén raised. Shén will be more thoroughly discussed in a later section.

There is another way to categorize the body's Qì: Fire Qì and Water Qì. As we discussed previously, the Qì generated from the food and air you take in warms the body, and so it is called Fire Qì. This Qì is associated with the emotions. The second type of Qì is called "Water Qì." It is also called "Original Qì" because it is generated from Original Jīng. It has its root in the kidneys, and it has a cooling effect on the body. It is associated with Yì and wisdom. As a Qìgōng practitioner you want Water Qì and Fire Qì to be balanced so your body and mind are centered and balanced. It is also said that your Yì should be in the center of your emotions. This way wisdom rules, and the emotions are controlled, not suppressed.

As a Qìgōng practitioner, in addition to paying attention to the food and air you take in, it is important for you to learn how to generate Water Qì and how to use it more effectively. Water Qì can cool down the Fire Qì and, therefore, slow down the degeneration of the body. Water Qì also helps to calm your mind and keep it centered. This allows you to judge things objectively. During Qìgōng practice, you will be able to sense your Qì and direct it effectively.

In order to generate Water Qì and use it efficiently, you must know how and where it is generated. Since Water Qì comes from the conversion of Original Jīng, they both have the kidneys for their root. Once Water Qì is generated, it resides in the Lower Dāntián below your navel. In order to conserve your Water Qì, you must keep your kidneys firm and strong.

Shén (神)

It is very difficult to find an English word to exactly express Shén. As in so many other cases, the context determines the translation. Shén can be translated as spirit, god, immortal, soul, mind, divine, and supernatural.

When you are alive, Shén is the spirit that is directed by your mind. When your mind is not steady it is said "Xīnshén Bùníng" (心神不寧), which means "the (emotional) mind and spirit are not peaceful." The average person can use his emotional mind to energize and stimulate his Shén to a higher state, but at the same time he must restrain his emotional mind with his wisdom mind (Yì, 意). If his Yì can control the Xīn, the mind as a whole will be concentrated and the Yì will be able to govern the Shén. When someone's Shén is excited, however, it is not being controlled by his Yì, so we say, "Shénzhì Bùqīng" (神志不清), which means "the spirit and the will (generated from Yì) are not clear." In Qìgōng it is very important for you to train your wisdom Yì to control your emotional Xīn effectively. In order to reach this goal, Buddhists and Daoists train themselves to be free of emotions. Only in this way are they able to build a strong Shén which is completely under their control.

When you are healthy you are able to use your Yì to protect your Shén and keep it at its residence: the Upper Dāntián (Shàng Dāntián, 上丹田). Even when your Shén is energized, it is still controlled. However, when you are very sick or near death, your Yì becomes weak and your Shén will leave its residence and wander around. When you are dead, your Shén separates completely from the physical body. It is then called a "Hún" (魂) or "soul." Often the term "Shénhún" (神魂) is used, since the Hún originated with the Shén. Sometimes "Shénhún" is also used to refer to the spirit of a dying person since his spirit is between "Shén" and "Hún."

The Chinese believe that when your Shén reaches a higher and stronger state, you are able to sense and feel more sharply, and your mind is more clever and inspired. The world of living human beings is usually considered a Yáng world (Yángjiān, 陽間), and the spiritual world after death is considered a Yīn world (Yīnjiān, 陰間). It is believed that when your Shén has reached this higher, sensitive state you can transcend your mind's normal capacity. Ideas beyond your usual grasp can be understood and controlled, and you may develop the ability to sense or even communicate with the Yīn world. This supernatural Shén is called "Líng" (靈). "Líng" is commonly used by the Chinese to describe someone who is sharp, clever, nimble, and able to quickly empathize with people and things. It is believed that when you die this supernatural Shén will not die with your body right away. It is this supernatural Shén (Líng) which still holds your energy together as a "ghost" or "Guǐ" (鬼). Therefore, a ghost is also called "Língguǐ" (靈鬼) meaning "spiritual ghost" or "Línghún" (靈魂) meaning "spiritual soul."

You can see from the above discussion that Líng is the supernatural part of the spirit. It is believed that if this supernatural spiritual soul is strong enough, it will live for a long time after the physical body is dead and have plenty of opportunity to reincarnate. Chinese people believe that if a person has reached the stage of enlightenment or Buddhahood when he is alive, after he dies this supernatural spirit will leave the cycle of reincarnation and live forever. These spirits are called Shénmíng (神明), which means "spiritually enlightened beings," or simply Shén (神), which here implies that this spirit has become divine. Normally, if you die and your supernatural spiritual soul is not strong, your spirit has only a short time to search for a new residence in which to be reborn before its energy disperses. In this case, the spirit is called Guǐ (鬼), which means "ghost."

Buddhists and Daoists believe that when you are alive you may use your Jīng and Qì to nourish the Shén (Yǎngshén, 養神) and make your Líng strong. When this "Língshén" (靈神) is built up to a high level, your will is able to lead it to separate from the physical body even while you are alive. When you have reached this stage, your physical body is able to live for many hundreds of years. People who can do this are called Xiān (仙), which means "god," "immortal," or "fairy." Since "Xiān" originated with the Shén, the "Xiān" is sometimes called "Shénxiān" (神仙), which means "immortal spirit." The "Xiān" is a living person whose Shén has reached the stage of enlightenment or Buddhahood. After his death, his spirit will be called Shénmíng (神明).

The foundation of Buddhist and Daoist Qìgōng training is to firm your Shén, nourish it, and grow it until it is mature enough to separate from your physical body. In order to do this, a Qìgōng practitioner must know where the Shén resides, and how to keep, protect, nourish, and train it. It is also essential for you to know the root or origin of your Shén.

Your Shén resides in the Upper Dāntián (Shàng Dāntián, 上丹田) (limbic system and brain) connection to the third eye. When you concentrate on the Upper Dāntián, the Shén can be firmed. Firm here means to keep and to protect. When someone's mind is scattered and confused, his Shén wanders. This is called Shénbù Shǒushè (神不守舍), which means "the spirit is not kept at its residence."

According to Qìgōng theory, though your Xīn (emotional mind, 心) is able to raise up your spirit, this mind can also make your Shén confused, so that it leaves its residence. You must use your Yì (wisdom mind) constantly to restrain and control your Shén at the residence.

In Qìgōng, when your Qì can reach and nourish your Shén efficiently, your Shén will be energized to a higher level and, in turn, conduct the Qì in its circulation. Shén is the force which keeps you alive, and it is also the control tower for the Qì. When your Shén is strong, your Qì is strong and you can lead it efficiently. When your Shén is weak, your Qì is weak and the body will degenerate rapidly. Likewise, Qì supports the Shén, energizing it and keeping it sharp, clear, and strong. If the Qì in your body is weak, your Shén will also be weak.

Once you know the residence of your Shén, you must understand the root of your Shén, and learn how to nourish it and make it grow. We have already discussed Original Essence (Yuánjīng, 元精), which is the essential life inherited from your parents. After your birth, this Original Essence is your most important energy source. Your Original Qì (Yuánqì, 元氣) is created from this Original Essence, and it mixes with the Qì generated from the food you eat and the air you breathe to supply the energy for your growth and activity. Naturally, this mixed Qì is nourishing your Shén as well. While the Fire Qì will energize your Shén, Water Qì will strengthen the wisdom mind to control the energized Shén. The Shén which is kept in its residence by the Yì, which is nourished by the Original Qì, is called Original Shén (Yuánshén, 元神). Therefore, the root of your Original Shén is traced back to your Original Essence. When your Shén is energized but restrained by your Yì it is called Jīngshén (精神), literally "Essence Shén," which is commonly translated "spirit of vitality."

Original Shén is thought of as the center of your being. It is able to make you calm, clear your mind, and firm your will. When you concentrate your mind on doing something, it is called Jùjīng Huìshén (聚精會神), which means "gathering your Jīng to meet your Shén." This implies that when you concentrate, you must use your Original Essence to meet and lift up your Original Shén, so that your mind will be calm, steady, and concentrated. Since this Shén is nourished by your Original Qì, which is considered Water Qì, Original Shén is considered Water Shén.

For those who have reached a higher level of Qìgōng practice, cultivating the Shén becomes the most important subject. For Buddhists and Daoists the final goal of cultivating the Shén is to form or generate a Holy Embryo (Xiāntāi, 仙胎) from their Shén, and nourish it until the spiritual baby is born and can be independent. For the average Qìgōng practitioner however, the final goal of cultivating Shén is to raise the Shén through Qì nourishment while maintaining control with the Yì. This raised Shén can direct and govern the Qì efficiently to achieve health and longevity.

In conclusion, we would like to point out that your Shén and brain cannot be separated. Shén is the spiritual part of your being and is generated and controlled by your mind. The mind generates the will, which keeps the Shén firm. The Chinese commonly use Shén (spirit) and Zhì (will) together as "Shénzhì" (神志) because they are so related. In addition, you should understand that when your Shén is raised and firm, this raised spirit will firm your will. They are mutually related, and assist each other. From this you can see that the material foundation of the spirit is your brain. When it is said "nourish your Shén," it means "nourish your brain." As we discussed previously, the original nourishing source is your Jīng. This Jīng is then converted into Qì, which is led to the brain to nourish and energize it. In Qìgōng practice, this process is called Fǎnjīng Bǔnǎo (返精補腦), which means "to return the Jīng to nourish the brain."

3-2. Yì and Xīn (Yì, Xīn, 意、心)

Chinese people will frequently use both Yì (意) and Xīn (心) at different times to mean "mind," often confusing people who are not familiar with the Chinese language. Before advancing any further, you should first be sure that you have a clear understanding of the subtle differences between these two words.

Yì is the mind which is related to wisdom and judgment. When Yì has an idea, it strives to bring it to actualization in the physical world as either an event you will seek to bring about, or as an object you will create. The Yì is focused and firmed by the will.

Chinese people also use the word "Xīn" to mean "mind," although the word literally means "heart." While Xīn also denotes the presence of an idea, this idea is much weaker than that expressed in Yì. Xīn is generated from and affected by the emotions. This mind is passive instead of active like the Yì. When someone says he has Yì to do something, this means he intends to do it. If he says he has Xīn to do it, this means his emotions intend to do it, he has within him the desire to do it, but he may lack the strength of resolve to actually commit himself. For example, your wisdom mind (Yì) knows you must do something before a certain deadline, but your emotional mind (Xīn) tries to convince you that it is not a big deal, and you needn't worry too much about it. In most people, the emotional mind is stronger than the wisdom mind. They act according to how they feel, instead of what they think. We've all heard the comment at one time or another: "You're your own worst enemy." Your emotional mind is your wisdom mind's enemy. The emotional mind is the source of laziness, bad temper, emotional upset, and so on. If your wisdom mind is able to dominate your emotional mind, you will surely be a success in whatever you attempt.

Sometimes people will put both words together and say "Xīnyì" (心意) to denote the mind which is generated from both emotion and thought. Since most of the thought was generated and given its primal nature by the emotions first, before being refined by the will, the word Xīn is placed before Yì. This is a good example of how Xīn is used to denote the emotional mind, and Yì is used for the mind of wisdom, intention, and will. In meditation society it is said: "Yǐxīn Huìyì" (以心會意), which means "modulate the Xīn (emotional mind) to match the Yì (wisdom mind)." This means that the emotional aspect and the wisdom aspect of your mind must work together in harmony during meditation. Only then will you be able to use your Yì to regulate your body, for it is also said: "Yǐyì Huìshēn" (以意會身), which means "use your Yì to meet the body."

Xīn and Shén are commonly used together as "Xīnshén" (心神). This refers to the emotional mind which affects or is affected by Shén. When a person is absent-minded or confused, people say "Xīnshén Bùníng" (心神不寧), which means "mind and spirit are not stable." Spirit is also related to Yì, or the wisdom mind. However, the Yì aspect of the mind is still the strongest, being generated from thought and will. This mind can firm the scattered emotional mind and the spirit, thereby raising the spirit. When the spirit is raised and firmed, the emotional mind (Xīn) will be steady. "Yì" is commonly used together with will—"Yìzhì" (意志). This implies that the wisdom mind and the will are working together. The wisdom mind is firmed by the will, and the will firms the wisdom mind.

In Chinese Qìgōng society it is believed that the emotional mind (Xīn) is mainly generated from the Post-birth Qì or Food Qì (Shíqì, 食氣), which is converted from the food essence, while the wisdom mind (Yì) comes from the Pre-birth Qì (Yuánqì, 元氣) which is converted from the Original Essence you inherited from your parents. The Post-birth Qì is considered to be "Fire" Qì, while the Pre-birth Qì is considered "Water" Qì. It is believed that your emotions and temper are closely related to the food you eat. It can be seen that the animals who eat plants are more tame and nonviolent than the animals which eat meat. Generally speaking, food which generates excessive Qì in the Middle Dāntián (Zhōng Dāntián, 中丹田) usually makes the body more positive and makes the person more emotional. This effect can also be caused by dirty air, dirty thoughts, or the surrounding Qì (for example, in the summer when it is too hot). Certain foods and drugs can also directly interfere with clear thinking. For example, alcohol and drugs can stimulate your emotional mind and suppress your wisdom mind. The Qì generated from food is normally classified as Fire Qì, and it can reside in the Middle Dāntián (solar plexus).

One part of Qìgōng training is learning how to regulate your Fire Qì and Water Qì so that they are balanced. This involves learning to use your wisdom mind to dominate and direct your emotional mind. One of the more common methods of strengthening the Water Qì (and wisdom mind) and weakening the Fire Qì (and emotional mind) is to greatly reduce or eliminate meat from the diet, and live mainly on vegetables. Daoists and Buddhists periodically fast in order to weaken the Fire Qì as much as possible, which allows them to strengthen their Water Qì and wisdom mind. This process of "cleaning" their bodies and minds is important in ridding the monks of emotional disturbance.

3-3. Elixir Field (Dāntián, 丹田)

Dāntián (丹田) is translated literally as "Elixir Field." In Chinese Qìgōng society, three spots are considered Dāntián. The first one is called "Xià Dāntián" (Lower Dāntián, 下丹田). In Chinese medicine it is called "Qìhǎi" (Co-6, 氣海), which means "Qì Ocean." It is located about one to one and a half inches below your navel and about one to two inches

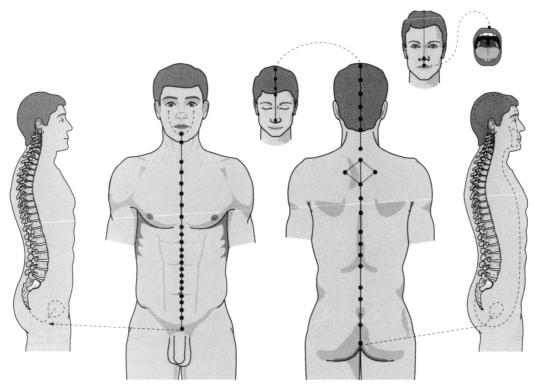

Figure 3-1. Conception and Governing Vessels

deep, depending of course on the individual. In both Chinese medicine and Qìgōng society, the Lower Dāntián is considered the well-spring of human energy. It is the residence of Original Qì (Yuánqì, 元氣), which has been converted from Original Essence (Yuánjīng, 元精).

The human body has twelve Qì channels (Jīng, 經) which are like rivers of Qì. They circulate Qì throughout the body, and connect the organs to the extremities. In addition to these twelve Qì rivers, there are eight "extraordinary Qì vessels" (Bāmài, 八脈) These are like reservoirs of Qì, and they regulate the flow of Qì in the rivers (the twelve channels). In order to be healthy, the Qì reservoirs must be full and the Qì must flow smoothly without stagnation in the rivers (see the detailed explanation of Human Qì circulation in Part Three).

Among the eight vessels is the Conception Vessel (Rènmài, 任脈), which is Yīn, and the Governing Vessel (Dūmài, 督脈), which is Yáng. They are located on the center line of the front and the back of the torso and head, respectively, and run into one another, creating a closed loop about the body (Figure 3-1). The Qì in these two vessels must be full and circulate smoothly in order to regulate all of the Qì in the twelve rivers properly. At any particular time, there is a section of this circle where the Qì flow is stronger than in the other sections. This section is called "Zǐwǔ Liúzhù" (子午流注), which means "midnight and noon major flow," and it keeps the Qì flowing in these two vessels. Qì behaves like water. If there is no difference in potential the Qì will stay still and become stagnant, and you are likely to become

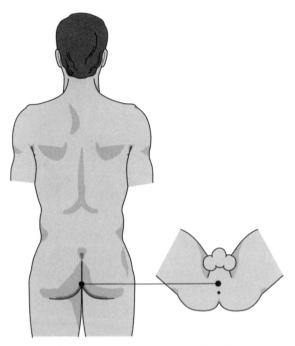

Figure 3-2. Huìyīn cavity (Co-1)

ill. Normally, this area of stronger Qì moves around the circle of these two vessels once every day.

Chinese Qìgōng practitioners believe that the Qì must be full and circulate strongly in these two vessels, for then they will be able to govern the entire body's Qì effectively. They also believe that as a child you continually move the abdomen while breathing, which keeps the path of these two vessels clear. However, as you get older and gradually lose the habit of this abdominal movement, the path becomes obstructed and the Qì circulation weakens. The most significant blockage can occur in the tailbone (Chángqiáng, Gv-1, 長強), connecting to the Huìyīn cavity (Co-1) (會陰) (Figure 3-2). Try an experiment. Use one finger to press firmly at your Huìyīn cavity while your abdomen is moving in and out. You will discover that the Huìyīn cavity moves up and down in sync with the in-and-out motion of the abdomen. It is this up-and-down motion of the perineum which keeps the Huìyīn cavity clear for Qì circulation. For this reason, exercises which move the abdomen in and out are called "Fǎntóng" (back to childhood, 返童) exercises.

Abdominal exercises not only open the Qì channels, they can also draw Original Qì from its residence in the Lower Dāntián to join the Post-birth Qì in its circulation. Original Qì is considered the original vital source of human energy. Therefore, in-and-out abdominal exercise is also called "Qǐhuǒ" (起火), which means "start the fire." This hints at the way the Daoists build up Qì energy. The Daoists consider the Dāntián to be the furnace in which they can purify and distill the elixir (Qì) for longevity.

The second of the three Dāntiáns is called the Middle Dāntián (Zhōng Dāntián, 中丹田), and it is located at the solar plexus. The Middle Dāntián is considered the center where the Post-birth Qì is produced and gathered. Post-birth Qì is the energy which is converted from the Jīng (essence) of air and food. Post-birth Qì is affected therefore by the type of food you eat and the quality of the air you breathe. The level of your Post-birth Qì is also influenced by such things as whether you are getting enough sleep, whether you are tired, irritable, nervous, sad, and so on.

It is believed in Chinese medical society that the lungs and the heart are the places where the Air Jīng is converted into Qì. The stomach and the digestive system are the center where the Food Jīng is absorbed and then converted into Qì. This Qì then resides at the Middle Dāntián, and follows the Conception and Governing Vessels to disperse throughout the entire body. The conversion of air and food to Qì is similar to the burning of wood to give heat. Therefore, the lung area is called the Upper Burner (Shàngjiāo, 上焦), the stomach is called the Middle Burner (Zhōngjiāo, 中焦), and the lower abdomen is called the Lower Burner (Xiàjiāo, 下焦). The three are referred to collectively as the Triple Burner (Sānjiāo, 三焦).

You can deduce from the above description that the Upper Burner is the burner which handles Air Qi, while the Middle and Lower Burners handle Food Qi. The Lower Burner, in addition to separating the pure from the impure and eliminating waste, also processes the Lower Dāntiánqì. When someone has eaten too much positive food such as peanuts or sesame seeds, the excess Qì will cause heat. This is called Shànghuǒ (上火), which means simply that the body is "on fire." When you don't get enough sleep, the body can also pass into the "on fire" state. When the Post-birth Qì is too positive, it is called Huóqì (火氣), which means "Fire Qì."

When the Post-birth Qì is too positive and is directed to the organs, the organs will become positive and degenerate faster. When the Post-birth Qì is too weak, for example because of starvation, there is not enough Qì to supply the organs and the body, and you will gradually become more unbalanced until you become ill. Most people get more than enough food, so their Post-birth Qì is too positive. For this reason, Post-birth Qì is usually called "Fire Qì." There is a Qìgōng practice which leads the Water Qì (Pre-birth Qì) at the Lower Dāntián up to mix with the Fire Qì (Post-birth Qì) at the Middle Dāntián in order to cool the Fire Qì. This process is called water-fire (坎-離, Kǎn-Lí).

The third Dāntián is located on the head and is called the Upper Dāntián (Shàng Dāntián, 上丹田). Your brain uses a lot of energy (Qì) for thinking. This Qì is supplied by one of the vessels called Chōngmài (Thrusting Vessel, 衝脈), which flows through the spinal cord up to the brain and limbic system. Your spirit resides in your Upper Dāntián, and when it is amply supplied with Qì, it is "raised," or energized. If the Qì stopped nourishing your brain and spirit, you would lose your mental center, your judgment would become faulty, and you would become depressed and mentally unbalanced.

You can see from this discussion that all three Dāntiáns are located on the Conception Vessel. The Conception Vessel and the Governing Vessel together form the most important Qì reservoir in the body, and it is important for it to be full.

3-4. THREE FLOWERS REACH THE TOP (SĀNHUĀ JÙDǏNG, 三花聚頂)

Daoists commonly call the three treasures (Jīng, Qì, and Shén, 精、氣、神) the three flowers. One of the final goals of Daoist Qìgōng training is to gather the three flowers at the top of the head (Sānhuā Jùdǐng, 三花聚頂).

The normal Daoist Qìgōng training process is: 1. to convert the Jīng (essence) into Qì (Yǐjīng Huàqì, 以精化氣); 2. to nourish the Shén (spirit) with Qì (Yǐqì Huàshén, 以氣化神); 3. to refine the Shén into emptiness (Liànshén Fǎnxū, 煉神返虛); and 4. crush the emptiness (Fěnsuì Xūkōng, 粉碎虛空). The first step is to firm and strengthen the Jīng, then convert this Jīng into Qì through meditation or other methods. This Qì is then led to the top of the head to nourish the brain and raise the Shén. When a Daoist has reached this stage, it is called "the three flowers meet on the top." This stage is necessary to gain health and longevity. Now the Daoist can start training to reach the goal of enlightenment.

3-5. FIVE QÌ'S TOWARD THEIR ORIGINS (WǓQÌ CHÁOYUÁN, 五氣朝元)

According to Chinese medical science, among the twelve main organs are five Yīn organs which have a great effect on the health. These five organs are: heart, lungs, liver, kidneys, and spleen. If any internal organ does not have the appropriate level of Qì, it is either too Yáng (陽) (positive) or too Yīn (陰) (negative). When this happens, it is like running the wrong level of electric current into a machine. If the condition remains uncorrected, the organs will run less efficiently. This will affect the body's metabolism, and eventually even damage the organs. Therefore, one of the most important practices in Qìgōng training is learning to keep the Qì in these five organs at the proper level. When the Qì of these organs has reached the appropriate levels it is called "Wǔqì Cháoyuán," which means "the five Qì's toward their origins." Your organs can now function optimally, and your health will be maintained at a high level.

There are twelve Qì channels and eight extraordinary Qì vessels. The Qì in the twelve channels should be at the levels appropriate for the corresponding organs. The Qì in these twelve channels changes with the time of day, the seasons, and the year. This Qì is affected by the food you eat, the air you breathe, and your emotions. Therefore, in order to keep your five Qì's at their right levels, you must know how Qì is affected by time, food, and air, and you must learn how to regulate your emotions.

CHAPTER 4

Qì and the Human Body

In order to understand human Qìgōng, you must understand the nature of the Qì in the human body, and how it functions. This includes understanding what kinds of Qì are in the body, what functions they perform, and how they carry out these functions.

In the first three chapters we have offered a general definition of Qì, discussed how Human Qì is included in and affected by Heaven Qì and Earth Qì, and shown how Qì relates to other aspects of our bodies, such as spirit and essence. In Part Three of this book we will review how Qì circulates in the human body.

In this chapter we will first focus on the general characteristics of Qì in our bodies. This will provide a foundation to help you understand the rest of the chapter. We will then concentrate on a number of subjects which will lead you to a deeper understanding of Human Qì, such as Qì's Yīn and Yáng, and the quality of Qì. Once you understand the traditional concept of Qì, we will discuss the modern concept of bioelectromagnetic energy. Following this, we will offer some hypotheses based upon this energy which Western science has recently discovered. Finally, we will discuss the theory of how Qì gates can be opened through Qìgōng practice.

4-1. ABOUT QÌ (GUĀNYÚ QÌ, 關於氣)

In this section, we will first discuss the natural characteristics of Qì and the relationship between Qì and the human body. Then we will explain how Qì's Yīn and Yáng are defined, and how the quality of Qì is determined.

The Nature of Qì

To understand the nature of Qì, you should first know where Qì originates. Something cannot come from nothing, so Qì (any type of energy) must come from matter, usually through some kind of chemical reaction. Matter is a physical form of energy, and energy is an unlocked potential (or an insubstantial form) of matter. For example, you may burn a piece of wood or gas and obtain Qì in the form of heat and light. Similarly, food and air are taken into your body, and through biochemical reaction are converted into Qì, which is commonly in the form of heat and bioelectromagnetic energy. Whenever you take in more food than your body requires, the unexcreted excess is stored in your body as fat.

Next you should understand that Qì generally manifests as heat, light, potential energy (e.g., gravity), and/or electromagnetic energy. Strictly speaking, heat (infrared) and light are alternative forms of electromagnetic waves, so, in effect, there are only two types of energy that we deal with in our daily lives—electromagnetic and potential energy. Often light and heat exist at the same time.

Finally, you should recognize that Qì moves from the area of higher potential to the area of lower potential, and this acts to naturally and automatically bring your system into balance.

Qì in the Human Body

Although, according to the general definition, heat is considered a type of Human Qì, heat is not the type of Qì which is circulating in your body. Oftentimes you will feel heat when Qì is circulating strongly, but the heat is not the circulating Qì itself. There is another type of Qì which circulates throughout your body to nourish the cells and keep them functioning, and even to repair damage.

Since electricity has become more familiar to people in China last century, many Qìgōng practitioners have come to believe that the Qì which circulates in the body is actually electromagnetic energy. If you run an electric current through a wire, the wire will heat up because of the resistance of the wire. The heat is an effect caused by the current, but it is not the current itself. According to this theory, as Qì circulates through your body, the resistance of your body causes part of the Qì to be converted into heat.

Qìgōng practitioners believe that the light which is sometimes perceived during meditation is also Qì. Light is a form of electromagnetic energy. Since all types of energy are convertible, heat can generate electromagnetic power and vice versa, and light can also generate heat, and vice versa. Once you have reached the higher levels of meditation, you will sense light in your eyes and mind. At an even higher level, your head will generate a glow like a halo. All of these can be considered transformations that the electric Qì undergoes when your training has reached a higher level.

The Behavior of Human Qì

Chinese doctors and Qìgōng practitioners have traditionally described the behavior of Qì as being similar to water. This is seen in a number of ways. First, just as water flows from higher areas to lower areas, Qì flows from areas of higher potential to areas of lower potential. In this way, Qì balances itself naturally. Second, if muddy water is left undisturbed, the sand will settle to the bottom, leaving the water above it calm and clear. However, if you stir up the water, the sand will rise up and dirty the water again. This is similar to how, when the mind is steady, the Qì will be calm and clear, but when the mind is scattered, the Qì will be disturbed and excited. Third, the Qì channels which supply Qì to the entire body are usually compared to rivers, and the vessels which store the Qì are compared to reservoirs. Water and Qì should both flow smoothly and continuously. When a river or channel is obstructed, the water/Qì flow will be agitated and uneven. In an obstructed channel, the water/Qì flow will be higher, and may overflow the banks.

Qì's Yīn and Yáng

When it is said that Qì can be either Yīn or Yáng, it does not mean that there are two different kinds of Qì like male and female, fire and water, or positive and negative charges. Qì is energy, and energy itself does not have Yīn and Yáng. It is like the energy which is generated from the sparking of negative and positive charges. Charges have the potential of generating energy but are not the energy itself.

When it is said that Qì is Yīn or Yáng, it means that the Qì is too strong or too weak for a particular circumstance. It is relative and not absolute. Naturally, this implies that the potential which generates the Qì is strong or weak. For example, the Qì from the sun is Yángqì (陽氣) and Qì from the moon is Yīnqì (陰氣). This is because the sun's energy is Yáng in comparison to Human Qì, while the moon's is Yīn. In any discussion of energy where people are involved, Human Qì is used as the standard. People are always especially interested in what concerns them directly, so it is natural that we are interested primarily in Human Qì and tend to view all Qì from the perspective of Human Qì. This is not unlike looking at the universe from the perspective of the Earth.

When we look at the Yīn and Yáng of Qì within and in regard to the human body, however, we must redefine our point of reference. For example, when a person is dead, his residual Human Qì (Guǐqì, 鬼氣 or Ghost Qì) is weak compared to a living person's. Therefore, the ghost's Qì is Yīn while the living person's is Yáng. When discussing Qì within the body, in the Lung Channel for example, the reference point is the normal, healthy status of the Qì there. If the Qì is stronger than it is in the normal state, it is Yáng, and, naturally, if it is weaker than this, it is Yīn. There are twelve parts of the human body that are considered organs in Chinese medicine; six of them are Yīn and six are Yáng. The Yīn organs are the Heart, Lungs, Kidneys, Liver, Spleen, and Pericardium, and the Yáng organs are Large Intestine, Small Intestine, Stomach, Gall Bladder, Urinary Bladder, and Triple Burner. Generally speaking, the Qì level of the Yīn organs is lower than that of the Yáng organs. The Yīn organs store Original Essence and process the essence obtained from food and air, while the Yáng organs handle the digestion and excretion. We will discuss this subject in more detail in Part Three of this book.

When the Qì in any of your organs is not in its normal state, you feel uncomfortable. If it is very much off from the normal state, the organ will start to malfunction, and you may become sick. When this happens, the Qì in your entire body will also be affected and you will feel too Yáng, perhaps feverish, or too Yīn, such as the weakness after diarrhea.

Your body's Qì level is also affected by natural circumstances such as the weather, climate, and seasonal changes. Therefore, when the body's Qì level is classified, the reference point is the level which feels most comfortable for those particular circumstances. Naturally, each of us is a little bit different, and what feels best and most natural for one person may be a bit different from what is right for another person. That is why the doctor will usually ask, "How do you feel?" It is according to your own standard that you are judged.

Breath is closely related to the state of your Qì, and therefore also considered Yīn or Yáng. When you exhale you expel air from your lungs, your mind moves outward, and the Qì around the body expands. In the Chinese martial arts, the exhale is generally used to expand the Qì to energize the muscles during an attack. Therefore, you can see that the exhale is Yáng—it is expanding, offensive, and strong. Naturally, based on the same theory, the inhale is considered Yīn.

Your breathing is closely related to your emotions. When you lose your temper, your breathing is short and fast, i.e., Yáng. When you are sad, your body is more Yīn, and you inhale more than you exhale in order to absorb the Qì from the air to balance the body's Yīn to bring the body back into balance. When you are excited and happy, your body is Yáng. You exhale longer than you inhale in order to get rid of the excess Yáng which is caused by the excitement.

As mentioned before, your mind is also closely related to your Qì. Therefore, when your Qì is Yáng, your mind is usually also Yáng (excited) and vice versa. In addition, as we discussed in the previous section, the mind can also be classified according to the Qì that generates it. The mind (Yì) that is generated from the calm and peaceful Qì obtained from Original Essence is considered Yīn. The mind (Xīn) that originates with the food and air essence is emotional, scattered, and excited, and it is considered Yáng. Finally, the Shén, which is related to the Qì, can also be classified as Yáng or Yīn based on its origin.

Do not confuse Yīn Qì and Yáng Qì with Fire Qì and Water Qì. When the Yīn and Yáng of Qì are mentioned, it refers to the level of Qì according to some reference point. However, when Water Qì and Fire Qì are mentioned, it refers to the quality of the Qì. This will be discussed in the next section.

The Quality of Human Qì

Some people think that Qì is of good quality when it is neither too Yīn nor too Yáng. However, they are wrong. When Qì is neither too Yīn nor too Yáng, this means that the level of the Qì is right. It is a quantitative statement rather than a qualitative one. The quality of Qì refers to its purity, as well as its contents. This quality depends on where and how the Qì originated. Usually, the quality of the Qì determines how it behaves and how it affects the body's Yīn and Yáng when it is circulating in your body.

Within the human body, Qìgōng practitioners have generally categorized Qì into "Fire Qì" and "Water Qì" to express the qualitative purity of the Qì. The terms "Fire" and "Water" indicate the effects that the Qì has on our body. For example, when Qì that is impure or of poor quality circulates in the human body, it may cause heat in the body and organs, and make the body too Yáng. It is therefore called "Fire Qì." If, however, the Qì is pure, clean, and circulating smoothly, it will enable the body to remain calm, keep the mind clear and steady, and allow the body to function properly. This Qì is called Water Qì because it is the Qì which enables the body to remain calm and cool, like water.

In the thousands of years that Qìgōng has been studied, practitioners have found that the Qì that comes from Original Jīng (and is therefore called Original Qì) is "Water Qì." It is pure and smooth, like sunshine in the winter, like crystal-pure water flowing smoothly in a stream, very comfortable and natural. This Qì makes it possible for the wisdom mind (Yì) to remain calm and grow stronger. When this Qì is circulating in the human body, it is smooth and will keep the physical body functioning in a steady, calm, and Yīn state.

Conversely, the Qì which comes from food and air is not of as high a quality as Original Qì. Because the body cannot discriminate between good and bad raw materials, many undesirable ingredients in the food and air are also converted into Qì. The quality of this Qì is dirty and nonuniform, like water that has been polluted. When this Qì goes to your brain, it can excite your emotions and upset your emotional balance. When this Qì is circulating in your body, the undesirable ingredients can change the body into Yáng and cause problems. For example, the Qì which was converted from fat can convert back into fat, and plug up the Qì paths. Plugged up Qì channels can have undesirable effects, such as high blood pressure, which speeds up the degeneration of the internal organs. For this reason, diet is a part of Qìgōng practice. Generally speaking, the Qì generated from food which comes from animal sources has more contaminants than the Qì generated from food obtained from plants.

You can see from this discussion that it is very important to distinguish both the level of Qì and its quality. The level of Qì (Yīn or Yáng) depends on the circumstances, and must have a reference point. The quality of Qì depends upon the essence from which it comes.

4-2. Qì and Bioelectromagnetic Energy (Qì Yǔ Shēnghuà Diàncínéng, 氣與生化電磁能)

In ancient China, people had very little knowledge of electricity. They only knew from acupuncture that when a needle was inserted into the acupuncture cavities, some kind of energy other than heat was produced which often caused a shock or a tickling sensation. It was not until the last few decades, when the Chinese people were more acquainted with electromagnetic science, that they began to recognize that this energy circulating in the body, which they called "Qì," might be the same thing as what today's science calls "bioelectricity."

It is understood now that the human body is constructed of many different electrically conductive materials, and it forms a living electromagnetic field and circuit. Electromagnetic energy is continuously being generated in the human body through the biochemical reaction of food and air, and circulated by the electromotive (or electromagnetic) forces (EMF) generated within the body by, for example, thinking or movement.

In addition, you are also constantly being affected by external electromagnetic fields such as that of the earth, or the electrical fields generated by clouds. When you practice Chinese medicine or Qìgōng, you need to be aware of these outside factors and take them into account.

Countless experiments have been conducted in China, Japan, and other countries to study how external magnetic or electrical fields can affect and adjust the body's Qì field. Many acupuncturists use magnets and electricity in their treatments. They attach a magnet to the skin over a cavity and leave it there for a period of time. The magnetic field gradually affects the Qì circulation in that channel. Alternatively, they insert needles into cavities and then run an electric current through the needle to reach the Qì channels directly. Although many experimenters have claimed a degree of success in their experiments, none has been able to publish any detailed and convincing proof of his results, or give a good explanation of the theory behind his experiment. As with many other attempts to explain the How and Why of acupuncture, conclusive proof is elusive, and many unanswered questions remain. Of course, this theory is quite new, and it will probably take a lot more study and research before it is verified and completely understood. At present, there are many conservative acupuncturists who are skeptical.

To untie this knot, we must look at what modern Western science has discovered about bioelectromagnetic energy. Many bioelectric-related reports have been published, and frequently the results are closely related to what is experienced in Chinese Qìgōng training and medical science. For example, during the electrophysiological research of the 1960's, several investigators discovered that bones are piezoelectric; that is, when they are stressed, mechanical energy is converted to electrical energy in the form of electric current.[1] This might explain one of the practices of Marrow Washing Qìgōng in which the stress on the bones and muscles is increased in certain ways to increase the Qì circulation (electric circulation).

Dr. Robert O. Becker has done important work in this field. His book *The Body Electric* reports on much of the research concerning the body's electric field.[2] It is presently believed that food and air are the fuel which generates the electricity in the body through biochemical reaction. This electricity, which is circulated throughout the entire body through electrically conductive tissue, is one of the main energy sources which keep the cells of the physical body alive.

Whenever you have an injury or are sick, your body's electrical circulation is affected. If this circulation of electricity stops, you die. But bioelectric energy not only maintains life, it is also responsible for repairing physical damage. Many researchers have sought ways of using external electrical or magnetic fields to speed up the body's recovery from physical injury. Richard Leviton reports that "Researchers at Loma Linda University's School of Medicine in California have found, following studies in sixteen countries with over 1,000 patients, that low-frequency, low intensity magnetic energy has been successful in treating chronic pain related to tissue ischemia, and also worked in clearing up slow-healing ulcers, and in 90 percent of patients tested, raised blood flow significantly."

Mr. Leviton also reports that every cell of the body functions like an electric battery and is able to store electric charges. He reports that: "Other biomagnetic investigators take an even closer look to find out what is happening, right down to the level of the blood, the organs, and the individual cell, which they regard as 'a small electric battery'."[3] This has con-

---

1. "Life's Invisible Current," by Albert L. Huebner, *East West Journal*, June 1986.
2. *The Body Electric*, by Robert O. Becker, M.D. and Gary Selden, Quill, William Morrow, New York, 1985.
3. "Healing with Nature's Energy," by Richard Leviton, *East West Journal*, June 1986.

vinced me that our entire body is just like a big battery which is assembled from millions of small batteries. All of these batteries together form the human electromagnetic field.

Furthermore, much of the research on the body's electrical field relates to acupuncture. For example, Dr. Becker reports that the conductivity of the skin is much higher at acupuncture cavities, and that it is now possible to locate them precisely by measuring the skin's conductivity. Many of these reports prove that the acupuncture which has been done in China for thousands of years is reasonable and scientific.

Some researchers use the theory of the body's electricity to explain many of the ancient "miracles" which have been attributed to the practice of Qìgōng. A report by Albert L. Huebner states: "These demonstrations of body electricity in human beings may also offer a new explanation of an ancient healing practice. If weak external fields can produce powerful physiological effects, it may be that fields from human tissues in one person are capable of producing clinical improvements in another. In short, the method of healing known as the laying on of hands could be an especially subtle form of electrical stimulation."[4]

Another frequently reported phenomenon is that when a Qìgōng practitioner has reached a high level of development, a halo would appear behind and/or around his head during meditation. This is commonly seen in paintings of Jesus Christ, the Buddha, and other Oriental gods. Frequently the light is pictured as surrounding the whole body. This phenomenon may again be explained by body electric theory. When a person has cultivated his Qì (electricity) to a high level, the Qì may be led to accumulate in the head. This Qì may then interact with the oxygen molecules in the air and ionize them, causing them to glow.

Although the link between the theory of the body electric and the Chinese theory of Qì is becoming more accepted and better proven, there are many questions still to be answered. For example, how can the mind lead Qì (electricity)? How actually does the mind generate an EMF (electromotive force) to circulate the electricity in the body? How is the human electromagnetic field affected by the multitude of other electric fields which surround us, such as radio and television waves, or the fields generated by household electrical wiring or electrical appliances? How can we readjust our electromagnetic fields and survive in outer space or on other planets where the magnetic field is completely different from earth's? You can see that the future of Qìgōng and bioelectric science is a challenging and exciting one. It is about time that we started to use modern technologies to understand the inner energy world which has been ignored by Western society.

4-3. SOME HYPOTHESES (YĪXIĒ JIĂSHÈ, 一些假設)

There are a number of questions which have puzzled Qìgōng practitioners and acupuncturists for many years. If Qì is the same thing as what is now being called "bioelectricity," which Western medical science is just discovering, then certain deductions or hypotheses can be made that might offer convincing explanations for many of these puzzles. In this section I will try to link together these aspects of Eastern and Western sciences, based on my

---

4.   "Life's Invisible Current," by Albert L. Huebner, *East West Journal*, June 1986.

understanding. In this section, I would like to raise some questions and draw some hypotheses concerning, for example, how a human body may react to and be influenced by external electromagnetic fields such as that of the Earth. I hope this section will stimulate your thinking and help the more conservative Qìgōng practitioners to accept this new science and participate in future analysis and discussion.

The Electromagnetic Field in the Human Body

How Is the Human Electromagnetic Field Formed? Since we and all other living things are formed and live in the Earth's magnetic field, our bodies also have a magnetic field of their own. The magnetic field of our body always corresponds with and is affected by the Earth's field. Modern science has shown that magnetic fields and electrical fields cannot be separated (Faraday's Law and Maxwell's equations), and indeed are aspects of the same force. Where there is one, there is also the other. This type of field is commonly called an "electromagnetic field."

Before we discuss how are we affected by the Earth's magnetic field, you must first understand the difference between four terms that are often confused: 1. the north and south poles of a magnet; 2. The north and the south magnetic poles of the Earth; 3. the geographic North and the South Poles of the Earth; and 4. the actual north and south poles of the Earth-magnet.

A piece of bar magnet has two poles, the north and south poles. The lines of force outside of the magnet start from the north pole and end at the south pole while the lines inside the magnet go from the south pole to the north pole (Figure 4-1). This is defined as the north and the south poles of a magnet.

Now let us take a look at the basics of the Earth's magnetism. If we place a bar magnet in the Earth's magnetic field, the magnet will align itself with the Earth's field. The "north" pole of this bar magnet is the "north-seeking pole," which points toward North of the Earth's magnetic field, which is called the "North Pole" (Figure 4-2). Naturally, the pole which points to the South is defined as the "South Pole." Therefore, the poles on a magnet are defined according to the directions they point to within the Earth's magnetic field.

Furthermore, we have defined the pole of the Earth toward which a magnet's north pole points as the Earth's "Magnetic North Pole" while the other end is the Earth's "Magnetic South Pole." Essentially, this means that, for ease of navigation and through convention, the Earth's Magnetic North Pole is for all intents and purposes considered to lie in the same direction as the Earth's Geographic North Pole. In fact, however, the geographic North and the South poles of the Earth do not actually coincide with the magnetic poles.

Let us take a closer look. We know that permanent magnets are collections of current loops (Figure 4-3). If the axis of the assumed current loop is more or less along the direction of the Earth's axis of rotation, the Magnetic North Pole will approximately coincide with the Geographic North Pole, as it actually does. In fact, the Magnetic North Pole is in northern Canada. This means that a compass needle does not point exactly north except at certain places. The difference between geographic north and magnetic north is called "magnetic

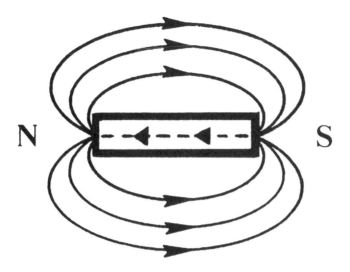

Figure 4-1. Magnetic field of a magnet

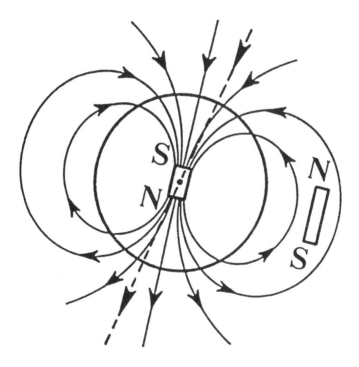

Figure 4-2. The Earth's magnetic field

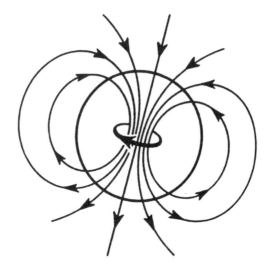

Figure 4-3. Current loop inside Earth

declination." This quantity varies from about 25 degrees east to 20 degrees west for different places in the United States, and also varies slowly from year to year (Figure 4-4).

We also know that the Earth's magnetic field has started at the Geographic South Pole and ended at the Geographic North Pole for at least the last million years (although evidence suggests that during the last several million years the magnetic poles of the Earth have reversed several times).

In 1570, an English court physician, William Gilbert, constructed a permanent magnet in the form of a large lodestone sphere. He used a small compass needle to survey the magnetic field near the surface of the sphere and discovered that his model successfully represented the main features of the Earth's magnetic field. In his survey, he discovered that in a point in the Northern Hemisphere, such as in England or the United States, the field is directed downward and to the north. Therefore, we can reasonably assume that a relatively short magnet, several hundred miles long, is buried deep inside the Earth. Since the lines of force are directed downward for an observer in the Northern Hemisphere, we may assume that the "Earth's magnet" has an S pole on the end which is beneath the North Magnetic Pole. Therefore, what we usually call the Earth's North Magnetic Pole is actually the south pole of the Earth's magnetic field. In other words, the actual magnetic poles of the Earth are the reverse of how they are shown on navigation maps (Figure 4-2).

The ordinary compass needle responds only to the horizontal component of the Earth's magnetic field, since it is pivoted in such a way as to prevent up-and-down motion. If a magnetized needle is mounted so as to be free to swing in a vertical north-south plane, it is free to point in the direction of the field, and in the Northern Hemisphere it will assume a position in which it points downward and to the north. Such an instrument is called a "dip

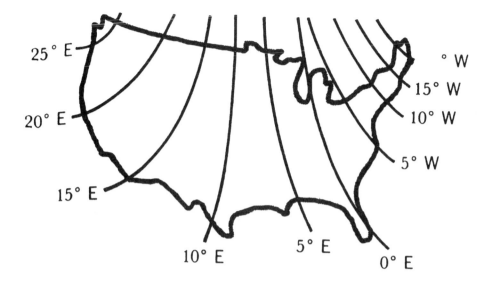

Figure 4-4. Lines of equal magnetic declination

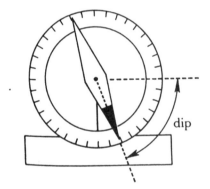

Figure 4-5. Dip needle

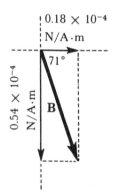

Figure 4-6. The Earth's magnetic field at Washington, D.C.

needle" (Figure 4-5). The angle of dip is measured from the horizontal. For example, values of the horizontal and vertical components of B for the Earth's field at Washington, D.C., have shown that the vertical component is about three times the horizontal component at this location (Figure 4-6).

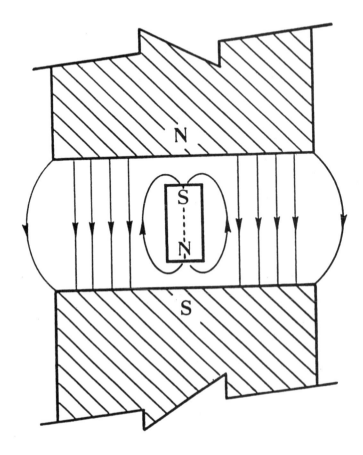

Figure 4-7. A piece of steel becomes a magnet when placed in a magnetic field

Now that we've assimilated the above concepts, let us now analyze our body's magnetic field. We know that when a piece of steel is placed inside a magnetic field, it becomes a magnet (Figure 4-7). Since our bodies are made up of conductive material, and we are in the magnetic field of the Earth, it is reasonable to assume that our bodies are like magnets. Since a magnet has two poles that must be located on the centerline of the magnet, we can easily guess that the poles of our bodies must be somewhere on the head and the bottom of the abdomen if we stand in either the Northern or Southern Hemisphere (note: the Earth's magnetic field passes through our bodies horizontally if we stand on the equator). The reason for this assumption is that the spinal cord is made of highly electric conductive fibers that connect the head to the sacrum. Thus, our task is to locate the poles of the human magnet.

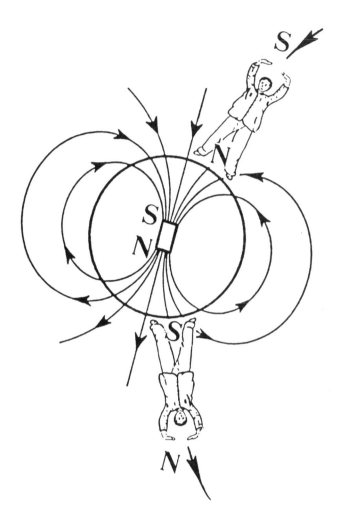

Figure 4-8. Human magnets in the Northern Hemisphere and the Southern Hemisphere

Since your body's magnetic field is formed under the influence of the Earth's magnetic field, the north and south poles of your body will be determined by whether you are in the Northern or Southern Hemisphere. For example, if you are standing near the North Pole, then the lines of force of the Earth's magnetic field will enter your body through your head and emerge from the bottom of your body. Naturally, if you are near the South Pole, then the lines of force of the Earth's magnetic field will enter the bottom of your body and exit from your head (Figure 4-8). This means that if you are at the Earth's North Pole your head will be a south pole while your abdomen will be a north pole. Naturally, the situation will be reversed if you are at the Earth's South Pole.

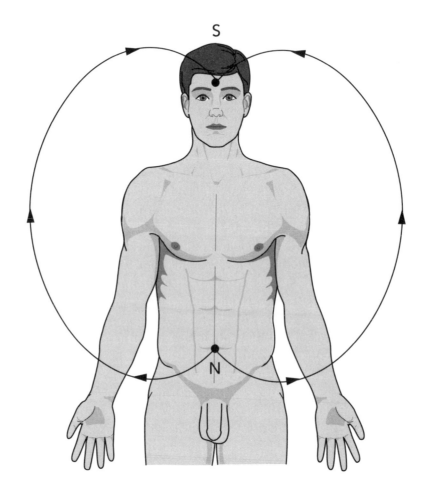

Figure 4-9. A human magnet in the Northern Hemisphere

I believe this means that if you live in the Northern Hemisphere, your brain (i.e., Upper Dāntián) is constantly being nourished and stimulated by the energy from the Lower Dāntián. However, if you live in the Southern Hemisphere, your Lower Dāntiánqì will be stronger, and naturally the sexual energy will also be strong. This may be a possible explanation for why more human technology was developed in the Northern Hemisphere.

When you are lying down or on the equator, the poles are on the sides of your body, and they change every time you move. This probably means that under these circumstances the Earth's magnetic field only has a minimal effect on your body.

Now let us discuss how this is related to Qìgōng. Assuming that you are in the Northern Hemisphere, your head should be a south pole while your abdomen is a north pole (Figure

4-9). Excluding all other factors such as location, weather, etc., the strength of your magnetic field depends on the natural qualities of your body. This may be what the Chinese mean by "Original Essence." It is analogous to the fact that when you place high-quality, refined steel in a magnetic field, the magnet formed will have a stronger magnetic field than if you had used poorly refined steel. Since this magnet is stronger, the magnetic energy will last longer. Similarly, if you received high quality Original Essence from your parents, your body's magnetic field will be strong, and the Qì or electrical energy circulating in your body will be strong and smooth. This means that your vitality will be great, and you will probably have a long and healthy life.

If this line of reasoning is valid, then we are able to explain something that has been confusing Qìgōng meditators. According to past experience (mostly from meditators in the Northern Hemisphere), when a person meditates facing south he is able to obtain a stronger Qì flow and is able to balance his Qì more quickly than if he were facing another direction. Facing south lines up the incoming energy with the "Small Circulation" of energy down the center of the front of the body and up the spine. Since the front of the body is Yīn, it absorbs energy more easily than the back or sides. Another possible explanation is related to the fact that we tend to turn and look at people who are talking to us as if this let us hear them better. Since your mind has a considerable influence on your body's energy, facing into the incoming energy may also help you to absorb and "digest" it. We can also explain why many Qìgōng practitioners claim that if they sleep with their head pointing north they sleep better, and feel more rested and balanced the next morning. (However, if you sleep sitting up, you should again face south.) These two claims become reasonable and understandable if we accept the concept of a bipolar human magnetic field.

It is clear that the energy patterns in the human body are affected by natural forces. It is also clear that the energy from the sun has a more significant effect than the energy from the earth. This leads me to believe that when you are meditating during the day you should face the east simply because the influence of the sun's energy is more significant than that of the Earth's magnetic field. During the night, when the influence of the sun has waned, it is probably best to face south if you are in the Northern Hemisphere.

Within the human magnet, we may again assume that there are millions of smaller magnets that correspond to the cells (Figure 4-10). Just as every cell has its own minute electrical field, so too does each cell have its own magnetic field. Indeed, the two are merely different aspects of the same force. When all of these small magnetic fields are combined together, they form a complete human magnetic field. All of these magnetic fields remain steady as long as there is no other energy source to disturb them. However, whenever any extra energy is generated either inside or outside of this field, the field will no longer be steady, and an electrical current will be generated. Each time this happens, the body's field must rebalance itself, and a new pattern of energy must be formed.

This means that if there is no energy source for the human magnet, the magnetic field will not be disturbed and naturally there will be no energy circulating in this field. In this

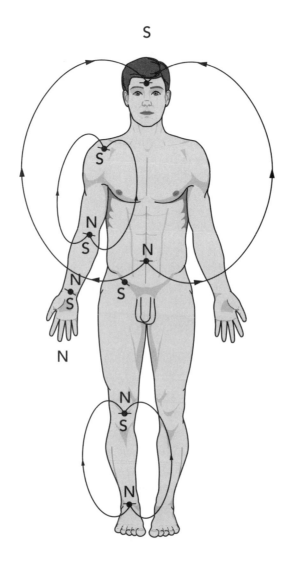

Figure 4-10. Human magnets in the Northern Hemisphere

case the body is dead. However, when you are alive, food and air essence generate energy inside your magnetic field through biochemical reaction. This energy builds up in your solar plexus, and then circulates throughout your body by way of the Qì channels, which are highly conductive paths through the fascial tissue. As the energy circulates in your body, it is important that every part, especially the organs, receives the right amount in order to function properly.

Let us take an even closer look. According to Chinese medical science, the electricity (Qì) circulates throughout your body from one channel to the next in a specific order. One end of each channel is therefore positive, and the other end negative. If an acupuncturist wishes to use a magnet to correct the Qì level of a channel, he must know how the magnetic field will influence the internal Qì circulation. He must know how Qì circulates and in what direction it circulates. He must also know how to orient the poles of the magnet. Wrong orientation will only worsen the situation. According to reports I have read about the use of magnets in acupuncture, sometimes it works and sometimes it doesn't. Possibly the failures are due to the acupuncturist's not taking the orientation of the magnets into account.

Time and the Human Electromagnetic Field. Since we are part of the Earth's electromagnetic field, our own fields are affected by variations in the Earth's energy field. These variations can be caused by such sources as the moon, the sun, or even the stars. The most obvious cycle that we are exposed to is that of the day. Every twenty-four hours our bodies should go through a cycle as the Earth rotates once and goes through a cycle of light and day. The rotation of the Earth is in turn affected by the sun's energy. It has been proposed that there is another cycle generated by the moon's influence on the Earth's energy pattern which repeats every twenty-eight days. Since the sun moves higher and lower above the southern horizon throughout the year, our bodies also go through a yearly cycle as well. The Chinese believe that the Earth and human beings go through other cycles every twelve and sixty years because of the influence of the stars. If you wish to study the human electromagnetic field, you must also take all of these cycles into your consideration.

Human Magnetic Model. Based on the above information, I would like to offer a magnetic model for a human being in the Northern Hemisphere on Earth. In Qìgōng society it is common knowledge that there are three energy storage areas from which energy can be taken and used without limit. These three places are called "Dāntián" or the "Fields of Elixir." The Lower Dāntián is thought of as the furnace of Original Qì. Let us consider it the north pole of the human magnetic field since the energy originates there. Let us consider the Upper Dāntián (the brain connecting to the third eye) to be the south pole because it receives energy (Figure 4-10). Science tells us that the lines of force in a magnetic field start from the north pole and end up at the south pole. In Qìgōng practice, the Qì originates at the Lower Dāntián and ends up at the Upper Dāntián to nourish the brain. The north pole is higher in energy and is in a relatively excited state while the south pole is lower in energy and is in a calm and steady state.

In his report on biomagnetics, Richard Leviton states: "One magnet practitioner, both a physician and a researcher, is Dr. Richard Broeringmeyer, a chiropractor, nutritionist, and publisher of the Bio-Energy Health Newsletter in Murray, Kentucky. 'Life is not possible without electromagnetic fields,' he said, 'and optimum health is not possible if the electromagnetic fields are out of balance for long periods of time. Magnetic energy is nature's energy in perfect balance.' Each of a magnet's two poles has a different energy and influence, says Broeringmeyer. The bipolar function is near the heart of biomagnetism."[5]

In regard to the two poles, I believe that it is the magnetic north pole at the Lower Dāntián which offers energy or Qì. It is able to increase the overall vital life force, strength, and development of a living system. In contrast, the south pole or the Upper Dāntián accepts energy or Qì. It acts to slow down, to calm, and to control the development of a living system.

You may understand now why I have located the poles of our magnetic field on either side of the Middle Dāntián (solar plexus). The Middle Dāntián can be considered the furnace where the essences of food and air are converted into electricity and generate an EMF for circulation.

The above assumptions are based on Chinese Qìgōng systems that were developed in the Northern Hemisphere of the Earth over the last several thousand years. I do not know if this theory is accurate, or how the poles affect living things in the Southern Hemisphere. The implication, however, is that people in the Southern Hemisphere have their magnetic poles reversed from how they are in the Northern Hemisphere. In other words, their Upper Dāntián will offer energy while the Lower Dāntián will receive it. Can this mean that, while the brains of people in the Northern Hemisphere are constantly being nourished, the brains of people in the Southern Hemisphere are being depleted? Does this explain why most technology was developed in the Northern Hemisphere? Do people in the Southern Hemisphere live longer because their Lower Dāntián is their south pole and it absorbs and retains Qì better than the Dāntián of a person in the Northern Hemisphere? I have heard of several doctors who recommend that patients who have lost their energy balance spend time on the equator, where the Earth's magnetic field has a minimal affect, and their bodies will be able to rebalance themselves. These are exciting and challenging ideas. It is time for a wide-scale study of human energy or Qìgōng in every corner of this world.

Channels

If Qì channels are areas where the electrical conductivity of the body tissue is higher than elsewhere, then we have answered one of the great questions of Qìgōng. In addition to explaining how Qì circulates, this can also enable us to learn what the ancients were never able to discover: the shape of the channels, and their exact location. In the past we have only been able to do Qì research on living people, but now we should be able to use cadavers and measure electrical conductivity throughout the body, and thereby determine the precise location and shape of the channels.

Vessels

We may assume that what are called the "Qì vessels" are tissues that can store electrical charges like a capacitor. The body has eight of these capacitors (called "the eight extraordinary vessels") that are responsible for regulating the current circulating in the twelve

---

5   "Healing with Nature's Energy," by Richard Leviton, *East West Journal*, June 1986.

channels. If this assumption is true, we should be able to determine the exact location and characteristics of these vessels with today's technology.

Cavities

Acupuncture cavities are small spots on the body where the electrical conductivity is higher than the surrounding areas.[6] Electricity is conducted between the main electrical channels (Qì channels) and the surface of the skin more easily at these locations than elsewhere. These cavities are the gates where needles, magnets, electricity, and other means such as lasers can be used to affect the flow of electricity in the Qì channels. The "Five Centers" or "Five Gates" (the Láogōng cavity at the center of each palm, the Yǒngquán cavity on the bottom of each foot, and the Bǎihuì cavity on the crown of the head) are probably larger openings where either the electric conductivity is higher or the conductive channels are larger.

Electromotive Force (or Electromagnetic Force) (EMF)

In order to have electric circulation, there must be an electromotive force (EMF). Without the EMF, the electric potential in the circuit will be the same throughout, and an electric current will not occur. The same principle applies to your body's electrical circuit. Generally, I can think of four possible causes for the generation of EMF in the human circuit: 1. Through the influence of natural energy. That means the EMF generated in the human body circuit can be affected by external energy interference, for example from the sun and the moon. Alternatively, you may expose your body to radioactive areas or even an electromagnetic field which can influence the electrical circulation in your body. 2. From the conversion of food and air essence. Whenever food and air are taken in, they are converted into bioelectric energy. This increase of the electricity will generate EMF for circulation. 3. From exercise. Whenever you move your muscles, part of the stored essence in your body is converted into electricity and generates an EMF in the exercised area. 4. From the mind and Shén (spirit). Your mind plays an important role in the generation of EMF. It might not be easy for the average person to understand this concept. However, if you understand that your thinking is able to affect the body's Qì circulation, you may be able to understand that the mind can generate an EMF. For example, your mind leads electricity to the limbs to energize the muscle tissues.

In Qìgōng training, you are training to increase your EMF through proper intake of food and air, Qìgōng exercises, and focused thought.

Stagnation

The flow of electricity can be reduced when the muscles are tightened or the structure of the channels (the conductive tissue) is changed. In Chinese medicine this is called "Qì stagnation." Tightening the muscles increases resistance to the flow of electricity and thereby causes an increase in temperature. It is still hard to say just how the resistance is increased. It may be due to a biochemical reaction generated by the mind, or possibly a change in the

---

6   *The Body Electric*, by Robert O. Becker, M.D. and Gary Selden, Quill, William Morrow, New York, 1985.

conductive tissue. The electric circulation can also be significantly affected when the conductive tissue is contaminated with material of low conductivity such as fat.

Obviously, relaxation is able to increase electrical circulation. In acupuncture, when a cavity is affected by a needle or magnet, the electrical field in that area is stimulated or sedated. It may possibly also convert the fat into heat and therefore open the path.

The Sensation of Heat

If Qì is electromagnetic energy circulating in the body, then the heat it produces is caused by the body's resistance to the electrical flow. If you run an electric current through a wire, when the current encounters resistance, electric energy is converted into heat. Therefore, the heat felt during acupuncture treatments and Qìgōng practice is not Qì, but rather a symptom of the presence of Qì. If this is true, then when practicing Qìgōng it is desirable to circulate the Qì so smoothly that it does not generate any sensation of heat. This is like running your current through a copper wire with low resistance instead of an iron one with high resistance. Whenever you generate too much heat in your body, especially in the organs, the tissue will begin to degenerate faster. Remember that the original Chinese symbol for Qì was constructed of two words: "no fire." Therefore, as a Qìgōng practitioner, you should not try to feel your Qì as heat. It is better to feel it as an electrical sensation. If you keep this in mind, you will be able to avoid making your body too Yáng during practice.

When we practice Qìgōng or Tàijíquán, it is common to experience warmth on the skin, especially in the centers of the palms (Láogōng, P-8, 勞宮), the bottoms of the feet (Yǒngquán, K-1, 湧泉), and on the face. We know that warmth is an indication of increased Qì circulation, but exactly how is this heat caused?

Before we continue, I would like to quote a report by Albert L. Huebner: "In England, doctors have discovered that children can regrow lost fingertips, perfect in every detail, when a procedure is followed that bears an interesting resemblance to limb regeneration in amphibians. A salamander won't regenerate its limb if the stump has become covered with skin, presumably because this blocks the 'current of injury' known to form there. Dr. Cynthia Illingworth of Sheffield found that if a child's fingertip is to grow back, the stump must also be left uncovered."[7]

This seems to indicate that the conductivity of muscle tissue is much higher than that of skin tissue. When skin has covered the injured area, it prevents the electric energy from extending beyond the stump and effecting the multiplication of cells and finally the regeneration of the finger.

I now believe that skin tissue is less conductive than muscle tissue, and both are less conductive than bone. When we have an injury deep in the muscle, the pain is more significant than when the injury is superficial. Likewise, the pain from an injury deep enough to reach the bone is even worse. The bone marrow and the brain are probably the two places where electric conductivity is the highest in the human body. However, it must be stressed that this

---

7.   "Life's Invisible Current," by Albert L. Huebner, *East West Journal*, June 1986.

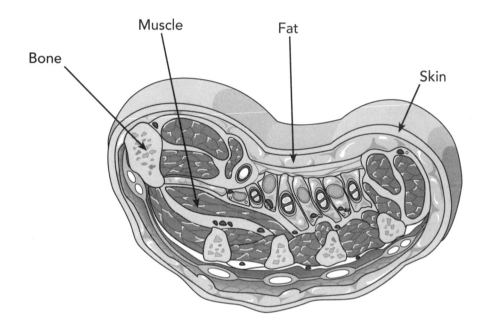

Figure 4-11. Cross section of a hand

is, in large measure, speculation. Experimentation and empirical evidence will be the only way to actually prove the correctness of the theory.

If you can accept these ideas, then it should be very easy for you to accept the explanation of how heat is generated in the skin during internal martial arts and Qìgōng. In these practices you often learn to relax and lead Qì to the ends of the limbs. The Qì or electricity will pass easily through the muscle and connective tissue, but when it reaches the skin the conductivity is suddenly lower. This means that resistance to the flow is increased. In combination with the fat (also of low electric conductivity) which normally accumulates between the skin and the muscle, the electricity is stopped and converted into heat (Figure 4-11).

You can see from this discussion why one of the purposes of Qìgōng is to reduce the heat and to open up the electrical blockages between the muscles and the skin and therefore increase the Qì flow to the surface of the skin. This ensures that the skin, hair, and nails receive an abundance of electricity to maintain health and increase growth.

Healing

The ideas we have discussed can also explain how some people can heal another person by touch. The average person can move only a limited amount of Qì through his body, and can bring only a very small amount to the surface of the skin. However, some people, including Qìgōng practitioners, can move Qì easily to the surface of the skin and beyond, and can even affect another person's Qì. If they can determine the status of the Qì throughout a person's body, they can supply energy to the areas that are low, and withdraw excess energy from areas that are oversupplied. Once they do this, it is important to rid their own bodies of the excess Qì through various Qì regulating methods.

Opening the Gates

One of the major goals of Qìgōng is "opening the gates" (Tōngguān, 通關). This means to remove any cause of electric (Qì) stagnation. Stagnation is when the flow of current is hindered in the Qì channels, usually around cavities. This is caused by improper food, poor-quality air, and aging of the body tissues. Various Qìgōng styles, which are based upon different theories, have various methods of opening the gates (this is discussed in Chapter 6). However, regardless of the style, the key to opening the gates is increasing the flow of current. This clears away obstructions and widens constricted areas ("gates" or "cavities"), smoothing the circulation. In order to increase the current flow, the EMF must be increased. This can be done by Qìgōng exercises and meditation in which the concentrated mind plays the main role.

The Measurement of Qì

If the theories discussed above can be proven to be valid, then we have finally answered the question of just what Qì is. We have also solved another problem, namely what unit of measurement to use. If Qì is bioelectricity, then we can simply use the same units of measurements we use with electricity. This is a great step forward, because with a standard unit of measurement we can now scientifically compare and evaluate results of tests and experiments.

Before we conclude this section, I would like to remind you of several things. Although we have used modern science's concepts of the magnetic field to draw comparisons with the magnetic fields which surround all living things, you should understand that the field around your body is much more complicated than the field around a simple magnet. Perhaps the main cause of this is due to your mind, which can affect your magnetic field. Exactly how the mind generates EMF is another one of the many mysteries of the brain. We also do not know exactly how food and air essences are converted into electric power.

Please remember also that many of the ideas discussed above are not proven facts. Although experimental evidence and scientific proof are accumulating, there are still many areas that are not understood. I have offered explanations for many of the big questions of Qìgōng, but they are personal theories and conclusions only. You should not take them as fact, because they still need more experimental proof. I hope that this section will stimulate people to think, and encourage a synthesis of the theories of Qì and bioelectricity.

4-4. OPENING THE QÌ GATES (KĀITŌNG QÌMÉN, 開通氣門)

The preceding discussion should give you an idea of some of the problems that need to be overcome in order to practice Qìgōng. To maintain your health, you must keep your Qì flowing smoothly in the proper pathways. Reducing the amount of bad food you eat, which is the main source of contaminated Qì, will help to maintain a smooth Qì flow. Then you must learn how to open all of the gates (cavities) that are obstructed and are causing Qì stagnation. This is a major part of the Qìgōng that is practiced for health.

In Qìgōng, opening the gates is called "Tōngguān" (literally, "to get through the gates," 通關). The theory of opening these gates is very simple. First think of what you would do if the drainpipe in your sink were partially blocked. You probably would run a lot of water through it to increase the pressure on the obstruction and wash it away. You would know when the pipe was clear because the water would pass through it quickly and strongly. You can use the same method with your Qì channels by running more Qì through them. But in order to move more Qì, you must first generate it. In Wàidān Qìgōng, when Qì is built up in the limbs it flows back into the body more strongly than before. As you continue to practice, the Qì will gradually widen the channels. Now, you might think that since increasing the Qì flow opens the gates, the more you increase the Qì, the more quickly you will open up the gates. However, you must remember one important thing. Your internal organs are designed to operate at certain levels of Qì, and if they receive too much Qì, they will become too Yáng and will degenerate more quickly.

It is very important in Qìgōng to do only enough to raise your Qì level just slightly above its normal level. As you continue to practice, the Qì channels will gradually widen so that the Qì level comes back down to normal, and the obstructed gates will slowly open. Then you can again increase the Qì level a little, the channels will become cleaner, and they will gradually become wider. Regular practice of the right exercises will smooth out the circulation, and keep the organs running properly. The proper amount of practice will maintain your health, too little practice will allow the channels to become plugged up, and too much practice will make your body too Yáng, and will shorten your life. This is the key theory of Wàidān.

There is no difference in the theory of Nèidān. However, in Nèidān training you normally open the gates in the Conception and Governing Vessels (Rènmài, Dūmài; 任脈、督脈) first. These two vessels are considered the major Qì reservoirs which govern the Qì, and so you must open them first if you want to regulate the Qì. Once this is done, you have completed Small Circulation (Xiǎozhōutiān, 小周天). There are three gates in this path which are considered the most difficult and dangerous when you practice. When you open these three gates, it is called Tōngsānguān ("to get through the three gates," 通三關). If you are interested to know more about Small Circulation, please refer to the book: *Qìgōng Meditation—Small Circulation*, by YMAA Publication Center (www.ymaa.com).

After you have completed the Small Circulation, you then lead the Qì to the limbs to open up all of the gates located on the Qì channels. Once you have completed this, you have accomplished Grand Circulation (Dàzhōutiān, 大周天). For further information, please refer to the author's books: *Qìgōng—The Secret of Youth* and also, *Qìgōng Grand Circulation*, by YMAA Publication Center.

CHAPTER 5

Categories of Qìgōng

Qìgōng is the study of your body's energy field, and it is directly related to your physical, emotional, mental, and even spiritual health. Both Eastern and Western religions influence the body's Qì, either indirectly through emotional or mental means, or directly through conscious manipulation. In the East, religion has been responsible for some of the greatest developments in Qìgōng. The Oriental religions have been more aware than the Occidental religions of the role Qì plays in our spiritual and emotional lives. Qìgōng starts with physical science (strengthening the body), then moves on to energy science (Qì), then to mental science (neutralizing the mind), and finally reaches spiritual science (enlightenment). When you study Chinese Qìgōng, you should be aware of the substantial role that religion has played in its development. As you learn more about Qìgōng, you will become more aware of the ways in which the Western religions have also practiced this science.

In this chapter we will first discuss the relationship between Qìgōng and the Chinese religions, and then we will discuss the different categories of Qìgōng.

5-1. QÌGŌNG AND RELIGION (QÌGŌNG YǓ ZŌNGJIÀO, 氣功與宗教)

It is part of the human condition that we frequently experience conflict between our hearts and our minds. So often we want to do things that we know we shouldn't. A part of us knows where our duties and moral obligations lie, but at the same time, our desires pull us in the opposite direction. All too often we find that wisdom and desire are in direct conflict. Desires we feel we cannot control drive us into acts of foolishness or even violence. When we do things we know we shouldn't, we feel an inner pain caused by the spiritual/moral conflict.

The Buddhists and Daoists say that there are seven human emotions: happiness (Xǐ, 喜), anger (Nù, 怒), sorrow (Āi, 哀), joy (Lè, 樂), love (Ài, 愛), hate (Hèn, 恨), and lust (Yù, 慾); and six desires which originate in the six roots: the eyes, ears, nose, tongue, body, and mind. These seven emotions and six desires are products of the emotional mind. Although some of the emotions, like love, can act to uplift us, most of the emotions and desires lead us to the evil and ugly side of life, the side of human disaster. If we learn to strengthen the wisdom mind we can gain calmness and peace, and this can help us to develop patience, perseverance, strong will, and a sense of justice and harmony. These virtues enable us to overcome the disasters created from the emotional mind. People need to be taught how to strengthen the good side and overcome the negative side of their nature. A proper education cultivates and matures the wisdom mind—the ability to judge, which can control the seven emotions and six desires.

Part of our nature is greedy and selfish, and causes us to struggle for money and power. When the moral part of our nature is suppressed, our minds seem to become evil—murder, theft, rape, anything becomes possible. Throughout history, many people have worshipped as heroes those who could kill, conquer, and enslave others. Today's movies and TV programs are filled with stories of killing and violence. The younger generations are continually being educated into this mindset when they watch these programs, and even in history classrooms. In this way the seed of the ugly side of human nature is planted and continually nourished. This seed will grow, and the next generation will perpetuate the violence, hatred, and greed.

These violent emotions can often suppress or distort the love and peace in people, but there is a cost. Since the longing for love and peace is an inborn part of human nature, the violent and hateful emotions constantly cause an inner conflict. It is this conflict that has generated the different religions of mankind. Religion brings a hope for peace, and encourages people to strengthen the good side of their natures. Many people gain peace and confidence, and overcome the sometimes crushing fear and uncertainty that surround us in this life.

All of the different religions seem to have one point of similarity—the believers must learn to meditate in order to gain peace of mind. Meditation (and prayer, which is a form of meditation) is able to bring spiritual consolation and calmness, and build self-confidence. Meditation regulates the mind, and balances the Qì which had been disturbed by emotional distress. Many people have found that prayer brings them an inner peace which has helped them recover from illness. With the increase of self-confidence, the spirit is raised and firmed. This raised spirit has become a major force in the fight to lessen the suffering in this world.

Buddhism and Daoism teach, like Christianity, that there is a heavenly kingdom and there is a hell. If you are good and have done good deeds while you were alive, you will be reborn as a human being, or you may even go to heaven as a Buddha or saint and leave the cycle of reincarnation behind. If you have been evil, you may end up in the hell of suffering and punishment, and/or be reborn as an animal. Almost everyone in ancient times was uneducated. They were worried and confused about their lives, and they were afraid of what might happen after death. Religions teach about heaven and hell to encourage people to be good instead of bad. Once people were trying to behave morally, religion taught them how to gain peace of mind through meditation.

Not surprisingly, a great number of meditation techniques were developed by religious practitioners, and the Chinese Buddhists and Daoists deeply researched the related field of Qìgōng. In fact, it was the religious Qìgōng practitioners who made the greatest achievements in the development of Qìgōng. This is especially true in the highest level of Qìgōng, which is enlightenment. At this level the study of human energy is spiritual science, and it becomes independent of religion.

From this discussion you can see that religion and Qìgōng are deeply intertwined. A thorough exploration of Chinese Qìgōng should also include the study of the historical background and theory of those religions which have influenced Chinese culture. It could also involve a comparison of Chinese Qìgōng with Western religious meditation techniques. I believe that this would help you to understand more clearly the relationship between human nature and Qìgōng.

5-2. CATEGORIES OF QÌGŌNG (QÌGŌNG ZHĪ FĒNLÈI, 氣功之分類)

In the several thousand years since Qì and its relationship to health were discovered, every level of the Chinese population has practiced Qìgōng at some time. There are four major schools or categories which were created by the different classes of people. The scholars, medical doctors, martial artists, and religious monks all had their distinctive categories of Qìgōng. The martial Qìgōng was again divided into external and internal styles, and the religious Qìgōng was divided into Buddhist, Daoist, and Tibetan styles.

In order to obtain a healthy body, you must cultivate both Xìng (Human Nature, 性) and Mìng (Physical Life, 命). A major part of Chinese philosophy has focused on the study of human nature, feelings, and spirit, as can be seen especially in Chinese scholarly and Buddhist (also Tibetan) religious society. Of all the different categories of Qìgōng, the scholarly and religious Qìgōng categories originated from and focused on the cultivation of human nature and spirit.

Human nature and spirit, as a matter of fact, were the most basic root of scholarly and religious philosophy in China. Physical life was considered to be not as important as the spiritual life. For this reason, most of the still meditation, which specializes in the cultivation of the spirit, was developed and studied by the scholars and Buddhist monks.

However, these two groups were striving for different goals. The scholars believed that the major illnesses were caused by emotional and spiritual imbalance. They used meditation to regulate the mind and spirit, and thereby gain good health. The Buddhist monks were aiming for spiritual independence and ultimately the stage of enlightenment or Buddhahood. Of these two groups, the Buddhist (including Tibetan) monks were able to reach the highest levels of meditation, which almost no other style in China was able to do. However, even though these two schools of Qìgōng emphasized spiritual meditation, they also used a limited number of Qìgōng exercises which trained the physical body, such as Dámó's Muscle/Tendon Changing exercises.

The Chinese medical doctors, on the other hand, thought that although spiritual meditation was important, physical cultivation was even more critical for health and healing. Furthermore, it was difficult to teach laymen still meditation, which was very hard to understand and practice. Therefore, the Qìgōng exercises created by the medical doctors focused on physical health and healing, and used mostly physical Qìgōng exercises. The physicians also relied heavily on acupuncture and herbs to adjust irregular Qì caused by sickness.

However, according to the available documents, many Qìgōng practitioners of different categories feel that the Daoist Qìgōng was probably the most complete both in theory and training because it emphasized the spiritual and physical equally. The Daoists also researched how different herbs affect the Qì circulation, and used these herbs to speed and smooth their progress. They even studied how one Qìgōng practitioner could share his Qì with his partners, or through mutual assistance help each other to speed up cultivation. The effect of diet on the Qì circulation was also deeply studied. Their research was extensive and practical. Their training methods therefore spread widely in Chinese Qìgōng society.

According to the available documents, we can roughly classify Qìgōng into five major categories, according to their purpose or final goal: 1. maintaining health, 2. curing sickness, 3. prolonging life, 4. martial skill, and 5. enlightenment or Buddhahood. Even though we show a different training purpose or aim for each category, you should understand that it is not possible to define all of the categories strictly according to their training purpose. This is simply because almost every style of Qìgōng serves more than one of the above purposes. For example, although martial Qìgōng focuses on increasing fighting effectiveness, it can also improve your health. The Daoist Qìgōng aims for longevity and enlightenment, but to reach this goal you need to be in good health and know how to cure sickness. Because of this multipurpose aspect of the categories, it will be simpler to discuss their backgrounds rather than the goals of their training. Knowing the history and basic principles of each category will help you to understand their Qìgōng more clearly. In this section we will discuss each category in more detail.

Scholar Qìgōng—for Maintaining Health (Xuézhě Qìgōng-Bǎoshēn, 學者氣功-保身)

In China before the Hàn dynasty (206 BCE, 漢前), there were two major schools of scholarship. One of them was created by Confucius (551–479 BCE, 孔子) during the Spring and Autumn Period (Chūnqiū, 春秋), and the scholars who practice his philosophy are commonly called Confucians. Later, his philosophy was popularized and enlarged by Mencius (372–289 BCE) (Mèngzǐ, 孟子) in the Warring States Period (戰國). The people who practiced this were called Rújiā (Confucianists, 儒家). The key words to their basic philosophy are Loyalty (Zhōng, 忠), Filial Piety (Xiào, 孝), Humanity (Rén, 仁), Kindness (Ài, 愛), Trust (Xīn, 信), Justice (Yì, 義), Harmony (Hé, 和), and Peace (Píng, 平). Humanity and the human feelings are the main subjects of study. Rújiā philosophy has become the center of much of Chinese culture.

The second major school of scholarship was called Dàojiā (Daoism, 道家) and was created by Lǎozi (老子) in the 6th century BCE. Lǎozi is considered to be the author of a book called the *Dào Dé Jīng* (*Classic on the Virtue of the Dào*, 道德經) which described human morality. Later, in the Warring States Period, his follower Zhuāngzhōu (莊周) wrote a book called *Zhuāngzi* (莊子), which led to the forming of another strong branch of scholarship. Before the Hàn dynasty, Daoism was not considered a religion, but rather another branch of scholarship. It was not until the Hàn dynasty that traditional Daoism was combined with the Buddhism imported from India, and it began gradually to be treated as a religion. Therefore, the Daoism before the Hàn dynasty should be considered scholarly Daoism rather than religious.

In regards to their contribution to Qìgōng, both schools of scholarship emphasized maintaining health and preventing disease. They believed that many illnesses are caused by mental and emotional excesses. When a person's mind is not calm, balanced, and peaceful, the organs will not function normally. For example, depression can cause stomach ulcers and indigestion. Anger will cause the liver to malfunction. Sadness will cause stagnation and tightness in the lungs, and fear can disturb the normal functioning of the kidneys and bladder. They realized that if you want to avoid illness, you must learn to balance and relax your thoughts and emotions. This is called "regulating the mind" (Tiáoxīn, 調心).

Therefore, the scholars emphasized gaining a peaceful mind through meditation. In their still meditation, the main part of the training is getting rid of thoughts so that the mind is clear and calm. When you become calm, the flow of thoughts and emotions slows down, and you feel mentally and emotionally neutral. This kind of meditation can be thought of as practicing emotional self-control. When you are in this "no thought" state, you become very relaxed, and can even relax deep down into your internal organs. When your body is this relaxed, your Qì will naturally flow smoothly and strongly. This kind of still meditation was very common in ancient Chinese scholarly society.

In order to reach the goal of a calm and peaceful mind, their training focused on regulating the mind, body, and breath. They believed that as long as these three things were regulated, the Qì flow would be smooth and sickness would not occur. This is why the Qì training of the scholars is called Xiūqì" (修氣), which means "cultivating Qì." Xiū in Chinese means to regulate, to cultivate, or to repair. It means to maintain in good condition. This is very different from the Daoist Qì training after the Hàn dynasty which was called Liànqì (練氣), which is translated "train Qì." Liàn means to drill or to practice to make stronger. Daoist Qìgōng after the Hàn dynasty will be discussed later.

Many of the Qìgōng documents written by the Confucians and Daoists were limited to the maintenance of health. The scholar's attitude in Qìgōng was to follow his natural destiny and maintain his health. This philosophy is quite different from that of the Daoists after the Hàn dynasty, who denied that one's destiny could not be changed. They believed that it is possible to train your Qì to make it stronger, and to reach the goal of longevity. It is said in scholarly society: "Rénshēng Qīshí Gǔláixī,"[1] which means "in human life seventy is rare." You should understand that few of the common people in ancient times lived past seventy because of the lack of good food and modern medical technology. It is also said: "Āntiān Lèmìng" (安天樂命), which means "peace with heaven and delight in your destiny"; and "Xiūshēn Símìng" (修身俟命), which means "cultivate the body and await destiny." Compare this with the philosophy of the later Daoists, who said: "Yībǎièrshí Wèizhīyāo,"[2] which

---

1. 人生七十古來稀。
2. 一百二十謂之天。

means "one hundred and twenty means dying young." They believed and have proven that human life can be lengthened and destiny can be resisted and overcome.

Confucianism and Daoism were the two major schools of scholarship in China, but there were many other schools which were also more or less involved in Qìgōng exercises. We will not discuss them here because there is only a limited number of Qìgōng documents from these schools.

To conclude, the basic characteristics of scholarly Qìgōng training include:

1. Spiritual and mental Qìgōng was emphasized more than physical Qìgōng.
2. The published documents which are related to Qìgōng discuss it in a random, unorganized, and unsystematic fashion.
3. Maintaining health was the goal of Qì cultivation. Overcoming death and destiny was considered impossible.
4. Before the Hàn dynasty, Daoism was considered a branch of scholarship, whereas after the Hàn dynasty it became involved in religion and became the Daoist religion. Therefore, the Qìgōng developed by the Daoists before the Hàn dynasty was considered scholarly Daoist Qìgōng.

Medical Qìgōng—for Healing (Yīxué Qìgōng-Liáobìng, 醫學氣功-療病)

In ancient Chinese society, most emperors respected the scholars and were affected by their philosophy. Doctors were not regarded highly because they made their diagnosis by touching the patient's body, which was considered characteristic of the lower classes in society. Although the doctors developed a profound and successful medical science, they were commonly looked down upon. However, they continued to work hard and study, and quietly passed down the results of their research to following generations.

Of all the groups studying Qìgōng in China, the doctors have been at it the longest. Since the discovery of Qì circulation in the human body about four thousand years ago, the Chinese doctors have devoted a major portion of their efforts to the study of the behavior of Qì. Their efforts resulted in acupuncture, acupressure or cavity press massage, and herbal treatment.

In addition, many Chinese doctors used their medical knowledge to create different sets of Qìgōng exercises either for maintaining health or for curing specific illnesses. Chinese medical doctors believed that doing only sitting or still meditation to regulate the body, mind, and breathing as the scholars did was not enough to cure sickness. They believed that in order to increase the Qì circulation, you must move. Although a calm and peaceful mind was important for health, exercising the body was more important. They learned through their medical practice that people who exercised properly got sick less often, and their bodies degenerated less quickly than was the case with people who just sat around. They also realized that specific body movements could increase the Qì circulation in specific organs.

They reasoned from this that these exercises could also be used to treat specific illnesses and to restore the normal functioning of these organs.

Some of these movements are similar to the way in which certain animals move. It is clear that in order for an animal to survive in the wild, it must have an instinct for how to protect its body. Part of this instinct is concerned with how to build up its Qì, and how to keep its Qì from being lost. We humans have lost many of these instincts over the years that we have been separating ourselves from nature.

Many doctors developed Qìgōng exercises which were modeled after animal movements to maintain health and cure sickness. A typical, well-known set of such exercises is Wǔqínxì (Five Animal Sports, 五禽戲) created by Dr. Jūnqiàn (君倩). Some say that the Wǔqínxì was created by Huátuó (華陀). Another famous set based on similar principles is called Bāduànjǐn (the Eight Pieces of Brocade, 八段錦). It was created by Marshal Yuè, Fēi (岳飛) who, interestingly enough, was a soldier rather than a doctor.

In addition, using their medical knowledge of Qì circulation, Chinese doctors researched until they found which movements could help cure particular illnesses and health problems. Not surprisingly, many of these movements were not unlike the ones used to maintain health, since many illnesses are caused by unbalanced Qì. When this imbalance continues for a long period of time, the organs will be affected, and may be physically damaged. It is just like running a machine without supplying the proper electrical current—over time, the machine will be damaged. Chinese doctors believe that before physical damage to an organ shows up in a patient's body, there is first an abnormality in the Qì balance and circulation. Abnormal Qì circulation is the very beginning of illness and physical organ damage. When Qì is too positive (Yáng) or too negative (Yīn) in a specific organ Qì channel, your physical organ is beginning to suffer damage. If you do not correct the Qì circulation, that organ will malfunction or degenerate. The best way to heal someone is to adjust and balance the Qì even before there is any physical problem. Therefore, correcting or increasing the normal Qì circulation is the major goal of acupuncture or acupressure treatments. Herbs and special diets are also considered important treatments in regulating the Qì in the body.

As long as the illness is limited to the level of Qì stagnation and there is no physical organ damage, the Qìgōng exercises used for maintaining health can be used to readjust the Qì circulation and treat the problem. However, if the sickness is already so serious that the physical organs have started to fail, then the situation has become critical and a specific treatment is necessary. The treatment can be acupuncture, herbs, or even an operation, as well as specific Qìgōng exercises designed to speed up the healing or even to cure the sickness. For example, ulcers and asthma can often be cured or helped by some simple exercises. Recently in both mainland China and Táiwān, certain Qìgōng exercises have been shown to be effective in treating certain kinds of cancer.[3]

---

3.   There are many reports in popular and professional literature of using Qìgōng to help or even cure many illnesses, including cancer. Many cases have been discussed in the Chinese Qìgōng journals. One book which describes the use of Qìgōng to cure cancer is *New Qìgōng for Preventing and Curing Cancer* (新氣功防治癌症), by Yè, Míng (葉明), Chinese Yoga Publications, Táiwān, 1986.

Over the thousands of years of observing nature and themselves, some Qìgōng practitioners went even deeper. They realized that the body's Qì circulation changes with the seasons, and that it is a good idea to help the body out during these periodic adjustments. They noticed also that in each season different organs had characteristic problems. For example, in the beginning of autumn the lungs have to adapt to the colder air that you are breathing. While this adjusting is going on, the lungs are susceptible to disturbance, so your lungs may feel uncomfortable and you may catch colds easily. Your digestive system is also affected during seasonal changes. Your appetite may increase, or you may have diarrhea. When the temperature goes down, your kidneys and bladder will start to give you trouble. For example, because the kidneys are stressed, you may feel pain in the back. Focusing on these seasonal Qì disorders, the meditators created a set of movements which can be used to speed up the body's adjustment. These Qìgōng exercises will be introduced in a later volume.

In addition to Marshal Yuè, Fēi, many people who were not doctors also created sets of medical Qìgōng. These sets were probably originally created to maintain health, and later were also used for curing sickness.

The characteristics of medical Qìgōng are:

1. Medical Qìgōng emphasizes moving meditative exercises more than sitting still meditation.
2. The major goals of medical Qìgōng are maintaining health and curing sickness.
3. Qìgōng exercises were only a small part of Chinese medical science. Herbal treatment, acupuncture, and acupressure remained the major methods of healing.

Martial Qìgōng—for Defense (Wǔxué Qìgōng-Fángshēn, 武學氣功-防身)

Chinese martial Qìgōng was probably not developed until Dámó's *Muscle/Tendon Changing Classic* (*Yìjīnjīng*, 易筋經) was developed in the Shàolín Temple (Shàolínsì, 少林寺) during the Liáng dynasty (502–557 CE, 梁). When Shàolín monks trained Dámó's Muscle/Tendon Changing Qìgōng, they found that they could not only improve their health but also greatly increase the power of their martial techniques. Since then, many martial styles have developed Qìgōng sets to increase their effectiveness. In addition, many martial styles have been created based on Qìgōng theory. Martial artists have played a major role in Chinese Qìgōng society.

When Qìgōng theory was first applied to the martial arts, it was used to increase the power and efficiency of the muscles. The theory is very simple—the mind (Yì) is used to lead Qì to the muscles to energize them so that they function more efficiently. The average person generally uses his muscles at under 40-percent maximum efficiency. If one can train his concentration and use his strong Yì to lead Qì to the muscles effectively, he will be able to energize the muscles to a higher level and, therefore, increase his fighting effectiveness.

As acupuncture theory became better understood, fighting techniques were able to reach even more advanced levels. Martial artists learned to attack specific areas, such as vital acupuncture cavities, to disturb the enemy's Qì flow and create imbalances which caused injury or even death. In order to do this, the practitioner must understand the route and timing of the Qì circulation in the human body. He also has to train so that he can strike the cavities accurately and to the correct depth. These cavity strike techniques are called Diǎnxuè (Pointing Cavities, 點穴) or Diǎnmài or Dim Mak (Pointing Vessels, 點脈).

Most of the martial Qìgōng practices help to improve the practitioner's health. However, there are other martial Qìgōng practices which, although they build up some special skill which is useful for fighting, also damage the practitioner's health. An example of this is Iron Sand Palm (Tiěshāzhǎng, 鐵砂掌). Although this training can build up amazing destructive power, it can also harm your hands and affect the Qì circulation in the hands and the internal organs.

Since the 6th century, many martial styles have been created which were based on Qìgōng theory. They can be roughly divided into external and internal styles.

The external styles emphasize building Qì in the limbs to coordinate with the physical martial techniques. They follow the theory of Wàidān (external elixir, 外丹) Qìgōng. In Wàidān Qìgōng, Qì is usually generated in the limbs through special exercises. The concentrated mind is used during the exercises to energize the Qì. This increases muscular strength significantly, and therefore increases the effectiveness of the martial techniques. Qìgōng can also be used to train the body to resist punches and kicks. In this training, Qì is led to energize the skin and the muscles, enabling them to resist a blow without injury. This training is commonly called Iron Shirt (Tiěbùshān, 鐵布衫) or Golden Bell Cover (Jīnzhōngzhào, 金鐘罩). The martial styles which use Wàidān Qìgōng training are normally called external styles (Wàigōng, 外功) or hard styles (Yìnggōng, 硬功). Shàolín Gōngfū is a typical example of a style which uses Wàidān martial Qìgōng.

Although Wàidān Qìgōng can help the martial artist increase his power, there is a disadvantage. Because Wàidān Qìgōng emphasizes training the external muscles, it can cause overdevelopment. This can cause a problem called "energy dispersion" (Sàngōng, 散功) when the practitioner gets older. In order to remedy this, when an external martial artist reaches a high level of external Qìgōng training he will start training internal Qìgōng, which specializes in curing the energy dispersion problem. That is why it is said "Shàolín Gōngfū from external to internal."

Internal Martial Qìgōng is based on the theory of Nèidān (internal elixir, 內丹). In this method, Qì is generated in the body instead of the limbs, and this Qì is then led to the limbs to increase power. In order to lead Qì to the limbs, the techniques must be soft and muscle usage must be kept to a minimum. The training and theory of Nèidān martial Qìgōng is much harder than those of the Wàidān martial Qìgōng. The interested reader should refer to the author's book: *Tài Chí Chuán and Martial Power—Advanced Yáng Style*. Several internal martial styles were created in the Wǔdāng (武當) and Éméi (峨嵋) Mountains. Popular styles are Tàijíquán (太極拳), Bāguàzhang (八卦掌), Liùhé Bāfǎ (六合八法), and Xíngyìquán (形意拳). However, you should understand that even the internal martial styles, which are commonly called soft styles, must on some occasions use muscular strength while fighting. Therefore, once an internal martial artist has achieved a degree of competence in internal Qìgōng, he should also learn how to use harder, more external techniques. That is why it is said: "The internal styles are from soft to hard."

In the last fifty years, some of the Tàijí Qìgōng or Tàijíquán practitioners have developed training which is mainly for health, and is called Wújí Qìgōng (無極氣功) which means "no extremities Qìgōng." Wújí is the state of neutrality which precedes Tàijí, which is the state of complimentary opposites. When there are thoughts and feelings in your mind, there is Yīn and Yáng, but if you can still your mind you can return to the emptiness of Wújí. When you achieve this state your mind is centered and clear and your body relaxed, and your Qì is able to flow naturally and smoothly and reach the proper balance by itself. Wújí Qìgōng has become very popular in many parts of China, especially Shànghǎi (上海) and Canton (Guǎngdōng, 廣東).

You can see that, although Qìgōng is widely studied in Chinese martial society, the main focus of training was originally on increasing fighting ability instead of health. Good health was considered a by-product of the training. It was not until this century that the health aspect of martial Qìgōng started receiving greater attention. This is especially true in the internal martial arts. Please refer to the in-depth Martial Qìgōng book: *The Essence of Shàolín White Crane*, available from YMAA Publication Center.

Religious Qìgōng—for Enlightenment or Buddhahood (Zōngjiào Qìgōng-Shéntōng, 宗教氣功-神通)

Religious Qìgōng, though not as popular as other categories in China, is recognized as having achieved the highest accomplishments of all the Qìgōng categories. It used to be kept secret, and it is only in this century that it has been revealed to laymen.

In China, religious Qìgōng includes mainly Daoist and Buddhist Qìgōng. The main purpose of their training is striving for enlightenment, or what the Buddhists refer to as Buddhahood. They are looking for a way to lift themselves above normal human suffering, and to escape from the cycle of continual reincarnation. They believe that all human suffering is caused by the seven emotions and six desires. If you are still bound to these emotions and desires, you will reincarnate after your death. To avoid reincarnation, you must train your spirit to reach a very high stage where it is strong enough to be independent after your death. This spirit will enter the heavenly kingdom and gain eternal peace. This is hard to do in the everyday world, so they frequently flee society and move into the solitude of the mountains, where they can concentrate all of their energies on self-cultivation.

Religious Qìgōng practitioners train to strengthen their internal Qì to nourish their spirit (Shén) until this spirit is able to survive the death of the physical body. Marrow/Brain Washing Qìgōng training is necessary to reach this stage. It enables them to lead Qì to the head, where the spirit resides, and raise it to a higher energy state. This training used to be restricted to only a few priests who had reached an advanced level. Tibetan Buddhists were also involved heavily in this training. Over the last two thousand years the Tibetan

Buddhists, the Chinese Buddhists, and the Daoists have followed the same principles to become the three major religious schools of Qìgōng training.

This religious striving toward enlightenment or Buddhahood is recognized as the highest and most difficult level of Qìgōng. Many Qìgōng practitioners rejected the rigors of this religious striving, and practiced Marrow/Brain Washing Qìgōng solely for the purpose of longevity. It was these people who eventually revealed the secrets of Marrow/Brain Washing to the outside world. If you are interested in Marrow/Brain Washing Qìgōng, please refer to the book: *Qìgōng—The Secret of Youth*, available from YMAA Publication Center.

Buddhist Qìgōng—for Buddhahood. Buddhism was created by an Indian prince named Sakyamuni (558–478 BCE). When he was twenty-nine years old, he became dissatisfied with his comfortable and sheltered life and left his country. He went out into the world among the common people to experience the pain and suffering in their lives. Six years later, he suddenly apprehended the "Truth," and started to travel around and spread his philosophy.

Buddhism was imported into China during the Eastern Hàn dynasty (58 CE, 東漢). The Hàn emperors became sincere Buddhists, and Buddhism became the main religion in China. Naturally, the Buddhist meditation methods were also learned by the Chinese Buddhist monks.

Buddhist Qìgōng training is very similar to Chinese scholarly Qìgōng. The main difference is that while scholarly Qìgōng aims at maintaining health, Buddhist Qìgōng aims at becoming a Buddha. Meditation is a necessary process in training the priest to stay emotionally neutral. Buddhism believes that all human suffering is caused by the seven passions and six desires (Qīqíng Liùyù, 七情六慾). The seven passions are happiness (Xǐ, 喜), anger (Nù, 怒), sorrow (Āi, 哀), joy (Lè, 樂), love (Ài, 愛), hate (Hèn, 恨), and lust (Yù, 慾). The desires are generated from the six roots which are the eyes, ears, nose, tongue, body, and mind (Xīn, 心). Buddhists also cultivate within themselves a neutral state separated from the four emptinesses of earth, water, fire, and wind (Sìdà Jiēkōng, 四大皆空). They believe that this training enables them to keep their spirits independent so they can escape from the cycle of repeated reincarnation.

The early priests were not so concerned with their physical health, and meditated in order to train themselves to stay emotionally neutral. Naturally, most of the priests did not have long physical lives.

This situation lasted until the Liáng dynasty (502–557 CE, 梁), when physical Qìgōng exercises began to be emphasized in a limited number of Buddhist temples. There is a famous story about Dámó (達摩). Dámó was an Indian Buddhist prince who was invited to China to preach by emperor Liáng. When the emperor did not favor his philosophy, Dámó went to the Shàolín Temple (少林寺). He discovered that all of the priests were weak and sickly, so he decided to help them. He shut himself away to ponder the problem, and stayed in seclusion for nine years. When he emerged he had written two books, the *Yìjīnjīng* (*Muscle/Tendon Changing Classic*, 易筋經), and the *Xǐsuǐjīng* (*Marrow/Brain Washing Classic*, 洗

髓經). The techniques taught in the *Muscle/Tendon Changing Classic* were practiced by many Buddhist priests. They believed that they needed strong and healthy bodies to complete their training.

The Shàolín priests learned that when they practiced these exercises, not only did their health increase, but their physical power also increased significantly. They naturally used this power in coordination with their fighting techniques when they had to defend themselves. This change marked one more step in the growth of Chinese martial arts: Martial Qìgōng. This was discussed earlier. Many sets of physical Qìgōng exercise have been developed over the years based on the principles expounded in Dámó's book on Muscle/Tendon Changing.

Although it was often necessary to defend oneself during that violent period, there were many priests who were against the martial training. They believed that as Buddhist priests they should avoid all violence. For this reason, most of the temples practiced only the still meditation for cultivating their Buddhahood.

Dámó's *Marrow/Brain Washing Classic* describes how a priest can strengthen his health and increase his longevity. Once he has finished this training he can go on to more advanced training which has the goal of attaining Buddhahood. Before a priest started his Marrow/Brain Washing training he had to first complete the Muscle/Tendon Changing, which was considered the foundation. Unfortunately, the theory of Marrow/Brain Washing is very difficult to understand, and the whole process was kept secret by the monks, so for many centuries it was thought to be lost. It was only in the last forty years that some of the documents have been revealed to the public.

Dámó is considered the ancestor of the Chinese Chán Zong (禪宗), or the Rěn (忍) sect of Buddhism. The traditional teaching philosophy which has been attributed to him is: "Jiàowài Biézhuàn, Bùlìwénzì, Zhízhǐ Rénxīn, Jiànxìng Chéngfó."[4] (Do not pass on to people outside of our religion, words should not be written down, point directly to the person's mind, to see and cultivate the personality, humanity, and becoming a Buddha.)

When Dámó died, it was said that he passed his Chán Buddhist philosophy and his *Marrow/Brain Washing Classic* techniques to his best and trusted disciple, Huìkě (慧可). Huìkě's name as a layman was Jìguāng (繼光). He was a scholar who gave up his normal life and became a priest in order to conquer himself. Huìkě passed the Buddhist philosophy on to Sēngcàn (僧璨). It then went to Dàoxìn (道信), Hóngrěn (弘忍), and Huìnéng (慧能). Including Dámó, these six are called "the Six Ancestors of Chán" (Chánzōng Liùzǔ, 禪宗六祖). Later, Chinese Buddhist society honored another monk, Shénhuì (神會) of the Táng dynasty of Kāiyuán (713–742 CE, 唐、開元), and subsequently referred to the Seven Ancestors of Chán (Chánzōng Qīzǔ, 禪宗七祖).

Since Dámó came from India, part of the Qìgōng training theory developed by him was identical to Indian Yoga (such as the still meditation), which had existed for some time in India. Later, Chán theory and training was brought to Japan by Chinese Buddhist monks, and became the Rěn (Zěn) meditation of Japan.

---

4.   教外別傳，不立文字，直指人心，見性成佛。

You can see that before the Liáng dynasty, the Buddhists used only still meditation. Since the Liáng dynasty, many priests learned Dámó's exercises, and then adopted the movements of various animals to use in Qìgōng sets, or even for martial purposes.
To summarize:

1. Before Dámó (527 CE), still meditation was the major part of Chinese Buddhist training. After Dámó, moving Qìgōng exercises—in the *Muscle/Tendon Changing Classic*—were introduced.

2. Muscle/Tendon Changing (Yáng, 陽) was the foundation of Marrow/Brain Washing. Muscle/Tendon Changing can change a person's physical body from weak to strong, and Marrow/Brain Washing (Yīn, 陰) is able to train a monk to use his Qì to keep his marrow clean and to nourish his brain for spiritual enlightenment, the way of reaching the goal of Buddhahood.

3. Because the Muscle/Tendon Changing training is able to increase the strength of the body, it has been used by Buddhists and non-Buddhists in their martial training. Since then, many martial Qìgōng styles have been created.

4. The *Marrow/Brain Washing Classic* is hard to understand and train, and has been kept secret for a long time.

5. Dámó was the ancestor of Chán or Rěn (Zěn) meditation.

Tibetan Qìgōng—for Buddhahood. Tibet was significantly influenced by both Indian and Chinese cultures. Buddhism had a great effect, so the root of Tibetan Qìgōng is similar to that of Indian Buddhism. However, over thousands of years of study and research, the Tibetans established their own unique style of Qìgōng meditation. The Tibetan priests are called Lǎmas (Lǎma, 喇嘛), and many of them also learned martial arts. Because of the different cultural background, not only are the Lǎmas' meditation techniques different from those of the Chinese or Indian Buddhists, but their martial techniques are also different. Tibetan Qìgōng meditation and martial arts were kept secret from the outside world, and were therefore called Mìzōng (密宗), which means "secret style." Because of this, and because of the different language, there are very few documents available in Chinese. Generally speaking, Tibetan Qìgōng and martial arts were not spread into Chinese society almost until the Qīng dynasty (1644–1911 CE). Since then, however, they have become more popular.

However, even though Tibetan Qìgōng training techniques are sometimes different from those of the Chinese and Indian Buddhists, they still have the same goal of all Buddhists—Buddhahood. According to the available documents, Tibetan Qìgōng training emphasizes spiritual cultivation through still meditation like the Buddhist meditation, although they use many physical Qìgōng exercises which are similar to Indian Yoga.

To summarize:

1. Tibetan Qìgōng is part of Buddhist Qìgōng, although it has developed its own unique system of cultivation.
2. Tibetan still meditation theory and training is similar to that of the Buddhists. However, they also have some physical Qìgōng training similar to Indian Yoga.
3. Documents on Tibetan Qìgōng are scarce. Hopefully someone who is specializing in researching Tibetan culture can fill this void.

Daoist Qìgōng—for Enlightenment. Daoism was created by Lǎozi (老子, or Lǐěr, 李耳) in the 6th century BCE. He wrote a book titled *Dào Dé Jīng* (*Classic on the Virtue of the Dào*, 道德經) which discusses natural human morality. Later, his follower Zhuāngzhōu (莊周) in the Warring States Period (Zhànguó, 戰國) wrote a book called *Zhuāngzi* (莊子). Soon, another branch of scholarship developed, which was separate from Confucianism. Before the Hàn dynasty, Daoism was purely a form of scholarship. It studied the human spirit and nature but, according to the available documents, it was not considered a religion.

In the Eastern Hàn dynasty (25–168 CE, 東漢), Zhāng, Dào-Líng (張道陵) created the Daoist religion (Dàojiào, 道教). Daoism worshipped primarily the deity Yuánshǐ Tiānzūn (The Primal Celestial Excellency, 元始天尊), also called "Yùhuáng Dàdì" (The Supreme Deity, 玉皇大帝) after the Sòng dynasty, and Lǎozi (popularly titled Tàishàng Lǎojūn, or Old Lord of the Ultimate, 太上老君). In Dàojiào philosophy, they believed there was a heavenly kingdom ruled by "The Primal Celestial Excellency." Only the immortals and the gods lived in this kingdom, which controlled everything on the earth. You can see that the original concept of Heaven Qì has been modified, and a religious color added. These religious Daoists also believed that when a person died, if he had done something very good, he would become a saint. Heaven would offer him a position which allowed him to rule the living. If a person did not do anything especially good while alive, when he died he would reincarnate as a human being. However, if a person had been bad, his soul would be sent to one of the eighteen levels of hell for punishment. There, the King of Hell (Yánluówáng, 閻羅王) would decide what kind of animal he should reincarnate as. If someone had been very bad, he would not reincarnate, but would stay in hell for an eternity of torture.

The religious philosophy and views on reincarnation of the Daoists were very similar to those of the Buddhists. This may be related to the fact that the Daoist religion was created only about one hundred years after Buddhism was imported into China. It is said that religious Daoism is a blend of Buddhism and traditional Daoism.

Like the Buddhists, the Daoists believe that if they can build up their spirit (Shén) so that it is independent and strong, they will be able to escape from the cycle of repeated reincarnation. When a Daoist or Buddhist has reached this stage, he has reached the goal of enlightenment or Buddhahood. It is said that he has attained eternal life. However, if he cannot build his spirit strong enough before he dies, his soul or spirit will not go to hell, and he will be able to control his own destiny and either stay a spirit or be reborn as a human. They believed that it is only possible to develop the human spirit while in a body, so that the continual cycle of rebirth is necessary to attain enlightenment.

The monks found that in order to enhance their spirit, they had to cultivate the Qì which was converted from their Jīng (essence). The normal Daoist Qìgōng training process is 1. to convert the Jīng (essence) into Qì (Liànjīng Huàqì, 煉精化氣); 2. to nourish the Shén (spirit) with Qì (Liànqì Huàshén, 煉氣化神); 3. to refine the Shén into emptiness (Liànshén Fǎnxū, 煉神返虛); and 4. to crush the emptiness (Fěnsuì Xūkōng, 粉碎虛空). The first step is to firm and strengthen the Jīng, then convert this Jīng into Qì through meditation or other methods. This Qì is then led to the top of the head to nourish the brain and raise up the Shén. When a Daoist has reached this stage, it is called "the three flowers meet on the top" (Sānhuā Jùdǐng, 三花聚頂). This stage is necessary to gain health and longevity. Finally, the Daoist can start training to reach the goal of enlightenment. However, the biggest obstacle to achieving this goal is the emotions, which affect the thinking and upset the balance of the spirit. This is the reason they hid themselves away in the mountains, away from other people and their distractions. They also abstained from eating meat, feeling that it muddied thinking and increased the emotions, leading the spirit away from self-cultivation.

While striving for enlightenment or Buddhahood, most Buddhist monks concentrate all their attention on the cultivation of the spirit. The Daoists, however, feel that in order to reach the final goal, you have to first be in good physical health. This may be the reason why more Daoists than Buddhists have lived very long lives. In their nineteen hundred years of research, they found many more ways to strengthen the body and to slow down the degeneration of the organs, which is the key to obtaining a long life. There have been many Daoists who have lived more than 150 years. In Daoist society it is said: "one hundred and twenty means dying young." Unfortunately, all of this Qìgōng training has been passed down secretly in the monasteries. It was not until the last twenty years that these secret theories and training methods were revealed to the outside world.

An important part of this training to prolong life is Marrow/Brain Washing Qìgōng. The basic idea of Marrow/Brain Washing Qìgōng is to keep the Qì circulating in your marrow so that the marrow stays clean and healthy. Your bone marrow manufactures your blood cells. The blood cells bring nourishment to the organs and all the other cells of the body, and also take waste products away. When your blood is healthy and functions properly, your whole body is well-nourished and healthy, and can resist disease effectively. When the marrow is clean and fresh, it manufactures an enormous number of healthy blood cells which will do their job properly. Your whole body will stay healthy, and the degeneration of your internal organs will be significantly slowed. Your body is not unlike an expensive car. It will run a long time if you use a high quality fuel; but if you use a low quality fuel, the car engine will deteriorate a lot faster than it needs to.

Although the theory is simple, the training is very difficult. You must first learn how to build up your Qì and fill up your eight Qì vessels (the twelve major Qì channels and eight Qì vessels will be discussed in Part Three), and then you must know how to lead this Qì into the bone marrow to "wash" the marrow. Except for some Daoist monks, there are very few people who have lived more than 150 years. The reason for this is that the training process is long and hard. You must have a pure mind and a simple lifestyle so that you can concentrate entirely on the training. Without a peaceful life, your training will not be effective. This is why the Daoist monks hide themselves in the mountains. Unfortunately, this is simply not possible for the average person. If you are interested in Marrow/Brain Washing Qìgōng training, please refer to the book: *Qìgōng—The Secret of Youth*, available from YMAA Publication Center.

Do not be misled into thinking that the Buddhist Chán (Rěn) meditation is inferior to the Daoist approach. In fact, the Buddhists often had much greater success in reaching enlightenment than the Daoists through their use of still meditation. Additionally, many of the Daoist Qìgōng practices originated with the Buddhists. The Daoists then modified them to suit their own circumstances and purposes, and some of the practices, like Marrow/Brain Washing, were practiced much more widely by the Daoists than the Buddhists.

Many Daoist Qìgōng styles are based on the theory of cultivating both the spirit and the physical body. In Daoism, there are generally three ways of training: Jīndān Dàdào (Golden Elixir Large Way, 金丹大道), Shuāngxiū (Dual Cultivation, 雙修), and Dàowài Cǎiyào (Herb Picking Outside of the Dào, 道外採藥). Jīndān Dàdào teaches the ways of Qìgōng training within yourself. This approach believes that you can find the elixir of longevity or even enlightenment within your own body.

In the second approach, Shuāngxiū (Dual Cultivation), a partner is used to balance one's Qì more quickly. Most people's Qì is not entirely balanced. Some people are a bit too positive, others too negative, and individual channels also are positive or negative. If you know how to exchange Qì with your partner, you can help each other out and speed your training. Your partner can be either the same sex or opposite.

The third way, which is called "Dàowài Cǎiyào," uses herbs to speed and control the cultivation. Herbs can be plants such as ginseng, or animal products such as musk from the musk-deer.

According to the training methods used, Daoist Qìgōng can again be divided into two major schools: Qīngxiūpài (Peaceful Cultivation Division, 清修派) and Zāijiēpài (Plant and Graft Division, 栽接派). This division was especially clear after the Sòng and Yuán dynasties (960–1367 CE, 宋、元). The meditation and the training theory and methods of the Qīngxiūpài (Peaceful Cultivation Division) are close to those of the Buddhists. They believed that the only way to reach enlightenment is Jīndān Dàdào (Golden Elixir Large Way), according to which you build up the elixir within your body. Using a partner for the cultivation is immoral and will cause emotional problems which may significantly affect the cultivation.

However, the Zāijiēpài (Plant and Graft Division) claims that in addition to Jīndān Dàdào, their methods of Shuāngxiū (Dual Cultivation) and Dàowài Cǎiyào (Herb Picking Outside of the Dào) make the cultivation faster and more practical. For this reason, Daoist

Qìgōng training is also commonly called Dāndǐng Dàogōng (丹鼎道功), which means "the Dào Training in the Elixir Crucible." The Daoists originally believed that they would be able to find and purify the elixir from herbs. Later, they realized that the only real elixir was in your body.

According to my understanding, the major difference between the two Daoist schools is that the Qīngxiūpài aims for enlightenment in a way similar to the Buddhists' striving for Buddhahood, while the Zāijiēpài uses the training to achieve a normal, healthy, long life. We will discuss these two major Daoist schools more extensively in a later volume.

You can see that Daoism has already been a religion and a scholarly study of Qìgōng methods. As a modern and scientific Qìgōng practitioner, you should only adopt the Qìgōng training methods which can benefit you. Superstition should be filtered out. However, you need to know the historical background so that you will understand the root and the motivation of the training.

To conclude, the characteristics of Daoist Qìgōng are:
1. Daoist Qìgōng and enlightenment theories were based on those of the Buddhists. It later developed into its own unique style.
2. Daoist religion was a mixture of Buddhism with traditional Daoism.
3. Original Daoist Qìgōng training aimed for enlightenment, and later was used for improving health and longevity.
4. There are two major schools of Daoist Qìgōng training, one of which is similar to Buddhist training.

CHAPTER 6

Qìgōng Theory

6-1. INTRODUCTION (JIÈSHÀO, 介紹)

Many people think that Qìgōng is a difficult subject to understand. In some ways, this is true. However, regardless of how difficult the theory and practice of a particular style of Qìgōng might be, the basic Qì theory and principles are very simple and remain the same for all of the Qìgōng styles. Basic Qì theory and Qìgōng principles are the roots of all Qìgōng practice, and it is from these roots that the different styles of training blossomed. Naturally, the results and the depth achieved are different from style to style. If, however, you understand the root of what you are doing, it does not matter which style you are practicing, because you will be able to grasp the key to the practice and grow.

As discussed in the last chapter, there are three major purposes of Qìgōng other than martial arts: health, longevity, and spiritual enlightenment. Although all three groups use the same basic Qì theory in their training, they use different training theories and methods to reach their goals. For example, people who are training for longevity use deeper, more advanced training methods than people who are practicing to improve their health, while the people who are striving for enlightenment use training theories and methods which are deeper still.

If you wish to understand the science of Qìgōng, you must understand the different categories and their respective training theories. This will be like a map of the terrain making it easier for you to select your goal and plan your route. Without this map, you will wander around confused, uncertain of your goal.

Previous sections have discussed general Qì theory, and some of the ways in which Qì affects human beings. Qì circulation theory will be discussed in greater detail later. Now, we will discuss general training theory and methods, and what each approach has to offer you.

Generally speaking, all Qìgōng practices, according to the training theory and methods, can be divided into two general categories: Wàidān (External Elixir, 外丹) and Nèidān (Internal Elixir, 內丹). Understanding the difference between them will give you an overview of most Chinese Qìgōng practices.

6-2. External Elixir (Wàidān, 外丹)

"Wài" means "external or outside," and "Dān" means "elixir." External here means the limbs, as opposed to the torso, which includes all of the vital organs. Elixir is a hypothetical, life-prolonging substance for which Chinese Daoists have been searching for millennia. They originally thought that the elixir was something physical which could be prepared with herbs or chemicals purified in a furnace. After thousands of years of study and experimentation, they found that the elixir is in the body. In other words, if you want to prolong your life, you must find the elixir in your body, and then learn to protect it and nourish it.

Sometimes Wàidān also refers to herbal pills which can be used to adjust or increase the Qì circulation in the body. In this book we will only discuss the Qìgōng Wàidān training theory and methods, and leave the discussion of herbal Wàidān theory to qualified herbal masters.

The human body has twelve major Qì channels (Jīng, 經) (actually pairs of channels, one on either side of the body), which are comparable to rivers. Six of these are connected to the fingers, and the other six are connected to the toes. All of these twelve are connected to internal organs. The body also has eight Qì vessels (Mài, 脈), which serve as reservoirs, and also regulate the Qì in the twelve channels. Millions of tiny channels (Luò, 絡) carry Qì from the major channels to every part of the body, from the skin to the bone marrow. Whenever the Qì is stagnant in any of the twelve major channels, the related organ will receive an incorrect amount of Qì. This will cause the organ to malfunction, or at least to degenerate sooner than normal, and this in turn will cause illness and premature aging if left uncorrected. Just as a machine needs the correct amount of current to run properly, your organs must have the right amount of Qì to function well. Therefore, the most basic way to maintain the health of the organs is to keep the Qì flow balanced and smooth. This is the idea upon which Wàidān (External Elixir) Qìgōng is based.

The theory is very simple. When you do Wàidān exercises you concentrate your attention on your limbs. As you exercise, the Qì builds up in your arms and legs. When the Qì potential in your limbs builds to a high enough level, the Qì will flow through the channels, clearing any obstructions and nourishing the organs. This is the main reason that a person who works out, or has a physical job, is generally healthier than someone who sits around all day.

There are many available Wàidān Qìgōng sets. A typical one is Dámó's *Muscle/Tendon Changing Classic* (*Wàidān Yìjīnjīng*, 外丹易筋經). In this set, the practitioner slightly tenses up the local limb muscles in specific postures, such as tensing up the wrist while holding both arms in front of the chest, and then relaxing completely. This repeated tensing and relaxing builds up a greater concentration of Qì in the area being exercised. When the practitioner finishes the exercise and relaxes, the accumulated Qì flows to the organs. In this category of Wàidān training, the specific stationary postures and the tensing and relaxing of the muscles are the two ways in which the Qì circulation is increased.

There are other Wàidān sets which, in addition to tensing and relaxing the muscles, also move the arms and legs in specific ways so that the muscles around certain organs are stretched and then relaxed. In addition to building up Qì in the limbs, these exercises increase the Qì circulation around and in the organs more directly than the *Muscle/Tendon Changing Classic* does. For example, you may raise your arms over your head and then lower them repeatedly, exercising the muscles around the lungs, extending and releasing them gently to massage the lungs and stimulate the flow of Qì and blood. A typical set of Wàidān which uses moving exercises is the Eight Pieces of Brocade (Bāduànjǐn, 八段錦).

Many Qìgōng beginners believe mistakenly that since Wàidān Qìgōng theory and training are simple, these sets are only for beginners. In fact, most people who train Nèidān Qìgōng later come back to Wàidān, and combine the two to increase their control over their Qì.

These two categories of Wàidān training methods, in addition to improving martial arts performance, also give you a healthy body, and can even cure some illnesses. Improved health may increase the length of your life, but not to the 150 years that was achieved by some of the Daoists and Buddhists. These results require deeper theory and training, under the supervision of a qualified master. Longevity Qìgōng exercises will be discussed in the section on Nèidān Qìgōng. I would like to conclude with three points about Wàidān Qìgōng:

1. Wàidān Qìgōng aims at maintaining health, and has only a limited effect on longevity. Many Wàidān Qìgōng exercises were created to increase martial ability.
2. Wàidān Muscle/Tendon tension and relaxation practice focuses on training the Qì in the limbs. The main purpose of increasing the Qì in the limbs is to energize the muscles to their highest efficiency. The specific postures also train the coordination of the muscles in the torso with those in the limbs. If you understand that one of the major purposes of Dámó's Wàidān exercises is to increase martial power, then you will see why the limbs are emphasized in the training. After Dámó, many sets were created from the same theory, mostly by martial artists. Naturally, these exercises will also improve health. However, many martial artists who trained the Dámó Wàidān exercises heavily for a long time found that they overdeveloped their muscles the way weight lifters often do. Although they were healthy as long as they were able to practice, once they got old their muscles degenerated much faster than normal. This is called Sàngōng (energy dispersion, 散功). Because of this, Dámó created a set of Nèidān exercises which is also included in the *Muscle/Tendon Changing Classic*. This set builds up and circulates the Qì internally, preventing the Qì channels from plugging up when the practitioner gets older.
3. The moving Wàidān practices focus on increasing the Qì circulation around the organs through specific movements. This category of Wàidān practice will not build the muscles like the last category. Wàidān exercises like this are used mainly for health.

6-3. INTERNAL ELIXIR (NÈIDĀN, 內丹)

"Nèi" means "internal" and "Dān" means "elixir." Thus, Nèidān means to build the elixir internally. Here, internally means in the body instead of in the limbs. Whereas in Wàidān the Qì is built up in the limbs and then moved into the body, Nèidān exercises build up Qì in the body and lead it out to the limbs.

Generally speaking, Nèidān theory is deeper than Wàidān theory, and its training theory and methods are more difficult to understand and practice. Traditionally, most of the Nèidān Qìgōng practices have been passed down more secretly than those of the Wàidān. This is especially true of the highest levels of Nèidān, such as Marrow/Brain Washing, which were passed down to only a few trusted disciples. There are a number of reasons for this:

1. Nèidān is hard to understand, so only the disciples who were intelligent and wise enough to understand it were taught.

2. Nèidān practice can be dangerous. Inaccurate practice may cause crippling, paralysis, or even death. This can happen especially to the disciple who does not understand the what, why, and how of his practice.

3. In much of Nèidān Qìgōng you are working with and guided by very subtle feelings and sensations. Under the guidance of a master you should be able to grasp the key to the training in a short time. However, if you try to figure it out by yourself, you may get confused, or injure yourself seriously.

4. In order to reach the higher levels of Nèidān Qìgōng, you must conserve your Jīng and restrain your sex life. Also, you must spend a lot of time in practice, which makes normal married life impossible. Furthermore, in order to reach a spiritual balance, you must train yourself to be emotionally neutral and independent. In order to preserve your Jīng and have a peaceful environment for your training, you almost have to go away to the mountains and become a hermit, or become a monk in a monastery. Still, though Nèidān is difficult to understand and practice, it is practiced by many laymen. They, however, can only reach a certain level of achievement, such as health and longevity, but not enlightenment.

Before we discuss the training categories of Nèidān, you should understand how Nèidān Qìgōng practice relates to the Qì circulation in the human body. As we have mentioned, the human body has twelve Qì channels which are considered Qì rivers. Each of these channels is connected to a finger or toe, and is also associated with an internal organ. In order to keep the twelve organs healthy, the Qì flowing in the Qì rivers must be smooth and continuous, and the Qì level running in each channel must be appropriate for that channel. Whenever the Qì flow is stagnant or the Qì level abnormal, the organs will not function properly and may eventually be damaged. Therefore, the first goal of this Qìgōng practice is to keep the Qì running smoothly and at the appropriate levels in the channels.

In addition to these twelve channels, there are eight vessels which are considered Qì reservoirs and which regulate the Qì running in the Qì rivers. In order to have the potential to supply and regulate the Qì, the vessels must be full. When there is enough Qì in the reservoirs to supply and regulate the Qì in the rivers, you will be healthy. Therefore, the second goal of Qìgōng practice is to learn to fill up the Qì reservoirs with Qì.

When you have attained these two goals, you have built a good foundation for a healthy body. The training methods you must practice to reach these two goals are explained clearly in Dámó's *Muscle/Tendon Changing Classic*. However, if you desire longevity, you must enter a deeper level of Nèidān Qìgōng exercises. This level is described in Dámó's *Marrow/Brain Washing Classic*.

In order to have a long life, you need to have not only a healthy physical body and smooth Qì circulation, but also training in two more disciplines. The first concerns your blood, the second your spirit. Your blood runs through your entire body. If your blood cells are not healthy, it does not matter how healthy and strong your physical body and organs appear to be, because your physical body will degenerate quickly. The marrow is the factory which makes your blood cells. If you know how to keep your marrow healthy and fresh, the quality of the blood cells will be high. When these healthy and fresh blood cells are running in your physical body, the degeneration process will slow down and your life span will increase.

When you train Marrow/Brain Washing Qìgōng, you must also learn how to lead Qì to your brain and raise your Shén. When the Shén is raised, you will have a center or headquarters which will be able to effectively control your Qì and strengthen your body's Guardian Qì (Wèiqì, 衛氣) so that it is better able to repel negative outside influences. The raised Shén will also direct the Qì so that the organs function properly. However, the most important benefit of Marrow/Brain Washing training is the fresh, nourishing Qì brought to your brain, which ensures its health. Marrow/Brain Washing training will keep your brain strong, calm, and peaceful.

Before we discuss Nèidān practice further, you should understand that there are many different methods of Nèidān practice. We will discuss the two major ones: Dámó's Muscle/Tendon Changing Classic (Yìjīnjīng), and his Marrow/Brain Washing Classic (Xǐsuǐjīng).

Dámó's Muscle/Tendon Changing Classic (Dámó Yìjīnjīng, 達摩易筋經)

As mentioned before, Dámó's Muscle/Tendon Changing Classic includes two parts. The first part is the Wàidān external Qìgōng exercises, and the second part is the Nèidān internal Qìgōng training. The Wàidān external Qìgōng has already been discussed, so we will discuss the Nèidān internal training here. Dámó's Nèidān training includes two major practices.

Small Circulation (Xiǎozhōutiān, 小周天)

One of the major purposes of Nèidān training is to fill up the Qì reservoirs, i.e., the eight vessels. When the Qì there is abundant, you will be able to supply enough Qì to the rest of

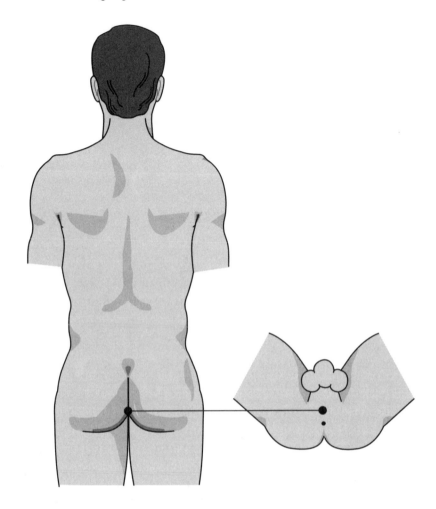

Figure 6-1. Huìyīn cavity (Co-1)

your body. Small Circulation has two major purposes. The first purpose is to build up Qì at the Lower Dāntián, and the second purpose is to store and circulate Qì in the two major reservoirs: the Conception and Governing Vessels.

You must learn abdominal breathing in order to build up Qì at your Lower Dāntián. Then you must lead this Qì to circulate in the vessels and open up the cavities which are plugged up or where the Qì flow is sluggish. For example, when you were a child, the Huìyīn cavity (Co-1) (會陰) (Figure 6-1) in the perineum was wide open. However, as you got older and abandoned abdominal breathing, it gradually plugged up so that the Qì circulation through it became sluggish. There are a number of other cavities where the Qì path narrows and the circulation slows down. Wherever the circulation is sluggish and not smooth, the Qì supply to the organs and the entire body will lose its balance and you may become sick.

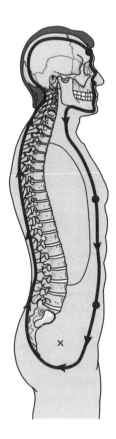

Figure 6-2. The Fire Path of Qì circulation

There are a number of ways in which Qì can be circulated in the body through the Small Circulation. However, there are two major ones which are commonly practiced: the "Fire Path" and the "Wind Path."

The Fire Path (Huǒlù, 火路). The Fire Path is the way Qì naturally circulates in the human body. The Qì moves down the Conception Vessel (Rènmài, 任脈) and up the Governing Vessel (Dūmài, 督脈) (Figure 6-2). The Conception Vessel is considered Yīn (negative), and runs down the center of the front of the body. The Governing Vessel is considered Yáng (positive). It runs from the Huìyīn, where it connects to the Conception Vessel, up along the outside of the spine to the back of the neck, passes over the head to the top of the inside of the mouth where it connects with the Yīn vessel on the tongue.

Normally, Post-birth Qì (Fire Qì, 火氣), is converted from the Jīng of food and air in the Sānjiāo (Triple Burner, 三焦). After this Qì is converted, it is stored in the Middle Dāntián. This Qì moves down to the Lower Dāntián and mixes with Water Qì. The mixed Qì moves down to the Huìyīn (會陰), and at the Huìyīn it divides into two Qì flows. One of them enters the Thrusting Vessel (Chōngmài, 衝脈) in the spinal cord and moves up to nourish the brain. This path is considered the Water Path (Shuǐlù, 水路) and is the path trained in Marrow/Brain Washing Qìgōng. The Water Path will be discussed later. The second flow passes the Huìyīn and moves up the back following the Governing Vessel (along the outside of the spine), passes over the crown and finally connects to the Conception Vessel to complete the cycle. This second path is the "Fire Path."

As Qì circulates through the Fire Path, there is always one part of the path where the Qì level is higher than elsewhere, and this area circulates around the path regularly over twenty four hours. It is this area of higher Qì potential which keeps the Qì flowing. (I believe that this potential is created by the earth's spinning inside the sun's electromagnetic field.) Just as water will only flow from a higher to a lower level, Qì will only move from a place of higher potential to one of lower potential. In Chinese medicine, this place of higher potential is called Zǐwǔ Liúzhù (子午流注). Zǐ (子) refers to the two hours between 11 pm and 1 am, and Wǔ (午) refers to the time between 11 am to 1 pm. Liú (流) means "flow," and Zhù (注) means "tendency." "Zǐwǔ Liúzhù" therefore means "the major Qì flow tendency which follows the time change." In the Fire Path, the place of higher potential normally starts at noon at the Middle Dāntián (solar plexus) and moves down to reach the Lower Dāntián and mix with the Dāntián Qì between 2 and 4 pm. Next, it goes down to the Huìyīn at sunset and moves to the back in the evening, reaching the top of the head at midnight. At sunrise the Qì is in the face, and by noon it has reached the Middle Dāntián to complete the cycle.

One of the major purposes of Small Circulation practice is to build up Original Qì at the Lower Dāntián. Original Qì is created from the Original Essence drawn from the kidneys, which mixes with and dilutes the Post-birth Qì which comes from food and air. Post-birth Qì, which contains undesirable products from the food and air, is considered Fire Qì because it has a heating effect on the body. Original Qì is considered Water Qì, and it is pure and cools down the Fire Qì. Diluting and cooling down the contaminated Qì is the first step in cooling down the fire in your physical body. This process will slow your body's degeneration. In the Fire Path, a practitioner usually learns to build or strengthen his Water Qì in the Lower Dāntián (Field of Elixir) through abdominal breathing or mental concentration. When the Qì is built up to a certain level, the mind leads the Qì to circulate through the Conception and Governing Vessels.

Another task in Small Circulation is the opening of cavities where the Qì flow is sluggish. In Fire Path Qìgōng training, there are three cavities which must be opened and are considered dangerous. If you do not understand this and do not proceed cautiously, you might cause yourself serious injury. If you are interested in Small Circulation Meditation,

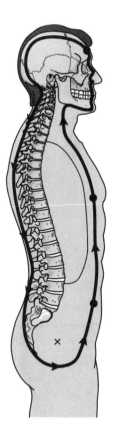

Figure 6-3. The Wind Path of Qì circulation

you may refer to author's book: *Qìgōng Meditation—Small Circulation*, by YMAA Publication Center.

The Wind Path (Fēnglù, 風路). Generally speaking, the Wind Path of Qì circulation is not as popular as the Fire Path. Because it circulates Qì in the direction opposite to the normal flow, many Qìgōng practitioners believe that it will disturb the natural Qì circulation and cause problems. There are very few documents which discuss this path. However, some discuss a portion of the complete cycle, usually from the Lower Dāntián up to the Middle Dāntián, and many Qìgōng practitioners have trained it.

In this portion of the Wind Path Qì circulation, once the Original Qì is built up in the Dāntián, the practitioner leads it up to circulate in the direction opposite to the one trained in the Fire Path (Figure 6-3). Normally, this is trained when you have completed your Fire Path Small Circulation. There are two reasons for circulating the Wind Path:

1. To slow down the natural Qì circulation in the Conception and Governing Vessels by circulating Qì against the flow. If the Qì flow in your Fire path is too Yáng

because of excitement, injury, sickness, or even eating poor food, your whole body will become too Yáng when this Qì is distributed through the twelve Qì channels. This Yáng Qì will damage your organs, and make your mind excited and scattered. The Wind Path can regulate the Qì circulating in your Fire Path, and rebalance the Qì in your body.

2. An important Qìgōng practice is raising up the Pre-birth Qì (Essence Qì or Water Qì) generated in the Lower Dāntián to cool down the Post-birth Qì (Food and Air Qì, or Fire Qì) which is generated in the Middle Dāntián at the solar plexus. When this is done, the clean Water Qì will be able to dilute the contaminated Fire Qì before it starts to circulate. This raising of the Water Qì is done through the Wind Path.

Wind Path circulation will be discussed in more detail in a later volume on Small Circulation Meditation.

Grand Circulation (Dàzhōutiān, 大周天). After you have opened up the path of the Conception and Governing Vessels, you have completed what is called Xiǎozhōutiān or "Small Circulation." This was the first step in the Nèidān part of Dámó's *Muscle/Tendon Changing Classic.* The second step is opening the twelve channels to keep the Qì flowing in the organs and limbs. As we mentioned before, Nèidān differs from Wàidān Qìgōng in that it builds up Qì in the body and then circulates it outward to the limbs.

Only after you have opened up all of the twelve channels and the Qì is able to flow to the extremities are you protected from the Qì blockages which are associated with the Wàidān Muscle/Tendon exercises. Once you have completed your Grand Circulation, you have completed Dámó's Nèidān Muscle/Tendon Qìgōng training. This training must be completed before a Qìgōng practitioner begins Dámó's Marrow/Brain Washing Qìgōng training.

Dámó's Marrow/Brain Washing Classic (Dámó Xǐsuǐjīng, 達摩洗髓經)

Dámó's *Marrow/Brain Washing Classic* was kept secret until 1980s. It explains the secret of longevity and of reaching the goal of enlightenment and Buddhahood. Both the theory and the training are deep. Normally, only those who thoroughly understood Qìgōng training theory and had long years of Qìgōng experience, especially of Dámó's *Muscle/Tendon Changing Classic*, were taught the *Marrow/Brain Washing Classic.*

The Chinese name of the work is *Xǐsuǐjīng.* "Xǐ" means "to wash, to keep clean and fresh." "Suǐ" means two things, the marrow which is called Gǔsuǐ (骨髓) and the brain which is called Nǎosuǐ (腦髓). Jīng is a treatise or classic. You can see from this that the main goal of Xǐsuǐjīng is to wash the bone marrow and the brain and keep them clean and fresh.

Generally speaking, Marrow/Brain Washing has two major purposes: longevity, and enlightenment or Buddhahood. Laymen usually strive for longevity, while monks sought enlightenment or Buddhahood as the culmination of their Daoist or Buddhist training. We will discuss these two purposes briefly here. The interested reader should refer to the YMAA book: *Qìgōng—The Secret of Youth.*

Longevity. According to Chinese medicine, your body deteriorates as you age mainly because your blood loses its ability to feed and protect your body. Your bone marrow produces the red blood cells and one type of the white blood cells, but as you grow older, the marrow becomes "dirty," and produces fewer and fewer useful blood cells. However, if you know how to "wash" the marrow, it will start once again to produce fresh, healthy blood. Your body will begin to rejuvenate itself, and restore itself to the glowing health of youth.

You should understand that in order to produce healthy blood cells, the marrow must be alive, fresh (clean), and active. To keep the marrow fresh and alive and functioning properly, Qì must be plentiful and continuously supplied. Whenever there is a shortage of Qì, the marrow will not function normally. In Marrow/Brain Washing Qìgōng, you must first learn how fill up the "eight extraordinary Qì vessels" with Qì. These vessels are your reservoirs of Qì. With plenty of Qì stored in them, you will have enough Qì to supply your muscles, organs, and marrow. In order to fill up the reservoirs, you must learn how to efficiently convert your essence into Qì. You must also learn how to increase your essence so that you will have enough material to convert into Qì. Essence is like the fuel, Qì is like the energy generated, and bone marrow is the factory. With plenty of energy supplied, the production line of the blood cells will be healthy. When the fresh and healthy blood cells are circulated throughout your body, they will carry out their mission efficiently. This will slow down the degeneration of your physical body so that it lasts a lot longer. It is just like running an expensive car with good quality fuel—the car will run more efficiently and last longer.

Enlightenment. For the Chinese monks, Marrow/Brain Washing is only a step necessary for reaching the final goal of enlightenment or Buddhahood. In order to reach this purpose, the Qì must be led up through the spinal cord to nourish the brain. When the brain is nourished, the Shén (i.e., spirit) is also nourished, and it will grow stronger and stronger until it is able to reach the final goal of spiritual independence.

According to Chinese medical science, the Chōngmài (Thrusting Vessel, 衝脈) is the major Qì reservoir which supplies Qì to the brain. The Chōngmài is located in the spinal cord. Therefore, in order to have plenty of Qì to continuously nourish the brain and Shén, the Chōngmài reservoir must be kept full.

You can see that religious Marrow/Brain Washing concentrates on the Qì circulation in the spinal cord. However, for good health and longevity you must wash the marrow in all of the bones so that all of the blood cell factories function properly. Many techniques have been developed by Qìgōng practitioners to achieve this purpose. However, the most complete and profound study both in theory and training is credited to the Daoists. Since ancient times, Daoists have practiced Qìgōng for both longevity and enlightenment.

Do not think that there is no health and longevity benefit when the Qì is led to nourish the brain and raise the Shén. As a matter of fact, your brain and spirit are the center and headquarters of your whole being. When your brain is healthy, you will be able to think clearly. You need to have a healthy brain if you want a healthy body. In the same way, your Shén is your Qì control center. When your spirit is high the Qì can be led efficiently to every part of the body, but when your spirit is low your energy level will be low and the Qì will not circulate smoothly.

Generally, there are three steps to Marrow/Brain Washing Qìgōng training:

1. **To increase the essence**

    The essence which is converted into Qì in Marrow/Brain Washing is not primarily from the kidneys, but rather from the sexual organs (testicles in men and ovaries in women). Essence here means the hormones. Many ways have been developed to increase this essence. This is discussed more fully in the YMAA book: *Qìgōng—The Secret of Youth*.

2. **To convert the essence into Qì**

    There are two vessels or Qì reservoirs in your legs which are called Yīnqiāomài (the Yīn Heel Vessel, 陰蹺脈). Their main Qì source is the essence which comes from your sexual organs. When the Qì that is in these vessels is withdrawn, more Qì will automatically be converted. Therefore, you must know how to draw Qì from these reservoirs. This is done in the next step.

3. **To sublimate the Qì upward**

    This means to lead your Qì upward into the Chōngmài (Thrusting Vessel), and then into the brain to nourish the brain and raise the Shén.

You can see that the processes discussed above include "converting the essence into Qì" (Liànjīng Huàqì, 煉精化氣) and "nourishing the Shén with the Qì" (Liànqì Huàshén, 煉氣化神). There are two more steps to reach the final goal of enlightenment. These two steps are: "to refine the Shén and enter emptiness" (Liànshén Fǎnxū, 煉神返虛) and "to crush the emptiness" (Fěnsuì Xūkōng, 粉碎虛空). This is discussed in the YMAA book: *Qìgōng—The Secret of Youth*.

The Water Path (Shuǐlù, 水路). Now that you have some idea of Marrow/Brain Washing Qìgōng training, it is time to discuss the Water Path of Qìgōng circulation. Water Path Qìgōng, which passes through the spinal cord, is one of the higher levels of Qìgōng practice. Once you have built your Pre-birth Qì in the Dāntián, you use your mind and special training to lead the Qì into the branch of the Thrusting Vessel (Chōngmài, 衝脈) which is located in the spinal cord (Figure 6-4). The Water Path, which is used in Marrow/ Brain Washing, uses the Water Qì generated from the Lower Dāntián, but it also generates Qì through a different method, for example, by using the sexual organs as mentioned above.

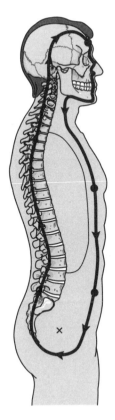

Figure 6-4. The Water Path of Qì circulation

The average person already has some circulation in the Water Path to nourish the brain. In the evening, when the Qì circulation is strongest in the Huìyīn (Co-1) (會陰), it divides into two flows. One flow circulates in the Fire Path outside of the spine, and the other passes through the spinal cord and moves up to nourish the brain and Shén. This usually happens at midnight while you are sleeping. Between midnight and early morning, the Qì also flows to the groin to energize the area and stimulate the generation of hormones and semen (Jīng or essence). A major part of Marrow/Brain Washing Qìgōng is increasing the efficiency of the conversion of semen into Qì and leading it to nourish the brain and energize the Shén (spirit). The energized mind is then able to adjust the Qì level in the organs and other parts of the body. This Qìgōng practice is difficult to do, but, once competence has been achieved, the practice is the most efficient. It is reported that priests who reach this level are able to slow down the aging process to a minimum, and some are able to live over two hundred years.

PART TWO

General Keys to Qìgōng Training

CHAPTER 7
General Concepts

7-1. INTRODUCTION (JIÈSHÀO, 介紹)

When the average person goes to an apple orchard, he will usually pay attention only to the fruit. If he goes to a nursery, he will notice only the beauty and fragrance of the flowers. Few people consider that the fruit and flowers are only the result of a great deal of planning, preparation, and hard work. In the same way, when most people see another person's success, few will stop to think about how that person could be so successful. Chinese people say: "When there is a result, there must be a cause," and "If you want to harvest rice, you must first plant rice." You have to know what you want and plan how to get it. Without this, there is no beginning. Next, your project must be patiently nourished, watered, and protected. If the root is not nourished and protected, the tree will not grow strong, and the harvest will not be bountiful.

Qìgōng training is not much different from growing a tree. In order for the Qìgōng tree to grow well and give an abundant harvest, you must plant a healthy seed. This means you must first do some research about the different kinds of trees so that you will know how to pick a seed which will grow into the kind of tree you want. In Part One we spread out all the seeds in front of you so that you could understand the background of the various Qìgōng training categories. Next, you must learn how to plant the seed, water it, protect it, and make it grow. If you nourish and protect it, the root of the plant will grow strong, and you can expect a good harvest. If the root is weak, your Qìgōng tree will wither and die.

The purpose of Part Two is to show you how to plant the seed, nourish it, and protect it. You should understand that it does not matter which type of tree you are growing, the general theory and methods for making the tree grow healthily remain the same. You always need sunshine, water, good soil, fertilizer, and protection from insects, and you always need to know where and when to plant your seed.

There are five things which you must know in order to make your Qìgōng tree grow well. These are: regulating the body (Tiáoshēn, 調身), regulating the breathing (Tiáoxí, 調息), regulating the mind (Tiáoxīn, 調心), regulating the Qì (Tiáoqì, 調氣), and regulating the Shén (Tiáoshén, 調神). You also need to know how they are interrelated. These are the foundation of successful Qìgōng practice. Without this foundation, your understanding of Qìgōng and your practice will remain superficial.

This gives you an idea of the How in Qìgōng training. However, knowing How is not enough. It only offers you the theory and principles of training which have been developed by previous Qìgōng practitioners. Following the past may lead you to great success in your Qìgōng training, but it will not help you to develop Qìgōng training any further. For this you must not only know How, you must also know Why. A farmer may know the How of growing apple trees well, but only someone who understands the Why of it all will be able to improve the growing techniques or develop new variety of apples. It is the same in Qìgōng training—you want to be a Qìgōng botanist instead of just a Qìgōng farmer. Why and How are the roots of understanding. They are the theory and principle of study.

Having an understanding of the Why of the training is especially important when you are just beginning. It lets you make an informed choice of a style which is best for you, and since you have a clear idea of where you are going, you can be confident, patient, and strong willed enough to complete the training.

The rest of this chapter will discuss the key parts of Qìgōng training, such as how to build up Qì and the importance of Kǎn (water, 坎) and Lí (fire, 離). Chapters 8 to 13 will discuss the general keys to Qìgōng training, such as how to regulate your body, breath, emotional mind, essence, Qì, and Shén (spirit, 神). Finally, Chapter 14 will review some important points in Qìgōng practice.

7-2. BUILDING QÌ (ZĒNGQIÁNG QÌLIÀNG, 增強氣量)

Before we go any further in our discussion of the keys to Qìgōng training, you should first understand how Qì is generated in your body. Generally, the Qì is generated or converted naturally and automatically from the essences within your body. These essences include the inherited Original Essence which goes to make Water Qì, and the essence from food and air which is transformed into Fire Qì. This natural Qì generation is the major source of your life force. If you eat more than you need and don't excrete the surplus, the extra food essence will be stored in your body as fat. If you do not eat enough to provide for your daily energy needs, the food essence stored as fat will be converted into Qì.

When you practice Qìgōng you are looking to build up the Qì in your body, to increase the efficiency of the conversion of essence into Qì, and to increase the smoothness of the Qì circulation. In order to increase the smoothness of the circulation you must build up the level of Qì and create Qì potential. When there is a difference in potential, the Qì will flow from the area of higher potential to the area of lower potential, thereby increasing the circulation. This will also clear up blockages that hinder the flow of Qì.

There are many ways to build up Qì in the body. Analysis of the Qìgōng practices known to the author shows that the methods of building up Qì can be divided into four categories: 1. physical stimulation, 2. mental stimulation, 3. energizing the Shén, and 4. others.

Physical Stimulation

Physical stimulation is probably the easiest and most basic method of building up Qì. The theory is very simple. Whenever you move, you need Qì to energize the muscles. If you keep moving for an extended period of time, Qì will have to be continuously supplied to the muscles. In order to keep supplying Yíngqì (i.e., managing Qì, 營氣), your body has to be continuously converting the essence stored in your body into Qì. The more you exercise, the more Qì will be converted, and the more Qì will be built up in the area you are exercising. Once you stop your exercises, part of this accumulated Qì will be dissipated into the air from your skin, and the remainder will flow into the body to increase the Qì circulation in the Qì channels.

We would like to remind you that if you over-exercise a particular area, your Qì may become too positive. As this Qì overflows into the channels, it may make your internal organs too positive, and speed up their degeneration. This is sometimes seen in people who do a lot of weightlifting. However, if you exercise properly, the Qì will circulate smoothly and your organs will receive only the proper amount of Qì. People who exercise correctly and regularly are usually healthier than people who do not exercise.

As discussed in the sixth chapter, exercises which build up Qì in the limbs are called "Wàidān." Wàidān Qìgōng exercises are simple. They are almost like any of the exercises which are common in the Western world. The only two differences are that when you practice you must concentrate your mind at the area being trained, and that the movements are designed for special purposes such as regulating specific organs. You should understand that it is your mind which leads the Qì to the area being trained. When you concentrate, you can build up and circulate the Qì more efficiently than when you don't concentrate. This is especially true right after exercising, when you are relaxed. When your muscles are relaxed and loose, the Qì channels are wide open. If you concentrate and use your Yì (i.e., wisdom mind) to lead the Qì you have built up to your body, in coordination with your inhalations, you will be able to reduce the amount of Qì dissipated into the air, and the Qì can more efficiently nourish your body.

Try the following experiment. It will help you to understand the key to building up and circulating Qì. It is a very simple Wàidān exercise called Gǒngshǒu (拱手), which means "Arcing the Arms." This exercise originated in Tàijíquán, where it is very widely practiced. It provides the Qìgōng beginner with a simple way to experience Qì flow.

For this exercise, stand with one leg rooted on the ground and the other in front of it, with only the toes touching the ground. Both arms are held in front of the chest, forming a horizontal circle, with the fingertips almost touching (Figure 7-1). The tongue should touch the roof of the mouth to connect the Yīn and Yáng Qì vessels (Conception and Governing Vessels respectively). The mind should be calm and relaxed and concentrated on the shoulders; breathing should be deep and regular.

When you stand in this posture for about three minutes, your arms and one side of your back should feel sore and warm. Because the arms are held extended, the muscles and nerves are stressed. Qì will build up in this area and heat will be generated. Also, because one leg carries all the weight, the muscles and nerves in that leg and in one side of the back will be tense and will thereby build up Qì. Because this Qì is built up in the shoulders and legs rather than in the Dāntián, it is considered "Local Qì" or "Wàidān Qì" (外丹氣). In order to keep the Qì build-up and the flow in the back balanced, after three minutes change your legs without moving the arms and stand this way for another three minutes. After the six minutes, put both feet flat on the floor, shoulder-width apart, and slowly lower your arms. The accumulated Qì will then flow into your arms naturally and strongly. It is just like a dam which, after accumulating a large amount of water, releases it and lets it flow out. At this time, concentrate and calm the mind and look for the feeling of Qì flowing from the shoulders to the palms and fingertips. Beginners can usually sense this Qì flow, which is typically felt as warmth or a slight numbness.

Naturally, when you hold your arms out, you are also slowing the blood circulation, and when you lower your hands the blood will rush down into them. This may confuse you as to whether what you feel is due to Qì or the blood. You need to understand several things. First, wherever there is a living blood cell, there has to be Qì to keep it alive. Thus, when you relax after the arcing hands practice, both blood and Qì will come down to the hands. Second, since blood is material and Qì is energy, Qì can flow beyond your body but your blood cannot. Therefore, it is possible for you to test whether the exercise has brought extra Qì to your hands. Place your hands right in front of your face. You should be able to feel a slight sensation, which has to come from the Qì. You can also hold your palms close to each other, or move one hand near the other arm. In addition to a slight feeling of warmth, you may also sense a kind of electric charge which may make the hairs on your arm move. Blood cannot cause these feelings, so they have to be symptoms of Qì.

Sometimes Qì is felt on the upper lip. This is because there is a channel (Hand Yángmíng Large Intestine, 手陽明大腸) which runs over the top of the shoulder to the upper lip (Figure 7-2). However, the feeling is usually stronger in the palms and fingers than in the lip, because there are six Qì channels which pass through the shoulder to end in the hand, but there is only one channel connecting the lip and shoulder. Once you experience Qì flowing in your arms and shoulders during this exercise, you may also find that you can sense it in your back.

This exercise is one of the most common practices for leading the beginner to experience the flow of Qì, and some Tàijíquán styles place great emphasis on it. A similar type of Qìgōng exercise is also practiced by other styles, such as Éméi Dàpénggōng (峨嵋大鵬功).

Mental Stimulation

In the third chapter we discussed how it is possible for your body to move. We said that in order to move, you must first generate an idea. This idea will lead the Qì to the muscles to energize them so that they execute the order from your brain. You can see that your mind plays a most important role in your Qìgōng practice. It is said, "Yǐyì Yǐnqì" (以意引氣), which means "Use your Yì (wisdom mind) to lead your Qì." Notice the word lead. Qì must be led. The word lead means that your mind must go first, and your Qì will naturally follow. If your mind is not ahead of your Qì, the Qì will not be led and your muscles will not be energized.

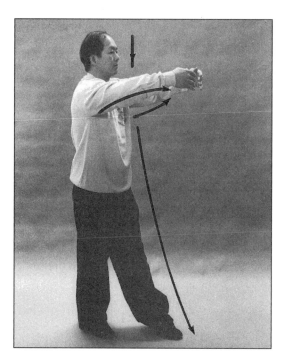

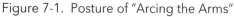

Figure 7-1. Posture of "Arcing the Arms"

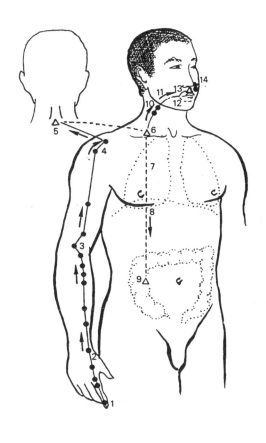

Figure 7-2. The Large Intestine
Channel of Hand-Yáng Brightness

For example, if you want to walk from one spot to another, you must first generate the idea of going to the second spot. This idea leads the Qì to the leg muscles and energizes them. If your mind stays at the first spot instead of going to the second one, you will not be able to move. You can see that it is your mind which you must activate first. Because of this, calming down and concentrating your mind is a very important part of Qìgōng training. The more you can concentrate, the stronger your Yì will be, and, naturally, the stronger your Qì will flow.

Generally speaking, building up Qì by using the mind alone without physical movement is much harder than using the mind and movement together. However, since the mind is so important in Qìgōng training, learning how to regulate your mind has become one of the major trainings.

The mental buildup of Qì is divided into Wàidān (external elixir) and Nèidān (internal elixir). In Wàidān, the mind focuses on the limbs. You must imagine that you are making an appropriate motion in order to generate the proper idea, because this idea will lead the

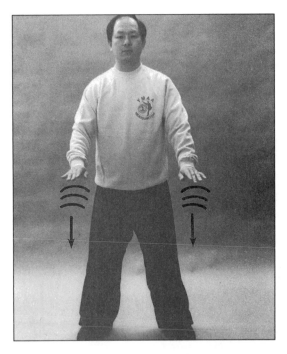

Figure 7-3. Feeling Qì on the palms by imagining pushing downward

Qì to the area. After you practice for a few minutes, the Qì will be built up in the area. The stronger you can concentrate, the more you will be able to feel the Qì.

Try this experiment. It will give you a feel for how Qì can be built up by your thinking. Hold your hands in front of you, where you feel that you can push downward most strongly (Figure 7-3). Your entire body must remain relaxed, especially your shoulders and arms. Inhale deeply, and as you exhale, image that you are pushing your hands down against a table. Do not actually move your body or arms, simply stand still with all of your muscles relaxed. If you are concentrating fully on what you are doing, after a few pushes your hands should start getting warm, and you may notice a sensation like air coming out of the center of your palms. This feeling will disappear when you inhale.

It is harder to feel the Qì in this exercise because there is no physical stimulation. However, if you concentrate and relax enough, you will soon be able to feel something happening in your palms. This is a typical experiment in which you use your Yì (the idea that you are pushing) to lead the Qì to the palms. The more you practice, the stronger you will be able to lead the Qì to your palms. Naturally, this is only an experiment. An experienced Qìgōng practitioner is able to lead Qì to any part of his body simply by thinking. This particular exercise is of course a Wàidān Qìgōng since the Qì is accumulated in the limbs.

In Nèidān mental Qì generation, the theory remains the same. The differences are first, you must concentrate your mind at the Lower Dāntián and build up the Qì there, and second, you do not imagine that you are moving. You can, however, use a different idea, such as that your Dāntián area is on fire. Your mind must stay at your Dāntián until you have built up the Qì. This training is called Yìshǒu Dāntián ("keeping your Yì on your Dāntián," 意守丹田). The more you can concentrate, the faster and stronger the Qì will be built up. This Dāntiánqì generation without physical stimulation is the source of Qì for Buddhist still meditation. Naturally, this exercise is much harder than the Wàidān one.

Energizing Shén

When you are excited because of happiness or joy, you will often feel that your body is hot. This is because you have energized your spirit to a higher state, making your body too Yáng, and your mind has directed the excess Qì to the skin to dissipate it so that the body can regain its energy balance. In the same way, when you are scared or nervous your body becomes too Yīn and you may start trembling. Your body will then automatically tense up to keep from losing Qì through the skin. Tensing the body narrows the Qì channels and cuts down the circulation. This tensing phenomenon is also common in the winter when you feel cold and are shivering. If, at such times, you relax and exhale as you lead Qì to your skin, you will be able to expand your Guardian Qì (Wèiqì, 衛氣) and stop feeling cold. Naturally, you will lose more Qì this way and will need to eat more to replenish the supply.

You may have guessed that your Qì is closely related to your feelings. But you should also know that your feelings are generated from your mind and directed by your spirit. In Qìgōng training, one of the most important practices is stabilizing and firming your spirit. This enables you to keep your emotions under control, and avoid extremes of excitation or depression. You are also able to build up or calm down your Qì by raising or calming your spirit. One of the final stages of Qìgōng training involves using your spirit to efficiently govern the Qì in your body.

Remember the times when you were tired both physically and mentally, and how easy it was to fall asleep then? When your mind is tired, your spirit gets weak, and loses control over your body. Your body seeks to recover from its fatigue, and let the Qì rebalance itself—i.e., you fall asleep so that your Yì gets out of the way and doesn't interfere with the rebalancing. However, if you are excited over something, or worried, your mind won't relax, and the Qì in your brain will keep your spirit high.

For example, suppose at work you are assigned an important project which must be completed by a certain deadline. Furthermore, your boss promises that you will have a two week vacation once the assignment is finished. While working on the project you cannot sleep well, you are thinking about it all the time, and you are worried and excited. Your mind is always busy and your spirit is continually in a highly excited state. You may find that even though everyone else in your office catches the flu, you don't. Finally, the project is completed and you have a two week vacation. All of the pressure is gone and at last you can relax. However, you find that when you start your vacation, you suddenly become ill.

This is a common phenomenon which is very easy to explain according to Qìgōng principles. When you are in an excited and nervous state, your spirit is high. The spirit governs the Managing (Yíngqì, 營氣) and Guardian Qì (Wèiqì, 衛氣), and when the spirit is high it allows the Managing Qì to run your body very efficiently, and it builds up a strong shield of Guardian Qì around your body which effectively protects you from illness. However, once you have completed your project, the pressure is gone and your mind is relaxed, and so your spirit weakens. This allows the shield of Guardian Qì to weaken, and you get sick easily. Perhaps you've heard people say: "I don't get sick because I'm too busy to get sick." As a matter of fact, this is true. When you are busy, your excited mind raises your spirit and increase its efficiency in governing the Qì.

Perhaps you have heard of someone who was desperately ill, and the doctors gave up all hope. However, because the patient had great faith and a strong will to live, he miraculously recovered. Again, his spirit played a role. His faith and strong will to live raised his spirit, which caused his Qì to repair the damage.

In the first example, the spirit was raised mainly by the emotional mind, and in the second example it was raised by the calm and firm wisdom mind. Raising the spirit with a calm mind and strong will is closer to the idea of how Qìgōng trains the spirit.

In Qìgōng training, you balance your Qì with your spirit, which is different from how your Qì balances during rest or sleep. In Qìgōng training you first train to regulate your mind, which makes your spirit steady, firm, and regulated. Then you use your mind and spirit to regulate the Qì in your body while you are meditating. When your emotional mind is regulated, you will be able to raise your spirit with your Yì without getting excited. This raised spirit will be able to govern the flow of Qì and regulate it efficiently.

Others

There are many other ways to build up the Qì or to increase its circulation in the body. Chinese medical society uses three: massage or acupressure, acupuncture, and herbal treatment. Massage and acupuncture use physical stimulation from outside of the body. Herbal treatment uses herbs either applied to the skin or taken internally. Controlling the diet is also considered an herbal internal regulating process. Acupuncture and herbal treatment are discussed in many books available today. If you are interested in Qìgōng massage, please refer to the book: *Chinese Qìgōng Massage*, available from YMAA Publication Center.

7-3. KǍN AND LÍ (KǍN HÉ LÍ, 坎和離)

The terms Kǎn and Lí (坎、離) occur frequently in Qìgōng documents. In the Eight Trigrams (Bāguà, 八卦) Kǎn represents "Water" while Lí represents "Fire." However, the everyday terms for water and fire are also often used. Kǎn and Lí training has long been of major importance to Qìgōng practitioners. In order to understand why, you must understand these two words, and the theory behind them.

Kǎn is Water and represents Yīn in relationship to Lí, which represents Fire and Yáng. Qìgōng practitioners believe theoretically that your body is always too Yáng unless you are sick or have not eaten for a long time, in which case your body may be more Yīn. When your body is always Yáng, it is degenerating and burning out. It is believed that this is the cause of aging. If you are able to use Water to cool down your body, you will be able to slow down the degeneration process and thereby lengthen your life. This is the main reason why Chinese Qìgōng practitioners have been studying ways of improving the quality of the Water in their bodies, and of reducing the quantity of the Fire. I believe that as a Qìgōng practitioner, you should always keep this subject at the top of your list for study and research. If your earnestly ponder and experiment, you will be able to grasp the trick of adjusting Fire and Water in your body.

The Origins of Fire and Water

First you must understand that Fire and Water mean many things in your body. The first concerns your Qì. Qì is classified as Fire or Water, which we have discussed earlier. When your Qì is not pure and causes your physical body to heat up and your mental/spiritual body to become unstable, it is classified as Fire Qì. The Qì which is pure and is able to cool both your physical and spiritual bodies is considered Water Qì. However, your body can never be purely water. Water can cool down the Fire, but it must never totally quench it. If the Fire in your body were put out, you would be dead. It is also said that Fire Qì is able to agitate and stimulate the emotions, and from these emotions generate a mind. This mind is called Xīn (heart, 心), and is considered the Fire mind or emotional mind. On the other hand, when Water Qì generates a mind, it is calm, steady, and wise. This mind is called Yì (intention, 意), and is considered the Water mind or wisdom mind. If your spirit is nourished by the Fire Qì, although your spirit may be high, it will be scattered and confused. Naturally, if the spirit is nourished and raised up by the Water Qì, it will be firm and steady. This will allow your mind to also be firm, calm, and steady. When your Yì is able to govern your emotional Xīn effectively, your will (firm emotional intention) can be firm.

You can see from this discussion that your Qì is the cause of the Fire and Water of your physical body, and of your mind and spirit. Therefore, adjusting the Water and Fire Qì to a healthy level has become a major study in Qìgōng society.

How to Adjust Water and Fire

There are many ways to adjust your Water and Fire. Among the more common ways are the following:

1. **Proper Food and Fresh Air**

   Since Fire Qì comes from the food and air you take in, you are able to control it from its source. Generally speaking, meat products are worse than vegetables and fruit, and add more impurities to your body. But you should be aware that eating vegetables alone does not mean that you are improving your health. As a matter of fact, if you do not know what you are doing, you might end up with a severe protein deficiency. For most people, meat is the main source of protein. Among the vegetables, nuts and beans have the most protein. Soybeans have become one of the major foods for Buddhist and Daoist priests as well as laymen Qìgōng practitioners because of its high protein content. However, although some nuts and beans are high in protein, if you eat too much, or if you cook them the wrong way, they can also significantly increase your Fire Qì. For example, roasting peanuts is worse than boiling them in water.

Daoists and Buddhists have studied this subject extensively. Not only have they studied vegetables, they have also investigated the use of herbs to improve the quality of the Qì in the body. They have even found that living in the mountains is better because the quality of the air is better. You can see that food, air, and herbs are of major importance in adjusting your Kǎn and Lí.

2. **Regulating the Mind and Breathing**

Regulating the mind and breathing are two of the basic techniques for controlling your Fire Qì. It is very important to remember that Fire Qì generates the emotional mind, and the emotional mind can increase your Fire Qì. Therefore, the first thing you must do is to learn how to regulate your mind. Once you can do this, your spirit will be firm and your emotions will be steady, and your Fire Qì will not be agitated to a high level. For example, if you have had too much alcohol, you will find that if you are able to keep your mind clear, and calm down your emotions, the Qì generated from the alcohol will not cause too much Fire in your body. However, if your wisdom mind is confused, your emotional mind will be agitated to a higher state and put your body on fire.

In addition, in order to keep your mind calm and steady, you must also regulate your breathing. Remember the trick is to use the Metal Lungs to cool down the Fire Heart.[1] When breathing is regulated, the Fire Qì residing at the Middle Dāntián (solar plexus) will be led to the lungs, which will dissipate the heat and cool down the body. Next time you have heartburn, before you reach for the antacids, first try deep breathing.

Regulating the mind and the breathing cannot be separated. When the mind is regulated, the breathing can be regulated. When the breathing is regulated, the mind is able to enter a deeper level of calmness. They help each other mutually. We will discuss regulating the mind and the breath in more detail later.

3. **Steadying the Spirit**

Fire Qì agitates and excites your emotional mind, which energizes your body and spirit. When you energize your spirit with your fiery emotional mind, the emotional mind will be scattered. On the other hand, when you raise your spirit with your watery wisdom mind, the wisdom mind becomes clearer. The emotional mind energizes and excites your spirit, while the wisdom mind raises and clears it.

---

1.   According to the Five Element theory (Wǔxíng, 五行) in Chinese medicine, lungs belong to the element of metal while the heart is associated with the element of fire.

In Qìgōng practice, once you have reached the higher levels, a large part of your efforts will be devoted to training your spirit. You want to raise your spirit, but you also want it to be firm. In Qìgōng training, it is said, "Yìshǒu yīdiǎn jīngāngqì",[2] which means literally, "Your mind keeps steady at one point metal steel Qì." The idea expressed here is that when you refine your Qì into one tiny point at the Upper Dāntián (i.e., the third eye), it can be as strong as steel. The Upper Dāntián, which is the residence of your Shén, is the point where you train yourself to keep your mind. When your mind stays there, it is calm and your will is firm. Your spirit is the headquarters for controlling the Qì in your body. When your spirit is firm and steady, the Qì will be controlled efficiently, and you will be able to regulate the Fire Qì and prevent it from energizing your body.

4. **Circulating the Wind Path**

   It was mentioned in the sixth chapter that one of the Qì circulation methods trained in Qìgōng is the Wind Path, in which you circulate the Qì in the reverse direction. This is done to slow down or cool down the Fire Qì. Normally, this exercise focuses on the front of the body, bringing Water Qì from the Lower Dāntián up the Conception Vessel to cool the Fire Qì in the Middle Dāntián. This cools down the Qì even before it starts to circulate. This will be discussed more extensively in a future publication.

5. **Leading the Qì to the Water Path**

   The major training of Marrow/Brain Washing Qìgōng is leading the Qì to the Water Path beginning at the Huìyīn cavity. When a portion of your Qì is led to the Water Path, it will weaken the Fire Qì and keep it from over-heating the body. This subject has been discussed briefly in the sixth chapter, and also covered more thoroughly in a subsequent volume, *Qìgōng—The Secret of Youth*, available from YMAA Publication Center.

2.　意守一點金鋼氣。

CHAPTER 8

Regulating the Body

8-1. INTRODUCTION (JIÈSHÀO, 介紹)

In Qìgōng training, you need to know how to regulate five things: your body, breath, Xīn (emotional mind), Qì, and Shén (spirit). In addition, in order to keep up a steady, adequate supply of Water Qì, you must also learn how to regulate the essence from which it is converted. We will discuss them separately, but you must remember that in practice they are all closely linked together.

Before we continue with this chapter, you should first understand the word regulating. Regulating means to adjust and tune constantly until the goal is reached. However, you should also understand that the real regulating happens only when you don't need to consciously regulate. This means that if your mind has to pay attention to the regulating, you have not reached the final goal. The real regulating happens naturally, when you do not have to regulate it at all. It is just like when you are driving. Before you can drive, you must first learn how. While you are involved in the learning process, your mind will be on regulating your new skills. Once you have mastered the skill of driving, it isn't necessary for your conscious mind to actually be on the act of driving, and you will be able to drive without driving. It is the same with Qìgōng training. When you start regulating the above five elements of your training, you may have to place all of your attention on it. After you have practiced and mastered the skills, regulating will no longer be necessary. Then, you have reached the real regulating without regulating.

Regulating the Body is called Tiáoshēn (調身) in Chinese. It means to adjust your body until it is in the most comfortable and relaxed state. This implies that your body must be centered and balanced posturally. If it is not, you will be tense and uneasy, which will affect the judgment of your Yì and the circulation of your Qì. In Chinese medical society it is said: "(When) shape (i.e., body's posture) is not correct, then the Qì will not be smooth. (When) the Qì is not smooth, the Yì (mind) will not be at peace. (When) the Yì is not at peace, then the Qì is disordered."[1] The relaxation of your body originates with your Yì. Therefore, before you can relax your body, you must first relax or regulate your mind (Yì).

1.　形不正，則氣不順。氣不順，則意不寧。意不寧，則氣散亂。

However, before you can do this, you must first regulate your Xīn (emotional mind). It is the main reason that your Yì has difficulty being calm and peaceful. When you have regulated both the emotional and the wisdom minds as well as the body it is called "Shēnxīn Pínghéng" (身心平衡), which means "body and heart (mind) balanced." The body and the mind are mutually related. A relaxed and balanced body doesn't distract your attention, and lets your Yì relax and concentrate. When your Yì is at peace and can judge things accurately, your body will be centered, balanced, and relaxed.

8-2. RELAXATION THEORY (SŌNGCHÍ DE YUÁNLǏ, 鬆弛的原理)

Relaxation is one of the major keys to success in Qìgōng. You should remember that only when you are relaxed will all your Qì channels be open. Relaxation includes two major parts: the mind (Yì and Xīn) and the physical body. Generally, mind relaxation must come before the physical body is able to relax. We discussed before the two kinds of mind: Xīn (emotional mind) and Yì (wisdom mind). The emotional mind affects your feelings and the condition of your physical body. The wisdom mind is able to lead you to a calm and peaceful state, which allows you to exercise good judgment. Therefore, in order to be relaxed, your Yì must first be relaxed and calm. Then, Yì is able to control the emotional mind and let it relax too. Finally, when the peaceful Yì and Xīn coordinate with your breathing, the physical body will relax.

In Qìgōng practice, there are three levels of relaxation. The first level is external, physical relaxation, or postural relaxation. This is a very superficial level, and almost anyone can reach it. It consists of adopting a comfortable stance and avoiding unnecessary strain in posture and movement. When you reach this level of relaxation, although you look relaxed, you are still tense internally. Of course, in order to reach this level of relaxation, the mind must first relax. Normally, your mind does not have to reach a very deep level to achieve this looking relaxed stage. Once you start to relax your mind, your body will follow naturally.

The second level involves relaxing the muscles and tendons. To do this, your meditative mind must be calm and peaceful enough to feel deep into the muscles and tendons. From this feeling, your mind will know how to gauge the level of your relaxation. Only when you have reached this level will your mind be able to feel the Qì flow in the muscles and tendons. This level of relaxation will help open your Qì channels, and will allow the Qì to sink and accumulate in the Dāntián.

The final stage is the relaxation which reaches the internal organs and the bone marrow, and every pore in your skin. In order to be relaxed in your internal organs, your Yì must first have reached a very deep level of calmness and peace. Only then will you be able to sense the organs and marrow. Remember, only if you can relax deep into your body will your mind be able to lead the Qì there.

Before we continue, you should understand the difference between feeling and sensing. The Chinese expression "Gǎnjué" (感覺) means "to feel" in the sense of touching and feeling something. The expression "Yìshì" (意識), which is translated "to sense," literally means

"Yì recognition" or "to recognize with your Yì." When you feel something, it happens physically. Feeling is direct and active, while sensing is more indirect. In feeling, your emotional mind is able to touch the object. When sensing, however, you must use your Yì to perceive the situation. To sense, therefore, you must collect the information generated by the object, and process it so that you can understand and realize what is happening. Sensing involves a deeper level of spiritual intuition, beyond feeling, in which the object and the mind can communicate directly.

In Qìgōng relaxation training, the deeper levels of relaxation include sensing the marrow and the organs. When you have reached this stage the Qì will be able to reach any point in your body. Then you will feel light and transparent—as if your whole body had disappeared. If you can reach this level of relaxation you will also be able to lead the Qì to your skin and strengthen your Guardian Qì. This will keep you from getting sick from outside causes. At this level of relaxation your Yì will also be able to adjust the Qì in your organs to cure Qì disorders. You will be able to protect your organs more effectively, and slow down their degeneration.

An important part of the training in Qìgōng involves "leading the five Qì's toward their origins" (Wǔqì Cháoyuán, 五氣朝元). This involves adjusting the Qì in the five Yīn organs (lungs, heart, kidneys, liver, and spleen) to the appropriate levels. Generally speaking, you are able to sense or even to feel the lungs much more easily than the other four organs. This is because your lungs move when you inhale and exhale. This obvious movement makes it very easy to be aware of them. The second organ that you can sense, once you have relaxed your lungs, is your heart. When you relax the heart, you can clearly sense and even feel it beating. The third organ is the kidneys. The kidneys can be sensed more easily than the liver and the spleen because there is liquid flowing constantly through them. The liver will be next, and then the spleen. Because the liver is much bigger than the spleen, it is easier to sense any movement, such as blood, inside it. We will discuss this idea further when we cover the regulation of organ Qì.

8-3. RELAXATION PRACTICE (SŌNGCHÍ DE LIÀNXÍ, 鬆弛的練習)

Relaxation practice can be done anytime and anywhere. It can also be done in any posture. The first key to relaxation is your mind, and the second key is your breathing. Remember: when you relax, you must first relax your mind. Only when your mind is relaxed will your body start to relax and your lungs loosen. When your lungs are loose, you will be able to regulate your breathing and slow down your heartbeat. When this happens, your mind will reach to a deeper level of calmness and peace. This deeper mind will relax your lungs again, slowing down your heartbeat a further step. These processes will lead you to a deeply calm state which allows you to feel and sense every cell of your body and every function of the internal organs. Only then may you say that you have relaxed your body completely.

Relaxing the Mind

The regulation of your mind and breathing will be discussed in detail later. At this point, in order to practice relaxation you must start to practice mind regulation. In practice, there are two steps in regulating your mind. The first step is to bring all of your thoughts from the outside world to your body. This is usually done by concentrating on your "third eye" or Upper Dāntián. Then regulate your concentrated mind until it is relaxed, easy, and natural.

First, let your thoughts be calm and peaceful, so that you can concentrate your mind on relaxing. Your wisdom Yì must be able to control the thoughts or ideas generated from the emotional Xīn. Only then will your mind be clear. Then you will be able to disregard surrounding distractions and focus on your body. When you have reached this stage, although your mind is clear, it may still be tense from concentrating. Therefore, you must learn to concentrate without mental tension. Remember: when your mind is tense, your physical body will also be tense. Therefore, the second step of practice it to relax your concentrated mind. Sometimes when people cannot sleep they concentrate all their attention on falling asleep. This only makes things worse. The trick is to concentrate on something else. Normally in Qìgōng you concentrate your mind on your breathing and on the sensation of your lungs expanding and contracting. Every time you exhale, feel your physical body relax to a deeper level.

Relaxing the Breathing

Once you have relaxed your mind, you will be able to relax your breathing. Your breathing is closely related to your thoughts, and especially to emotional feelings. Once the mind is calm and peaceful, breathing can be independent of thought. The first step toward relaxing your breathing involves neutralizing the effect your emotions have on the breathing process. Normally, once you have relaxed your mind, you have reached this stage. Next, you must understand that breathing is caused by the physical motion of the body. For the average, untrained person, this means moving the chest. Since it is the muscles of the chest and the diaphragm which draw the air into your body and push it out, you must learn to relax all of the muscles which relate to your breathing.

Bring your calm and concentrated mind to your chest. Take in air and push it out slowly without holding your breath. While you are doing this, pay attention to how the muscles of the diaphragm move. The more you can feel them, the more your Yì is able to lead the relaxation to a deeper level.

When you do this breathing training, you will notice that the area around your solar plexus starts loosening up. When your chest is loose, you have reached the fundamental stage of relaxation.

Relaxing the Body

Relaxing the body is the first step in regulating your body. Only when your body is relaxed are you able to sense your physical body's center, root, and balance, and reach the goal of body regulation.

Relaxing the body includes relaxing the muscles, skin, marrow, and organs. Remember: only when you are able to relax all of these will the Qì flow smoothly and freely. Then you will be able to lead the Qì and feel that your body is transparent.

Because you use your mind to control your muscles whenever you move, relaxing your muscles is easiest. Your mind is able to feel them. Once your mind is calm, the mind will be able to effectively lead the muscles into a state of relaxation.

Relaxing the skin is the next easiest. Your skin is the interface between your body and your surroundings. Every time your skin feels something, the message is sent to your brain for evaluation. Because communication between the skin and the brain is happening all the time, it is easy for your Yì to reach the skin and lead it to a relaxed state.

Relaxing the organs is the next step. In order to reach this stage, your mind must have reached a deeper level of calmness and peace. There are five Yīn organs which are most important in Qìgōng relaxation training. These organs are: lungs, heart, kidneys, liver, and spleen. Except for the lungs, which can be controlled by the mind directly, all the other organs must be reached or sensed indirectly. In order to sense the last four organs, you must first be able to feel the muscles surrounding them for clues about their condition. Once your mind is able to reach all of these muscles, your mind will be led to the organs and sense them clearly.

There is an important point to be aware of. When you practice communication between your mind and organs, the Qì will be led to those organs in order for your brain to sense them. If you are not careful, excess Qì will be led to them and make them too Yáng, which will cause problems. This is especially true of the heart. Your heart is very sensitive to Qì, so the Qì level must be correct. When you place your mind on your heart, the heart will become Yáng, and the heart beat will increase. Therefore, when you relax an organ, you must be very careful to avoid leading your mind directly to it. Instead, notice the area around the organ, as well as the organ itself. Do not zero in too intensely on an organ, or you will upset its natural balance. Organs must function normally while you are relaxing them. Organs are not like your skin or muscles. They are vital and more sensitive to Qì. You should be able to see from this why leading the five Qì's to their origins is considered one of the hardest and highest stages of Qìgōng practice.

Relaxing the bone marrow is the hardest relaxation exercise. Your mind does not communicate directly with it as it does with the skin and muscle. Also, since there are no muscles connected to the marrow, you cannot use motion to sense it. The hardest discipline in Chinese Qìgōng is Marrow/Brain Washing, because your mind has such great difficulty communicating with the marrow. This will be discussed in a later book.

Postures for Practicing Relaxation

There is no specific posture which you must use for relaxation training. In fact, no matter which posture you use, part of your body will be tensed to support your body. For example, your legs will be tensed when you stand, your thighs are pressed when you sit down, your back is pushed down by your body's weight when you lie down. Obviously, there is no relaxation posture which is absolutely good for the entire body. The prerequisite to relaxing your mind and body is feeling comfortable and natural. Your body should be centered and balanced. You also need to consider how the environment might affect you. Is it too noisy, or is the surface you are lying or sitting on too hard? For the beginner, we suggest that you lie on your back. When you are lying down, you don't have to pay attention to your root, center, and balance, so it is easier for you to regulate your mind. Lying down for relaxation practice also has a disadvantage. When you lie down, your back muscles are pressed down by your weight, which restricts their ability to loosen up.

Once you are familiar with the relaxation exercises, you should also learn to relax while you are sitting. This is harder than lying down because part of your mind must be kept in your body's center to prevent your falling over. Sitting relaxation, however, is better for your trunk and upper limbs. You can see that the different postures have their advantages and disadvantages. Remember, it does not matter which posture you are using, as long as you feel comfortable and natural.

Suggested Procedures for Relaxation Exercises

There are many methods of relaxing. Once you have some experience with one method, you may find another exercise or set of exercises which are easier and better for you. Here, we will only suggest some procedures which will help you start out. We recommend that the beginner start lying down.

Bring Your Mind to Your Shén. Relax your body with a few comfortably deep breaths. Normally, most people can do this easily. Next, bring your mind from outside of your body to your Upper Dāntián, where your Shén resides. When your mind is on the Shén, your spirit will be centered, and thoughts generated by outside distractions will start to disappear. Your mind will now be able to concentrate on feeling your body.

Relax Your Mind. When you concentrate your attention on relaxing your mind, you will find that your mind stays tense. You have to relax it by moving the focus of your consciousness away from your mind. One of the best ways is to pay attention to your breathing.

Feel and Sense Your Middle Dāntián. Move your mind to the Middle Dāntián (Solar Plexus), which is the center and residence of your Fire Qì. Feel the physical location of your solar plexus, and sense the Qì there. Remember, Fire Qì stimulates the emotional mind and emotional feelings, and increases tension. When you move your mind to the Middle Dāntián, you will be able to feel what is happening with your Fire Qì.

Use Breathing to Cool Down the Fire Qì. In Qìgōng, the lungs are considered Metal and the heart is considered Fire. Metal is able to absorb heat and cool down Fire. Whenever you have heartburn or an uneasy feeling in your chest, use deep breathing to cool down the Fire and release the pressure. Similarly, when you want to relax, you must first cool down your chest Fire and relax the chest area. Smooth, relaxed deep breathing will enable you to extend your relaxation from your chest to your entire body. When you reach this stage, you have completed the first step of relaxation.

Use Your Mind to Direct the Body. Once you have relaxed your body at the surface level, you must enter a deeper level of relaxation. At this level, use your concentrated mind to feel and relax deep into the muscles and tendons. This stage allows you to open the Qì channels by relaxing any muscular tension which is constricting the channels and restricting Qì circulation. When you do this, your breathing is deeper, your pulse is slower, and your meditating mind reaches a deeper level.

When you relax your whole body, start at the toes. Concentrate your mind on each of your toes and relax them. Next, move your mind up to your feet, ankles, calves, thighs, and hips. You may feel your lower body disappear, and feel as if you were floating. Keeping your lower body relaxed, move your mind to your fingers and repeat the same procedure—from your fingers to the hands, wrists, forearms, elbows, and shoulders. Then concentrate your mind on your stomach, and move up to the chest and neck. Finally, focus on your head. After your head is relaxed, keep your mind relaxed while concentrating on feeling your whole body. When you have reached this level, you will be able to feel your muscles, tendons, and skin. The more you practice, the better your mind will be able to concentrate on the local areas and relax them. When you relax your body starting from the extremities, you are also relaxing and clearing the Qì channels. To relax the channels, you have to relax the ends first, then work your way down their length. If you start in the middle, you will relax in one direction, but the other side will be tense.

If you are able to practice twice a day, the Qì in your body will be able to rebalance itself easily and naturally. Your mind will be peaceful and you will be able to maintain your health. The best time to practice is two hours after lunch, when the Fire Qì is strongest at your Middle Dāntián. If you can practice your relaxation at this time, you will be able to cool down and help your body. The second best time is just before you sleep. After a long day of physical and mental exercise, you will be able to relax your mind as well as your body. This will enable you to have a more relaxing sleep, with fewer dreams, and you will be able to effectively recover from fatigue. If you would like to know more about the relaxation practice at this level, refer to the audio tape: *Self Relaxation—A Chinese Qìgōng Meditation* (YMAA Publication Center).

Relaxing Your Organs. If you are a Qìgōng practitioner, you will want to relax all the way into your organs in order to regulate the Qì in them. Generally, this stage is much harder for the person who does not know the theory and does not have the above relaxation training. In order for your mind to reach your organs, you will need to reach a much deeper level of meditation. The five Yīn organs are considered the most vital. Generally speaking, to feel or sense the lungs is the easiest, followed by the heart, kidneys, liver, and spleen. When you are able to feel and sense these organs, you will be able to evaluate their status, and use your mind to regulate their Qì.

Relaxing Your Marrow. After you have reached the level of organ relaxation, you have come to the third level of relaxation. This final stage involves relaxing your body deep into the marrow. Your marrow manufactures your blood cells. The marrow is alive, and must have a constant supply of Qì to keep functioning. Your conscious mind does not normally sense the Qì in the marrow and control it. In Marrow/Brain Washing Qìgōng training, however, you want Qì to be supplied to the marrow with maximum efficiency so that the blood will be kept fresh and healthy. In order to do this, your mind must be able to reach the marrow. Again, you may refer to the book: *Qìgōng—The Secret of Youth*, available from YMAA Publication Center.

You can see that relaxation is not as simple as many people think. Your final goal is to relax until you feel transparent. Only when you are at this stage will your Qì be able to flow smoothly and fluidly to every cell of your body.

8-4. ROOTING, CENTERING, AND BALANCING (ZHĀGĒN, ZHŌNGDÌNG, PÍNG-HÉNG, 紮根、中定、平衡)

When you regulate your body, in addition to relaxing it you are also seeking its root, center, and balance. In order for you to feel natural, comfortable, and stable you must first have a firm root. The way of rooting for standing and sitting are different. When you stand, you build your root from your feet into the ground, while when you are sitting on a chair you build your root from your hips down to the ground. In every posture or movement, there is a root for that form or movement. Rooting includes rooting not just the body, but also the form and movement. Every posture or form has its unique way of rooting which is determined by its purpose or principle.

For example, in certain Qìgōng exercises you want to lead the Qì to your palms. In order to do this, you must image that you are pushing an object forward while keeping your muscles relaxed.[2] In this exercise, your elbows must be down to build the sense of root for the push. If you raise the elbows, you lose the sense of intention of the movement because the push would be ineffective if you were pushing something for real. Since the intention or purpose of the movement is its reason for being, you now have a purposeless movement, and you have no reason to lead Qì in any particular way. In this case, the elbow is the first root of the movement. This root must be connected to the root of your body which is in the ground in order to be firm and complete. Therefore, the root of the arms is built upon the body's root. In order to connect these two roots strongly, your chest must be arched in to form the support (Figure 8-1). Furthermore, your stance cannot be straight up. When you push a heavy object, you have to lean slightly forward. When you are standing up, you will not have a pushing root. You must have a bow-and-arrow stance (Gōngjiànbù, 弓箭步) in order to push backward and generate forward pushing power. When you have all of these, you can say that you have a firm root for pushing. In order to push with maximum power, you must also seek your center and balance. When you have your root, center, and balance,

---

2. The verb *image* as used here means to mentally create something that you treat as if it were real. If you image that your are pushing something heavy, you have to adjust your posture exactly as if you were in fact pushing something heavy. You must feel its weight and resistance as you exert force against it, and realize the force and counter force in your legs. If you mentally treat your actions as real, your body will too, and the Qì will automatically move appropriately for those actions. If you only "pretend" or "imagine" that you are pushing something heavy, your mind and body will not treat your actions as real, and the Qì will not move strongly or clearly.

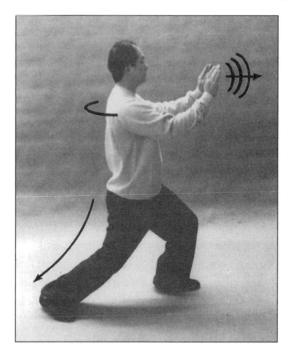

Figure 8-1. Feeling Qì on the palms by imagining pushing forward

your posture will be natural and comfortable, and your Yì will be strong enough to direct the pushing.

You can see that in order for a posture to have a root, you must first understand the purpose of the posture. When you understand the Why of the posture, your mind will not wander and you will know what you are looking for. Understanding the purpose and the theory is the root of everything. It firms your mind so that it can lead your body to a posture which offers you the best root, center, and balance. Naturally, in order to reach this stage, you must first have a relaxed mind and body.

Before you can develop your root, you must first relax and let your body settle. As you relax, the tension in the various parts of your body will dissolve, and you will find a comfortable way to stand. You will stop fighting the ground to keep your body up, and will learn to rely on your body's structure for support. This lets the muscles relax even more. Since your body isn't struggling to stand up, your Yì won't be pushing upward, and your body, mind, and Qì will all be able to sink. If you let dirty water sit quietly, the impurities will gradually settle down to the bottom, leaving the water above it clear. In the same way, if you relax your body and let it settle, your Qì will sink to your Dāntián and the Bubbling Wells (Yǒngquán, K-1, 湧泉) in your feet, clearing your mind. Then you can begin to develop your root.

After you have gained your root, you must learn how to keep your center. The center includes the mind's center and the physical body's center. You must have your mind centered first in order to lead your body to its center. Naturally, in order to have your mind centered, you must first relax your body, which allows your mind to feel and sense every part of it. Although your root is important to the process of locating your center, many times you are able to find your center without even having a root. For example, when you ski you do not have a root but you must have your center in order to balance. In stationary Qìgōng practice, however, having a root will help you to locate your center more easily; and when you have the center, the root will be even firmer. Both of them are related and cannot really be separated.

A stable center will make your Qì develop evenly and uniformly. If you lose this center, your Qì will not be led evenly. In order to keep your body centered, you must first center your Yì, and then match your body to it. It is very important for you to understand that very often your mind's center and your body's center do not match each other. For example, while standing in a bow and arrow stance you may lean slightly forward so that the center of your body is over your front foot. If you keep your mental center back further, you can still keep you body centered, even though someone looking at you would think that you are off balance to your front. If, however, your mental center is also off and moves forward, you will lose your center and balance. Naturally, if your physical center is off too much, you will not be able to use your mental center to balance it. The closer together your mental and physical centers stay, the more stable you will be. In Qìgōng practice, your mental and physical centers are keys which enable you to lead your Qì beyond your body.

Finally, after you have a relaxed body, firm root, and center, you will be able to balance your Yì, Qì, and physical body. Balance is the product of rooting and centering. Regardless of which aspect of balance you are dealing with, you must balance your Yì first. Only then can you balance your Qì and your physical body. If your Yì is balanced, it can help you to make accurate judgments, and to correct the path of the Qì flow. When your Yì is balanced, your Qì will be led evenly. Remember the trick to expanding your Qì is to expand it evenly. It is like when you push a car, you need a backward force in order to generate forward power.

Normally, a person's Qì is not balanced in both sides of the body simply because he uses one hand more than the other. For example, if you are right handed, your mind can lead the Qì to the right hand much more easily than it can to the left hand. You will find sometimes that one side of the sole of your shoe is flatter than the other. As a Qìgōng practitioner, you are looking for your mental center in this unbalanced situation. In order to do this, your mind must be very clear and able to judge the environment and your body's condition. For example, if you place your right arm into warm water and your left arm into cold water for three minutes, and then place both hands immediately into another container of water, one hand will feel warmer than the other. This kind of outside influence scatters your Yì and causes it to lose its center. In Qìgōng practice, therefore, you are looking for the practice which develops the Yì and body evenly. For example, practice the same form with both hands the same number of times.

In order to help you analyze rooting, centering, and balancing, we will discuss two of the most common stances. Once you understand these two, you should be able to use the same method to analyze any other stance.

Horse Stance (Mǎbù, 馬步)

The horse stance is the most common stance used by Qìgōng practitioners and martial artists. The horse stance is used by martial artists to develop their root, center, and balance, as well as to strengthen the legs. For the non-martial Qìgōng practitioner, however, although rooting is important, it is not as critical as it is for marital artists who need a strong root for fighting. In Qìgōng, rooting is helpful in finding your center and balance, which in turn lets you feel relaxed, natural, and comfortable. Since the martial arts horse stance is harder and is the basis for the non-martial horse stance, we will discuss it here. Once you understand it thoroughly, you may adjust it to fit your situation.

There are many ways to stand in the horse stance. For example, the width of the feet in the horse stance used by Southern Chinese martial styles is narrower than the one used in Northern styles (Figure 8-2). This is because the Southern styles emphasize short range fighting, and the wider stance is more open and dangerous in short range techniques. The situation is different for the Northern styles. Because they emphasize long range techniques, a larger posture is more advantageous, so they use a much wider horse stance (Figure 8-3). You should understand that regardless of which style of horse stance is trained, the purpose, training principles, and theory remain the same.

In the horse stance, both legs share your weight equally. In Qìgōng training, the width of the stance depends on your feeling. If you are standing too narrow or too wide, you will have a uncomfortable feeling. You should try different widths to see which one is most comfortable and natural for you. Remember, when you feel comfortable and natural you will be able to relax and find your center and balance more easily.

If you are training a martial arts horse stance, how high you stand depends upon the style. For Qìgōng practice, how high you stand depends on your feeling. For example, if you stand lower, your leg muscles will be more tensed and it will be harder for the Qì to flow to the bottom of your feet. If you stand too high, your center of gravity is higher and your root will be shallower and less stable. However, since the leg muscles are more relaxed, you can lead the Qì to the bottom of your feet more easily. In Chinese internal martial styles such as Tàijíquán, when a beginner's Qì cannot be efficiently directed to the bottom of the feet, the stance is lower. In this case, the beginner is able to lower his physical center of gravity to increase his root. When, however, a Tàijíquán practitioner has reached a high level, he will stand higher and keep the leg muscles relaxed, allowing his Qì to reach the bottom of his feet.

In Qìgōng horse stance training, the best way to build a firm root is to begin with a height at which you get the strongest feeling of pushing upward. In other words, try out different heights, and at each one pretend you are pushing a heavy object upward. At one particular height you will feel that you can push upward most strongly. At this height your Yì can exert the strongest push upward, and it can therefore also exert the strongest push

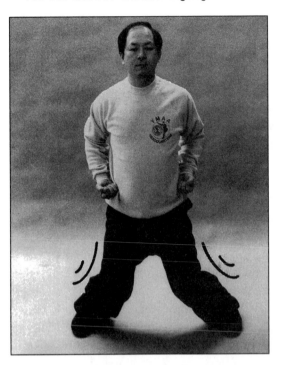

Figure 8-2. Horse Stance of the southern martial styles

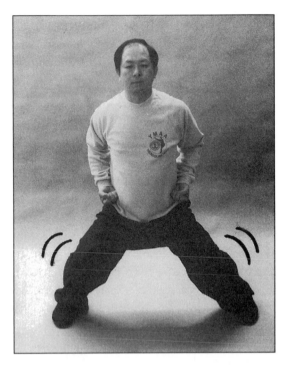

Figure 8-3. Horse Stance of the northern martial styles

downward. It is this downward pushing of your Yì that builds your root. If you keep practicing, you will eventually start to feel that your Yì is leading your Qì into the ground, and that your root is starting to grow.

To root your body, you must imitate a tree and grow an invisible root beneath your feet. Naturally, your Yì must grow first, because it is the Yì which leads the Qì. Your Yì must be able to communicate with the ground in order to lead your Qì beyond your feet and build the root. This means your Yì must feel or sense the ground, noticing whether it is soft or hard, how flat the ground is, how slippery it is. Try different ways of standing, shift your weight on your feet, and notice the ground. With practice your Yì will be able to sink further into the ground, and you will develop a strong root. The more you practice, the deeper the root will grow (Figure 8-4). After practicing for a period of time, you will start to stand higher in order to relax the leg muscles more. In turn, this will help you to lead the Qì to the bottom more effectively. The Bubbling Well cavity is the gate which enables your Qì to communicate with the ground.

There is one more thing to remember when you build your root. A tree's root is very strong because it has many branches and spreads out far to the sides. You must do the same thing, and spread your roots to the sides as well as downward.

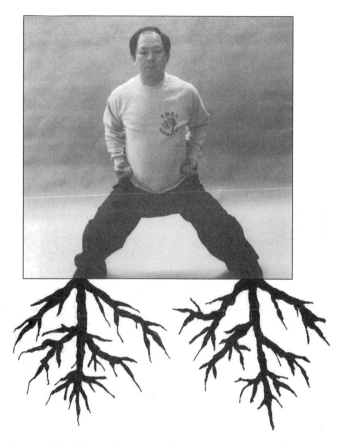

Figure 8-4. Horse Stance with the root growing like a tree's

Once you have built your root, you can consider being centered and balanced. You can be centered physically and you can be centered mentally. When you are centered physically, a vertical line from your center of mass falls between your feet, so your root comfortably supports your weight. Being centered mentally is a matter of feeling. If you are mentally centered, you can be physically balanced even when you are not physically centered. An example of this is the person who cannot be pushed over even when he is standing in a very awkward position. When you start practicing, stand so that you are physically centered and have a good root, and be centered mentally in the same way. After a while, change your stance slightly so that you physical stance becomes less centered and less stable, and practice maintaining your balance and stability mentally. Remember, if you are not centered physically or mentally, you will not be able to maintain your balance.

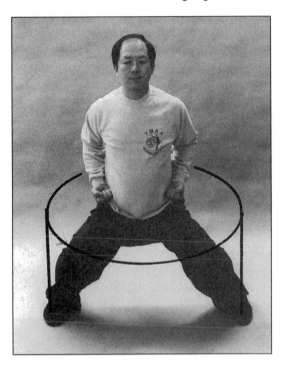

Figure 8-5. In a low stance, your body is stable within this area

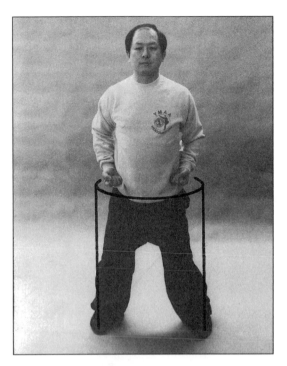

Figure 8-6. In a high stance, your body is stable within this area

The degree to which your physical body's center can be separated from the mind's center without losing balance depends on how you stand. Generally speaking, it depends on how wide you build your root. For example, if you stand low with a firm root, your body's center can be moved in the space between the two roots built by your feet (Figure 8-5). If you stand higher, the width is narrower, and the circle of movement you can allow your body will be smaller (Figure 8-6).

A highly skilled martial artist can defend himself even in a high, narrow stance. His range of movement is limited, but if he has strong Qì he will be able to build a strong root, and if his technique is good enough, he will be able to fight effectively. Remember, in order to reach this stage, you must start with a low, wide stance, and gradually narrow and raise it. The Chinese have a proverb: "Yǎngāo Shǒudī" (眼高手低), which means, "Eyes are high and the hands are low." This scoffs at those people who keep dreaming of high levels of mastery while they are still at a very low level.

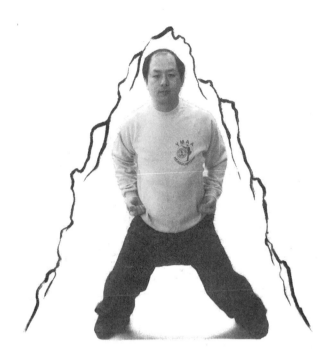

Figure 8-7. In the Horse Stance, stand like a mountain

The final goal in developing your root is to make your stance like a mountain. Your stance must be wide and firm, and you must also train your Qì to cover your body and spread out as it goes down to the ground. Your mental image of yourself and your Qì should be shaped like a mountain or cone—narrow on top and wide on the bottom (Figure 8-7). Once you can do this, it will be extremely difficult for anyone to push you over or make you lose your balance.

Bow and Arrow Stance or Mountain Climbing Stance (Gōngjiànbù or Dēngshānbù, 弓箭步、登山步)

The bow and arrow stance is another common stance used by both martial artists and non-martial artists. Generally speaking, this stance is harder than the horse stance. Because the weight of the body is not divided evenly, therefore, the mind is also uneven. The bow and arrow stance is commonly used in moving and in exerting force forward. Normally, the front leg is used to stabilize the body and the rear leg is used to generate the forward power.

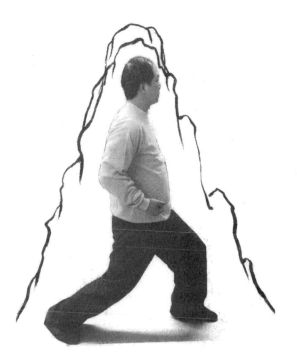

Figure 8-8. In the bow and arrow stance, stand like a mountain

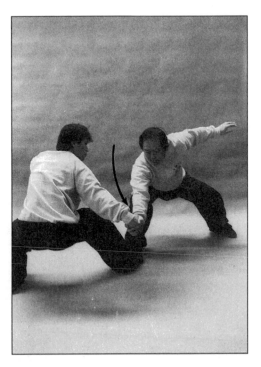

Figure 8-9. Rooting and balance competition

In this stance, as your rear leg pushes your body forward, you must keep your body straight up in order to keep your center and balance. Sometimes the body can lean forward slightly; in which case, however, you must keep your mind at the original center or you will easily lose your balance.

In this stance, the trick to building the root lies in keeping the center and balance just as you did in the horse stance. Your root must be firm, deep, and wide. Again, your body must be low so you can build a foundation like a mountain (Figure 8-8). Finally, your mental and physical centers must actively adjust with each other to keep the body steady.

Once you have built your root and stability, there is a very common exercise you can do to test and strengthen them. You and your partner face each other in a bow and arrow stance. Then clasp your leading arms, and try to unbalance each other (Figure 8-9). This practice will help you to build your root, to coordinate your mental and physical centers, to build your own mountain, and finally to destroy the root of your partner. If you continue this practice you will find that, in order to win, you must stand low. Your body must be very soft to keep your partner from finding your center and root. When your body is tense, he can locate your center easily and destroy your balance. In addition, you must also learn how to feel and sense your partner's center. Once your mind and power are able to reach his center, you will be able to dislodge his root.

CHAPTER 9
Regulating the Breath

9-1. BREATHING AND HEALTH (HŪXĪ YǓ JIÀNKĀNG, 呼吸與健康)

Right after your birth, you started to rely on the two major sources of essence to supply your body's needs. Once these two essences, of food and air, are absorbed into your body, they are converted into Qì. The Qì obtained from food is called Shíqì (Food Qì, 食氣), while the Qì obtained from air is called Kōngqì (空氣). (The Chinese call air "Kōngqì.") The Qì from these two sources is called "Post-birth Qì" or "Fire Qì." Although your body needs Fire Qì, if it is of a poor quality it will cause your body to degenerate. In order to have good health and a long life, you must be serious about the quality of these two sources. The search for the right kinds of food and the correct quality of air has been an important part of Qìgōng practice. In this chapter we will discuss Air Qì and how we benefit from practicing methods of regulating the breath.

In order to know how to regulate your breath, you must first know how you take in and expel air during inhalation and exhalation. You must understand that your lungs themselves cannot bring in and push out air. In order for the air to reach the lungs and then be pushed out, the muscles around the lungs and the diaphragm must expand and contract, sucking the air into and pushing it out of the chest cavity. When this process is going on, the oxygen will mix with the blood in the lung cells, and the blood will release the carbon dioxide it carries. When the diaphragm moves up and down during respiration, it massages the internal organs and increases the Qì circulation.

Once the oxygen is mixed with the blood, it is carried to every cell of the body to keep them functioning. Normally, when there is a shortage of oxygen, your brain will sense it first. According to experiments, the oxygen required for your brain cells is many times more than that which is required for muscle cells. Whenever the oxygen is insufficient, you feel dizzy, heavy, and cannot think clearly.

Normally after a baby is born, it retains the habit of breathing from the lower abdomen. The breathing is deep. Since a child takes in plenty of oxygen, its mind is usually clearer than an adult's. When a person reaches 30, his breathing becomes shallower and generally takes place around the stomach rather than the lower abdomen. At this age, a person still has enough oxygen to supply body, and the diaphragm still moves up and down actively. This movement maintains health. When he is older, the breath becomes progressively shallower as the person relies on moving his chest to breath. Now the person starts losing his memory, his thinking ability, and his mental clarity. Because of the shallowness of the breathing, the diaphragm does not move up and down actively any more, and it does not massage the internal organs. The Qì becomes stagnant, and the organs degenerate. Also, the degeneration of the cells of the body is speeded by the shortage of oxygen.

You can see how important breathing is to your health. In Qìgōng practice, regulating the breathing is the most important training. The first step toward maintaining your health involves increasing your oxygen supply. You must resume breathing deep down in your abdomen like a baby does. This exercise is called Fǎntóng (返童), which means "Back to Childhood." Once you have a sufficient supply of oxygen, you are able to relax, clear your mind, and circulate the Qì.

9-2. REGULATING THE BREATH (TIÁOXÍ, 調息)

It is important to learn how to regulate your breath so that you can obtain enough essence from the air, and so that you can learn how to prevent the Air Qì from overstimulating your body and making it too Yáng. You need to be concerned with the quality of the air you breathe, and you need to learn the different methods of breathing which are used to achieve different goals. In the first stage of regulating your breath, it becomes calm, smooth, and peaceful. Once you have reached this point, the next step is to make your breathing deep, slender, long, and soft. This is the prerequisite for successful Qìgōng practice.

In order to make your breathing calm, smooth, and peaceful, you must first regulate your mind. Remember, your mind is the headquarters of your whole being. When your mind is not steady and calm, your emotions will be agitated. Your emotions are closely related to your breath. For example, when you are angry or excited, you exhale more strongly than you inhale. When you are sad, you inhale more strongly than you exhale. When your mind is peaceful and calm, your inhalation and exhalation are relatively equal.

Therefore, in Qìgōng breathing training, you first have to regulate your emotional mind. This, in turn, will allow you to regulate your breathing, which in turn will allow you to regulate your mind more deeply. Again, the calmer and deeper your mind is, the calmer and deeper your breathing will be. After you have trained for a long time, your breathing will be full and slender, and your mind will be very clear. It is said: "Xīnxī Xiāngyī" (心息相依), which means "Heart (mind) and breathing (are) mutually dependent." When you reach this meditative state, your heartbeat slows down, and your mind is very clear: you have entered the sphere of real meditation.

Normally, when your emotional mind is agitated, not only is your breath affected, but your Qì circulation as well. Understand that your emotions are related to your internal organs. For example, anger can make your liver Qì supply lose its balance. Happiness can make your heart too Yáng. Fear can make the Qì supply to your bladder deficient. Obviously, in order to regulate the Qì in your body, you must first regulate your emotional mind. Regulating your breathing will help you to do this.

The other side of the coin is that you can also use your breathing to control your Yì. When your breathing is uniform, it is like you are hypnotizing your Yì, which helps to calm it. But there is another way in which you can use breathing to control your Yì. Whenever you take in poor food or air you tend to get heartburn from the over-accumulation of Fire Qì, which normally resides in the Middle Dāntián (solar plexus), stirring up your emotions and disturbing your wisdom mind (Yì). As you regulate your breath to dissipate the heart fire and calm your emotional mind (Xīn), you will also be calming your Yì.

We have established that Yì and breathing are interdependent. Deep and calm breathing relaxes you, keeps your mind clear, and fills your lungs with plenty of air so that your brain and entire body have an adequate supply of oxygen. In addition, deep and complete breathing enables the diaphragm to move up and down, which massages and stimulates the internal organs. For this reason, deep breathing exercises are also called "internal organ exercises."

Finally, one additional point: regulating the breath is not only the key to leading the mind into a deeper and calmer stage of meditation, it is also the key to leading the Qì to the extremities and the skin. When the Qì is led to the limbs, it can open up the channels in the limbs and complete the Grand Circulation (Dàzhōutiān, 大周天), as well as increase the efficiency of the muscles to the higher power state needed by a martial artist. When the Qì is effectively led to the skin, you are able to strengthen and enlarge your Guardian Qì shield, which can keep you from sickness caused by outside negative influences.

Next we will discuss the thirteen methods of regulating the breath used in Qìgōng, starting with the most basic and ending with the most advanced. However, since the more advanced methods are difficult, both in understanding and practice, it is impossible to discuss them thoroughly here. A more detailed discussion of these advanced techniques will be presented in later volumes.

9-3. THE DIFFERENT METHODS OF QÌGŌNG BREATHING (BÙTÓNG DE TIÁOXÍ FĀNGFǍ, 不同的調息方法)

In the last four thousand years of study and experimentation, many ways have been developed to regulate the breath. Each technique has its unique theory and goal. These techniques are called Tiáoxí (調息), which means "to regulate the breathing." It is also often called Tǔnà (吐呐), which means "to utter and to take in." The latter name is used especially when the nose is used to inhale and the mouth is used to exhale. Since there are many levels of Qìgōng practice, the methods of regulating the breath are classified according to their difficulty, from the easiest to the most difficult. Here we will list and explain thirteen breathing techniques used in Chinese Qìgōng.

Natural Breathing (Píngcháng Hūxī, 平常呼吸)

Frequently people who are just starting to practice Qìgōng will start right away to use advanced breathing methods. However, the best way to grasp the key to the deeper breathing methods is to start by regulating the method of breathing you use every day.

You should understand that your natural breathing is constantly affected by your thoughts and emotions. For example, when you feel tense or excited, you breathe faster, and when you feel sad and depressed, you breathe slower. The lengths of inhalation and exhalation are also affected by your emotions. When you are happy, your exhalation is longer than your inhalation, but when you are sad, your inhalation is longer. So you can see that although you have always regulated your breathing, you have usually done it unconsciously.

People breathe in different ways. Little children and some adults still have the habit of abdominal breathing. Most middle-aged people breathe with their stomachs, and older people breathe with their chests. Regardless of how you breathe, the purpose is to bring oxygen into the lungs and expel carbon dioxide. Though we talk of abdominal breathing, in fact the air does not, or at least should not, go any lower. If air goes into your digestive system, it will cause pain, so it should be expelled immediately.

To regulate your natural breathing means to regulate your current pattern of breathing. You should not intentionally change your breathing habits while doing this training, because you would put your Yì on the new method and be distracted away from what you normally do and experience. Regulating the natural breath means concentrating your mind to understand your natural way of breathing, to feel the way you breathe, and finally to guide your breathing to a more relaxed and smoother stage.

In order to regulate your natural breathing, you must first be natural and comfortable, and your mind must get rid of emotional disturbances. Then, learn how to feel the muscles which are related to your breathing. Finally, your mind leads the muscles into a more relaxed stage, and you can feel or sense the Qì flow.

Choose any posture you like, as long as you feel comfortable and natural. Breathe through your nose. Do not actively control the breath, but simply pay attention to it and feel it. Breathe softly and gently. The final goal of the process involves training your natural breathing to be: 1. Calm (Jìng, 静), 2. Slender (Xì, 細), 3. Deep (Shēn, 深), 4. Continuous (Yōu, 悠), and 5. Uniform (Yún, 勻). We will discuss these in more detail at the end of this chapter. After a while you will reach the stage of regulating your breathing without conscious effort, when your breathing will enter a new stage. Most important of all, however, is the experience you gain through practicing the technique of regulating your natural breathing. This experience becomes the seed which produces the deeper understanding you need to fathom the more difficult breathing techniques.

Chest Breathing (Xiōngbù Hūxī, 胸部呼吸)

Chest breathing, or breathing by expanding and contracting the rib cage, is one of the main methods of regulating the breath, especially in the external martial Qìgōng styles, as well as deep sea diving.

Chest breathing increases the capacity of your lungs, and therefore increases the amount of oxygen and carbon dioxide exchanged. It also allows you to hold your breath longer. External martial artists use this method to increase the amount of Air Qì they take in, which is used to support their muscular exercise. Weight lifters and people who do heavy labor also do this.

When you practice chest breathing, keep your mind and chest muscles relaxed. If they are tense, you will use more oxygen. In the training used by the external martial arts such as Tiger style, when you exhale you lead the Air Qì to your limbs. The more you practice, the more efficiently you will be able to do this. Although when you practice chest breathing your abdomen moves up and down slightly, you should understand that external martial artists generally do not pay attention to the abdomen until they get older. Once they pass 30, they will start to practice breathing lower and lower in the abdomen.

Practitioners of the internal martial arts do not consider increasing the lung capacity as important as the external stylists. Internal practitioners believe that the more you increase lung capacity, the more Fire Qì (Air Qì) you will take in, which may scatter and confuse the mind and increase the Fire in the body. For an internal Qìgōng practitioner, regulating the breath means breathing lower down in the abdomen in the Dāntián, instead of emphasizing the chest.

Before we finish discussing chest breathing, I would like to point out that your lungs behave like a rubber band: the more you stretch them the larger they will become. However, after you have practiced chest breathing for a long time, or even if you have done a good deal of heavy exercise, you should not stop exercising completely and suddenly. Once your lungs have expanded to a larger size, a sudden stop may cause part of your lungs to collapse, causing problems such as pneumonia. If you want to stop practice, you should cut down the exercises gradually and allow your lungs to adjust themselves. In external martial Qìgōng society, we often see that when a practitioner gets old and loses the ability to do the same exercises, he loses the ability to expand his lungs, and his lung capacity lessens. Consequently, the muscles that used to obtain a large amount of oxygen degenerate faster than normal. This is called Sàngōng (energy dispersion, 散功).

You can see that if you are not an external martial artist, you have no need to form the habit of chest breathing. Still, there are advantages to doing chest breathing from time to time. First, you will enliven the cells in the parts of the lungs which are not commonly used, and keep them from degenerating. Second, heavy chest breathing increases the supply of Air Qì, so that you can send a lot of Qì to the skin. This helps to open the tiny Qì channels in the skin and strengthens your Guardian Qì.

Normal Abdominal Breathing (Zhèng Fùhūxī, 正腹呼吸)

Abdominal Breath is the key to the Nèidān (internal elixir) Qìgōng exercises. In abdominal, or Dāntián breathing, there are two common ways of breathing: Normal Abdominal Breathing (Zhèng Fùhūxī, 正腹呼吸) and Reverse Abdominal Breathing (Fǎn Fùhūxī, 反腹呼吸). We will discuss Normal Abdominal Breathing first.

Normal Abdominal Breathing is the next step after chest breathing for the Qìgōng beginner. Abdominal Breathing is a deep breathing exercises, but it is not like the breathing you do in the chest. Correct deep breathing involves slow, deep breaths that seem to go all the way down to your Dāntián. It requires that your mind be relaxed and concentrated. This kind of breathing is called Fǎntóng (返童) breath, or "Back to Childhood" (Fǎntóng Fùhūxī, 返童呼吸) Breathing, because it is deep, soft, and natural like a child's. It is the first step in Nèidān Qìgōng training.

In abdominal breathing the lungs are expanded and contracted by the muscles of the diaphragm and abdomen, rather than the chest muscles. There are several benefits to Normal Abdominal Breathing:

1. **Internal Organ Massage.** In abdominal breathing, the diaphragm and the muscles of the lower abdomen are constantly moving back and forth. This movement massages the internal organs, increasing the circulation of Qì and blood in and around them. This keeps them healthy and strong, avoiding the Qì stagnation which is one of the major causes of illness.

2. **Invigorating the Abdominal Muscles.** Because babies naturally do deep abdominal breathing, their abdominal muscles are constantly moving. Not only does this keep the Qì circulating around the organs, but it also loosens up the Qì channels which connect the front of the body to the legs and to the back. Usually, once you have given up your abdominal breathing, the Qì flow to the Governing Vessel (Dūmài, 督脈) in your back becomes sluggish. This weakens the ability of the Governing Vessel to regulate Qì throughout the body and allows a number of problems to arise.

3. **Increasing the Efficiency of the Qì Flow from the Kidneys to the Lower Dāntián.** One objective of Qìgōng practice is the strengthening of your Water Qì (Original Qì), which is converted from the essence residing in your kidneys. As we have discussed, the Lower Dāntián is the residence of this Qì. The muscular movement of the muscles in abdominal breathing help to lead Qì from the kidneys to your Lower Dāntián and keep it there. The more abdominal breathing you do, the more Qì is led, and the more efficiently the essence is converted. Abdominal breathing acts like an engine which is able to convert fuel into energy more efficiently than normal engines can, and thereby conserve more fuel.

4. **To Increase the Water Qì.** Once you are able to increase the efficiency of the Essence-Qì conversion process, you will be able to create more Water Qì (Original Qì). Strong Water Qì is the key to successful Qìgōng practice. Water Qì is able to calm down your mind, strengthen your will, and firm your spirit. Since Water Qì is the major source of coolant for your Fire Qì, you are able to maintain your health and lengthen your life.

   Normal Abdominal Breathing is an important part of Buddhist Qìgōng training, and so it is often called "Buddhist Breathing." To practice it, you must first use your Yì to control the muscles in your abdomen. When you inhale, intentionally expand your abdomen, and when you exhale, let it contract. In addition, when you inhale you should gently push out your Huìyīn (Co-1) (會陰) cavity or anus, and when you exhale, hold it up. If you practice for ten minutes three times a day, in a month you should be able to resume the abdominal breathing you did as a baby.

There is a very important rule when you practice: do not hold your breath. Your breath must be smooth, natural, continuous, and comfortable. Abdominal deep breathing is done in the lower abdomen, so you should not be expanding and contracting your chest. Instead, you should feel like you are drawing the air deep into your lower abdomen.

Reverse Abdominal Breathing (Fǎn Fùhūxī, 反腹呼吸) (Nì Fùhūxī, 逆腹呼吸)

The Reverse Abdominal Breathing method is commonly used by Daoist Qìgōng practitioners, and so it is often called "Daoist Breathing." Since you are moving your abdomen, you gain the same health benefits that you do with the Normal Abdominal Breathing. However, in Reverse Abdominal Breathing, when you inhale, you draw the abdomen in and hold up your Huìyīn (Co-1) cavity or anus. When you exhale, gently push out your abdomen and Huìyīn cavity or anus. There are many reasons for this. The major ones are:

1. **Greater Efficiency in Leading Qì to the Extremities.** Whenever you exhale, you are expanding your Guardian Qì. When you inhale, you are conserving your Qì or even absorbing the surrounding Qì into your body. Experience teaches that when you intentionally try to expand your Qì during exhalation, it is easier to expand your abdominal muscles than to relax them. Try blowing up a balloon, and hold one hand on your abdomen. You will find that when you blow out, your abdomen expands rather than withdraws. Or imagine that you are pushing a car. In order to express your power, you have to exhale while you are pushing. If you pay attention to your abdomen while you are doing this, you will realize that your abdomen is expanding again. If you pull your stomach in when you are doing this, you will find that there is less power and that it feels unnatural.

    Now imagine that you feel cold, and want to absorb energy from your surroundings. You will find that your inhalations are longer than your exhalations, and that your abdomen withdraws when you inhale, rather than expands.

    Daoist Qìgōng practitioners have found that whenever you try to intentionally expand or condense your Qì, your abdomen moves opposite to the way it moves during normal breathing. They realized that reverse breathing is a tool and a strategy that you may use to lead the Qì more efficiently. You can see that the foremost advantage to the Daoist Reverse Abdominal Breathing is its ability to lead Qì to the extremities more naturally and easily than is possible with Normal Abdominal Breathing. Once you have mastered the coordination of Yì, breath, and Qì, you will be able to lead Qì to any part of your body.

2. **For Martial Arts.** The internal martial arts training of the Daoists is more advanced than that of the Buddhist or any other style. This is simply because the Daoists learned how to lead Qì to any part of the body more efficiently than any of the others. The key to this success is Reverse Abdominal Breathing.

3. **For More Effectively Raising the Qì in Marrow/Brain Washing Qìgōng.** In Marrow/Brain Washing Qìgōng, Reverse Abdominal Breathing is able to raise Qì from the legs to the brain more efficiently than the Buddhist methods.

Although there are many advantages to Reverse Abdominal Breathing, there are also several disadvantages or problems which arise during training. Qìgōng practitioners who use Daoist breathing should be aware of these potential problems, especially during the early period of training. The major problems are:

1. **Tensing the Chest.** In the reverse training, when you inhale the diaphragm moves down while the abdomen is withdrawing. The drawing in of the abdomen generates pressure upward, which makes it harder for the diaphragm to move down. This can cause pressure and tension below the solar plexus, which leads to Qì stagnation. This is especially common with people who have just started doing reverse breathing.

   This pressure below the solar plexus may cause problems such as stomach ache, diarrhea, or even chest pain. The tension and pressure may cause the heart to beat faster. When this happens, the body becomes positive, the mind is scattered and confused, you become impatient, and your will is unsteady. Enduring this does not advance your Qìgōng—it makes you sick and hinders your training.

   Many Qìgōng masters will encourage their students to practice Normal Abdominal Breathing until it feels natural and comfortable. Only then will they encourage Reverse Abdominal Breathing. Reverse Abdominal Breathing starts with a small abdominal motion in coordination with the breathing. During practice you must always pay attention to the Middle Burner (from the solar plexus to the navel), keeping this area relaxed and comfortable. After a few months of practice, you will find that there is a point of compromise which allows your reverse breathing to be deep and which also keeps the chest area relaxed. When you reach this stage, you will have grasped the key to Daoist breathing. After you have practiced for a long time, you will realize that your mind does not have to be in conscious control of your breathing. It happens naturally whenever you are practicing Qìgōng.

   The final stage of Reverse Abdominal Breathing is moving your abdominal muscles like a rotating ball (Figure 9-1). Because the ball is round, your breathing no longer causes any tension in the Middle Burner area. If you train patiently, you will eventually be able to use reverse breathing naturally all the time.

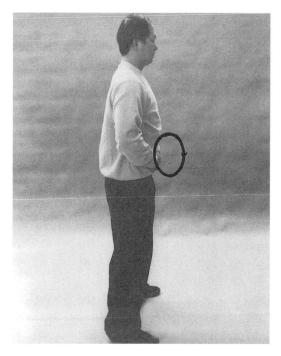

Figure 9-1. Move your abdomen like a ball

2. **Holding the Breath.** Because reverse breathing can cause tension and generate pressure in the chest area, people will sometimes unconsciously hold their breath. It is very important that the Qìgōng beginner understand that holding the breath while practicing is very harmful. There are some exercises in which you hold your breath, but unless you are doing these specific exercises, you should be careful to keep your breathing smooth and steady.

Holding the Breath Breathing (Bìxí, 閉息)

Holding the breath breathing is a training technique for when a Qìgōng practitioner wishes to lead his Qì to a specific area and hold it there. For example, martial artists, especially in the external styles, will generate Qì in their limbs and then hold their breath. This causes the Qì to stay in the limbs so that they can use it for fighting. To use a more prosaic example, when pushing a car you will find sometimes that after you have exerted your power you hold your breath in order to make the power last longer. In internal Qìgōng practice, practitioners will often lead Qì to a specific spot and then gently hold their breath. This may be done to raise the potential in a cavity in order to dissolve a block. When an internal martial artist has an internal injury, he will often lead Qì to the injury and keep it there for a short time to energize the area and speed up the healing process. When he does this, he must hold his breath gently while keeping his body relaxed so that he can feel and lead the Qì.

You can see that holding the breath Qìgōng training is a higher level than those discussed above. Before you train this, you must have acquired mastery of the right breathing techniques and you must understand your body's Qì, otherwise you will make the situation worse. You should also understand that if you do not know the Why and How of the practice thoroughly, holding the breath is very dangerous—especially in Nèidān Qìgōng. When you hold your breath, the Qì will accumulate and stagnate. If this accumulated Qì stays in a cavity or in the organs, it may affect the normal functioning of your body. It is very easy for a beginner to hold his Qì in his solar plexus and heart, which may cause damage to the heart or even death. Before starting holding the breath training, you must complete Small Circulation and Grand Circulation.

In the external Qìgōng styles, holding the breath is not as dangerous as it is in the internal styles. Most of the external Qìgōng styles work with Qì in the limbs. Qì stagnation in the limbs is not as dangerous as stagnation in the body, where it can affect the internal organs.

In Nèidān Qìgōng training there are three major purposes for holding the breath:

1. **To Lead Qì to the Ends of or Even Beyond the Body.** Remember that when you practice Nèidān you must remain relaxed and calm, then you will be able to lead Qì to your skin. Normally, without special training it is very hard to move Qì to the hair or beyond the skin. Nèidān Qìgōng practitioners found that, once they led Qì to their skin, if they gently held their breath they could use their mind to lead the Qì further. When Qì is held at the skin, the Qì potential is raised and the millions of tiny Qì channels are opened. This makes it easier for the Qì to reach past the skin. The more you train, the further beyond your body you will be able to expand it. It is said: "Transport Qì as though through a pearl with a hole with nine curves, not even the tiniest place won't be reached."[1] You should be able to transport Qì to every part of your body, from deep inside the marrow to beyond the surface of the skin.

2. **To Move Qì Without Coordinating It with the Breath.** You know that when you move the abdomen in and out the Qì is led out from the Dāntián. Beginners usually have to coordinate this with their breathing in order to do it effectively. After several years of practice you may wish to lead the Qì (or as it is commonly said, generate the Qì) solely with your mind without coordinating it with your breathing. In order to do this, hold your breath for a short time, while keeping your body completely relaxed. Move your abdomen in and out, leading the Qì either upward or downward without coordinating it with your breathing. When you reach this stage, it is said that you have "picked up the little herb" (Cǎixiǎoyào, 採小藥). This means both that the student is starting to be able to use his Qìgōng (as in picking up something to use it), and that he is bringing Qì (the herb) up his back. This exercise is done in the beginning stages of Qìgōng training, when most students still need to

---

1.　行氣如九曲珠，無微不到。

move the abdomen in order to coordinate the movement of Qì with the opening and closing of the Huìyīn cavity and the anus.

3. **Hibernation Training.** One of the highest Qìgōng practices is training yourself to use oxygen more efficiently. Holding the breath is the most basic step of this training. You must train yourself to stay calm and relaxed even when your air supply is cut off. Your meditative mind should reach a level of sleeping meditation, like hibernating animals, in which your heart beat slows down. Once you have learned to use oxygen more efficiently, you will breathe less and less and be able to enter a deep sleep. We will discuss hibernation breathing later.

Full Inhale and Exhale Breathing (Quánmiànxí, 全面息)

In this type of abdominal breathing, you practice inhaling and exhaling to the maximum in coordination with the in-and-out motion of your abdomen. You also try to extend the length of each breath. When you practice this, you make a slight sound as you inhale and exhale. This training has several aspects:

1. Like the chest breathing discussed above, full inhale and exhale abdominal breathing increases the amount of oxygen you take in and the amount of carbon dioxide you put out. However, this exercise is one step ahead of chest breathing because the abdominal movement causes Qì to accumulate in the Dāntián. This exercise also trains the abdominal muscles to expand and contract to their maximum.

2. When you make a slight sound while doing full inhale and exhale breathing, you raise your Yì and spirit to their maximum. This can help you in leading Qì to the surface of the skin and condensing it in the center of your body or into the marrow.

When you practice this type of breathing, keep your body as relaxed as possible. Your mind must be calm and clear, so that you can lead the Qì to the skin and condense it in the marrow. Do not make a habit of doing this full inhalation and exhalation all the time. Practice it only occasionally in order to enliven the lung cells which are not generally used. Full breathing is the key to skin breathing, which will be discussed next.

Body Breathing (Tǐxí, 體息) or Skin Breathing (Fūxí, 膚息)

Body breathing or skin breathing is one of the main goals of Qìgōng breathing. It means that when you breathe, your entire body is also breathing Qì through your skin. When you exhale you move Qì to your skin, and your pores open; and when you inhale you draw in Qì from outside, and your pores close. When you are able to lead Qì to your skin when you exhale, it feels like when you expose your skin to the sun on a winter day. In the sun, your pores open up to absorb and expel energy more easily. In Qìgōng training, however, you use your mind to lead the Qì to the skin to energize your pores from inside your body. Once the pores are energized they open wide, and when you inhale, the Qì is led inward and the pores close. After you have practiced Qìgōng for a while, you will want your Qì to reach every cell of your body, especially the skin. Skin breathing allows you to open your pores so that the air can come in and remove the waste that accumulates in them. Leading Qì to the skin is a required step if you want your Qì to expand beyond your body. If you are able to reach this stage, your Qì will be able to reach anywhere your will leads it. You will have plenty of Qì, and your Qì circulation will be smooth everywhere. This is the key to maintaining health and lengthening your life.

When you train body breathing, center yourself in your Dāntián and imagine that your body and Qì are like a big beach ball. Every time you inhale, your Yì brings all of the Qì to the center and the ball shrinks, and when you exhale, the imaginary ball expands. If you catch the trick, you will discover that this Qì ball gradually expands to cover your entire body. When you breathe, this Qì ball also breathes (Figure 9-2).

In the Daoist books, this body breathing or skin breathing method is considered one of the "Fúqìfǎ" (Yield Qì Methods, 伏氣法) and is included in the Língbǎo Bìfǎ (Spiritual Treasure to Reach the End Method, 靈寶閉法). In this training, start with a full inhalation and intentionally hold the air in your body. Then, slowly let the air out. When you practice this method, you are also beginning to do skin or body breathing. After you train for a long time, you will be able to extend the duration of the breaths and reach the goal of the "Guīxí" (Turtle Breath, 龜息). It is believed that the turtle is able to live for several hundred years because it is able to exchange air directly through its skin.

Five Gates Breathing (Wǔxīnxí, 五心息)

In Chinese meditation there are five places or centers (Wǔxīn, 五心) which are considered to be the gates through which the Qì in the body communicates with the Qì which surrounds you. These centers are the face (or crown, Bǎihuì, Gv-20, 百會), the two Bubbling-Wells (Yǒngquán, K-1, 湧泉) on the bottom of your feet (Figure 9-3), and the two Labor Palaces (Láogōng, P-8, 勞宮) in the center of your palms (Figure 9-4). Daoist Hánxūzǔ (涵虛祖) said: "The feet breathe, continuously and unbroken, existing softly."[2] Zhuāngzi (莊子) said: "The normal person breathes in his throat, a real person (an immortal) breathes through his feet."[3]

The major purposes of these centers or gates are:

1. **To Regulate the Body's Qì Level.** For example, when the body is too positive because of fever, these five gates will release Qì to cool down the body. A very common treatment for fever in Chinese medicine is to place the feet in cold water, and to put alcohol in the center of the palms and blow on it. This speeds the lowering of the body's Qì level and, consequently, cools down the temperature of the body. You

---

2.　涵虛祖曰：「踵也者，相接不斷，綿綿若存也。」
3.　莊子曰：「常人之息以喉，真人之息以踵。」

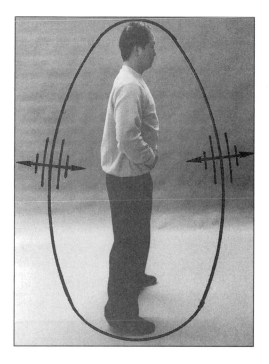

Figure 9-2. Expanding the Qì ball

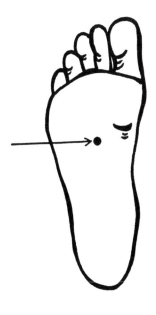

Figure 9-3. The Bubbling Well
cavity (Yǒngquán, K-1)

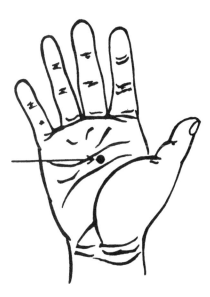

Figure 9-4. The Labor Palace cavity (Láogōng, P-8)

know that in the summertime when you are very hot, you can cool down by washing your face and hands in cold water. And remember how good it feels to immerse your feet in a nice cold stream?

2. **To Sense Your Surroundings.** Frequently you will first sense hot or cold on your face or the centers of your palms. This is because they are the centers or gates which allow you to communicate most directly with the environment. You have to be able to sense what is going on with the Qì around you before your body can adjust its Guardian Qì level to protect itself. Although the centers of the feet are also designed for this, these gates are not as sensitive as they used to be because of the use of shoes.

3. **To Absorb Qì from Outside of Your Body.** When you feel cold, you use warm water to wash your face, hands, and feet. When you have a cold, placing your feet and hands in warm water will keep you warm because it allows you to absorb environmental Qì through the gates to nourish your body. In Chinese Qìgōng, it is very important to train yourself to absorb environmental Qì. When you are able to do this efficiently, you will be able to cut down on the amount of food and air that your body requires.

Generally speaking, the face center (or crown) is the most important and sensitive gate among the five. The gates work in both directions: you are able to sense what is going on outside of you, but they also reveal what is going on inside you. Your face is the first part of you to sense whether the air is warm or cold, and four of your five senses are located in your face and head. On the other hand, your face clearly reflects your emotions, and often indicates what you are thinking. In the centers of your palms are the Láogōng cavities. They are the gates which lead Qì to the skin of the entire palm and fingers. The more Qì you have flowing through your palms, the more Qì flows to the skin of the whole hand, and the greater your sensitivity of touch. Good Qì flow in the hands is also important for manual labor, which is why the cavities are called "Labor Palaces" (Láogōng). The cavities in the bottom of the feet play a similar role. The are called "Bubbling Wells" (Yǒngquán) because the Qì is continually coming out of them.

Because these five gates are keys to adjusting the Qì in your body, Qìgōng meditators train until they are able to govern the Qì in these five areas efficiently. They are not only learning how to release excess Qì, but they are also learning how to absorb Qì from the environment. This practice will allow them to regulate their bodies' Qì by using the natural, environmental Qì which is considered more pure and clean than the Post-birth Qì converted from the food and air essences. Medical Qìgōng practitioners train with the two gates in the palms so that they can increase their effectiveness in adjusting their patients' Qì. Martial artists train these two gates so that they can lead Qì to the hands more efficiently and energize the muscles. This also increases their ability to sense their opponent's energy, which is called "skin listening" (Tīngjìng, 聽勁) in the internal martial styles. They also train the gates in the feet so that they can jump high, run fast, and kick powerfully. You can see from these

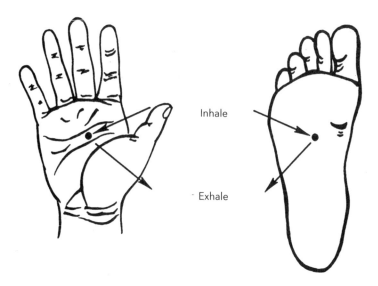

Figure 9-5. Exchanging Qì through the Qì gates

examples that governing the Qì in the five gates is a serious concern in every style of Chinese Qìgōng.

In the previous section we discussed how the pores in the skin are millions of tiny Qì gates which allow you to sense the environment and exchange Qì with it. Unfortunately, since people have protected their bodies from the natural environment for so long by wearing clothes, we have lost a lot of the sensitivity that we used to have, and that animals still have. However, the hands and the face still have a lot of their sensitivity.

In order to govern the Qì in the gates, you must learn to breathe through the centers of your palms and feet. Breathing here means to exchange the Qì of the body for the Qì of the environment through special breathing techniques. Generally speaking, Daoist Reverse Abdominal Breathing is the easiest way. In Daoist training, when you inhale you draw Qì from your limbs into the center of your body. While you are doing this, imagine that you are absorbing Qì from the environment through the gates. When you exhale, lead the Qì to the gates and release it into the air (Figure 9-5). After you train for a long time, you will be able to feel that, when you breathe, these five gates are also breathing. You must train until it becomes natural and you do not have to concentrate on it to do it. Remember: regulate your breathing until you no longer need to do it consciously. Naturally, before you can breathe through these gates, you must have mastered all of the basic breathing techniques which we have discussed before.

Thread Breathing (Guànqì, 貫氣)

Thread breathing is a higher level breathing technique. Usually, before you reach this stage, you should already feel that your physical body has become transparent. That means you can transport your Qì easily and smoothly without any stagnation. Thread breathing teaches you to lead the Qì anywhere in your body in coordination with your breathing. There are two major purposes to this training:

1. **To Adjust the Qì in the Body.** Very often after you practice Qìgōng you will find that the Qì in one area is higher than in another. The thread breathing method, however, allows you to lead the Qì to other areas very effectively, whenever you want. This practice can also be used to adjust abnormal Qì levels caused by sickness.

2. **To Raise Clean, Pure Qì and to Sink Dirty, Contaminated Qì.** In Qìgōng training, in order for you to reach the higher meditative stages, you must settle or sink your contaminated Fire Qì and raise up your pure Water Qì. The thread breathing method is also used to reverse the positions of the Water Qì and Fire Qì. This method is called Kǎn-Lí (Water-Fire, 坎-離). When the Fire Qì sinks to the Dāntián, it will be controlled and settled. In Qìgōng training, it is also common to sink the Fire Qì to the bottom of the feet and to raise the Water Qì to the top of your head—a process which threads your entire body together.

3. **To Open the Qì Channels and the Blood Vessels.** The thread breathing method can not only help you to complete Grand Qì Circulation, but it can also open up all of the other Qì branches in addition to the twelve major Qì channels.

You can see that thread breathing training involves leading the Qì to move within your body, a process which is different from the skin and gates breathing methods, in which Qì is exchanged with the natural environment. You should understand that the first requirement is that your body must be relaxed completely into the third level of relaxation, which will allow the Qì to move freely. The second requirement is that your mind must be within your body instead outside of your body. If your mind is not in your body, how will you be able to sense and lead the Qì? We will discuss regulating the mind later. Finally, you must learn how to coordinate your breathing with your mind and Qì. Naturally, it is impossible for a beginner to reach this stage. It normally takes at least ten or more years of correct training.

We would like to remind you that many of the subjects discussed in this volume are presented as information, as a guide for understanding Qìgōng. It is almost impossible for anyone to grasp the keys simply by reading this book. As long as you remember: do not look high and walk low, sooner or later you will reach your goal.

Hibernation Breathing (Dōngmiánxí, 冬眠息)

One of the highest levels of Qìgōng involves disciplining your spirit to leave your body and travel around. Often your spirit will leave your body for long periods of time, sometimes even for several months. In order to keep your physical body alive without food while your spirit is gone, your heartbeat must slow down, your body's use of energy must be kept to a minimum, and the energy must be used most efficiently. Hibernation breathing makes this possible, slowing your breathing rate down almost to a stop, and making it very shallow. Hibernation breathing is also trained in Indian Yoga.

In order to reach the stage of hibernation breathing, you must first have a deep level of experience with still meditation. You need to train your body, through fasting and other techniques, to slowly and efficiently convert stored food essence (i.e., fat) into Qì. Your body must be completely relaxed and transparent to the flow of Qì. Naturally, before you are able to freely separate your spirit from your physical body, you usually need to complete the training for spiritual enlightenment. According to the Marrow/Brain Washing documents it usually takes twelve years of proper training as a hermit or priest.

Shén Breathing (Shénxí, 神息)

In religious Qìgōng, Shén breathing is one of the final practices in leading the Shén to separate from the body. Once the mind has been regulated into a deep, calm, and peaceful level, Shén breathing unites the Shén with the breathing so that they correspond to each other. Because breathing is your strategy in guiding and governing the Qì, your Shén can govern the Qì effectively only when your Shén and breathing are able to work together as one. This is called "Shénxí Xiāngyī, 神息相依) in Qigong practice.

Naturally, you must first learn how to keep your Shén (Shǒushén, 守神), and then how to firm it (Gùshén, 固神). "Keep" here means to protect, to nourish, and to keep the Shén at its residence. "Firm" means to solidify, to strengthen, and to control it effectively in the Upper Dāntián. After you have reached this level, you learn how to use your Yì to move your Shén away from its residence and finally separate from the physical body. In order to reach this final stage, you must first learn Shén breathing. When you start moving your Shén, it first stays close to its residence, the way a small child stays near its home when it first starts to walk.

It is said in Daoist society: "Shén is the master of Qì, and it moves and stops with the Qì. Breathing is the secret key to the Qì's forward and backward. The secret key must have the master (Shén), and the master must have the Yì. Three things (Shén, breathing, and Yì) must be used at the same time. Then it will be the really marvelous and tricky Gōngfū of heavenly circulation. When one is missing, it is hard to reach the final goal."[4] You can see that Shén is the headquarters of the Qì and moves together with it. The secret to controlling the movement of the Qì is the breathing. However, most important of all is what is behind the Shén. It is the Yì which ultimately controls the entire training. It is also said: "Shén and Qì move and stop together and not separately. The Yì stays at the center palace like a cart's axle. Wheels (Shén and Qì) and the axle (provide) mutual support. The axle does not move, but lets the wheels turn by themselves."[5] Shén and Qì move together like the wheels. However, these wheels are directed and controlled by the axle. This axle is your mind (Yì). The mind

4. 神是與氣同行同住之主宰，息是進氣退氣之機關，機不可少主，主不可少意，三物並用，方為真正玄妙周天之功夫，缺一難成正果。
5. 神氣同行同住而不離，其意主中宮如軸心，輪軸互用，軸不動而任輪之自轉也。

keeps to the center so that it can direct what is happening, but it should not get involved in the turning of the wheels. The Daoist Zǐyángzǔ (紫陽祖) said: "Slowly tend the herb furnace and watch the (cooking) timing, but keep peace in your Shén breathing and let nature be."[6] This sentence means that when you are building your Qì at the Dāntián, take it slow and easy. Pay attention to the timing to notice when the herb is done. However, you must keep your Shén breathing peacefully and let it happen naturally. The deep meaning of this sentence is that you must train until your Shén breathing becomes natural and you do not need your Yì to regulate your Shén any longer. It is also said in one of the Daoist classics: "Breathing is hidden in the Shén and Shén is hidden in the eyes. The large Dào (has) no shape and no appearance."[7]

Real Breathing (Zhēnxí, 真息)

Real breathing, or Zhēnxí, comes from regulating normal breathing. From real breathing is born embryonic breathing. Once you have regulated your normal breathing, you start abdominal breathing, whereby Qì is led from the kidneys to the Lower Dāntián. This lays the foundation of real breathing. Then what is real breathing? It is said: "The inner scenery of 'real breathing' is (that) there is Qì moving up and down a few inches under the navel (Dāntián)."[8]

It is also said: "The 'real breathing,' one close and one develop, on the top, it does not conflict with the heart; on the bottom, it does not conflict with the kidneys. The 'real person' (is able to) dive into the deep water, float swiftly (but) keep the regular center."[9] "One close and one develop" means that the Qì is contracting and expanding. This saying explains that in real breathing, the Qì is generated in the Dāntián and moves up and down. When it moves up it will not disturb the functioning of the heart, and when it moves down it will not affect the normal functioning of the kidneys. The heart and the kidneys are the most vital organs and must have normal Qì levels. It is therefore important when you do Qìgōng that you do not let the extra energy you develop interfere with the normal functioning of your body. A "real person" is someone who has reached the stage of real breathing, and Qì is able to reach deep into every part of his body. Regardless of how this Qì moves, the mind (Yì) must remain at the Dāntián, which is the "regular center."

It is also said: "The real breathing, like there like gone, soft and nonstop, one name 'internal breathing.' (Though) the external normal breathing is stopped, there is an up-and-down internal scenery at the Dāntián."[10] The Daoist song, "Língyuángē" ("Spiritual Source Song," 靈源歌) says: "Concentrate on the (training) of Qì until it reaches softness, and the Shén is able to stay long, to and fro of the 'real breathing' naturally leisurely."[11] This sentence leads you to the key to real breathing. In order to reach the stage of real breathing, you must

---

6. 紫陽祖曰：〝謾守藥爐看火候，但安神息任天然。〞
7. 經曰：〝息隱神中神隱眸，大道無形固無相。〞
8. 真息之內景為臍下四五寸處，有氣上下往來。
9. 真息者，似有似無，綿綿不斷，一名內呼吸。外面之凡息雖斷，而丹
10. 田之中猶有一上一下之內景。
11. 靈源歌曰：〝專氣致柔神久留，往來真息自悠悠。〞

concentrate on training your Qì flow to be as soft as possible, and your spirit must concentrate and stay in one place, then someday you will sense the Qì's up-and-down movements and attain "real breathing."

The Daoist Sānfēngzǔ (三豐祖) said: "Do not forget the Qì, regulate 'real breathing,' but keep Xūwú (nothing), transport Kǎn (water) and Lí (fire)."[12] This sentence means that in Qìgōng training you must always pay attention to the Qì and learn to regulate the 'real breathing.' Keep your mind at the Upper Dāntián where your Shén resides. Xūwú (虛無) means "nothing," and represents the place where the spirit resides because spirit was generated from nothing. If you are able to do this, you will be able to transport the Water Qì up to cool the Fire Qì.

Embryonic Breathing (Tāixí, 胎息)

We mentioned in the first chapter that there are two major kinds of Qì: Pre-birth Qì or Original Qì (Yuánqì, 元氣), and Post-birth Qì. Original Qì is converted from the Original Essence you inherited from your parents, and Post-birth Qì is converted from the food and air essence. Original Qì is generally considered to be Yīn Qì or Water Qì, while Post-birth Qì is thought to be Yáng Qì or Fire Qì.

It is said: "Producing the large herb is not different from growing things between heaven and earth. In all, it is only Yáng and Yīn, two Qì's. When the two Qì's provide each other and become one, the heaven and the earth will mutually interact."[13] This means that in order to generate the herb (elixir), you must have both Yīn Qì and Yáng Qì. Both Qì's must mutually interact with each other, then a living thing or herb will be produced. The herb or living thing here means the embryo, which represents the beginning of a new life. Daoist Zhāng, Zǐ-Qióng (張紫瓊) said: "Not assisting, not forgetting, the marvelous breathing. To cultivate human nature (the Dào), (you) must comprehend this Gōngfū. Regulate the two Qì's to originate the embryonic breathing. Then build your (herb or elixir) furnace in it."[14] This sentence means that when you cultivate your Dào, you should not concentrate on (assist) nor ignore (forget) the marvelous strategy of breathing. In order to reach the embryonic breathing stage, you must learn to regulate the Yáng and Yīn Qì. After you can regulate your Yáng and Yīn Qì, you will be able to generate the elixir in it.

What then is embryonic breathing? It is said: "(When) the Shén is hidden at the Qì cavity, it is called the embryo. (When) the (Post-birth) Qì is able to reach to the cavity, it is called breathing. With embryonic Shén and breathing Qì, when Gōngfū advances to embryonic breathing, then no exit and no entrance. (One) will no more have normal breathing."[15] Before we continue, you should first understand what cavity is meant here. In Qìgōng, several places

12. 三豐祖曰：“休忘氣，調真息，但守虛無運坎離。”
13. 圭旨曰：“大藥之生，與天地生物不異，總只是陰陽二氣，二施一化，而玄黃相交矣。”
14. 張紫瓊曰：“非助非忘妙呼吸，修行要解這功夫，調停二氣生胎息，而向中間設鼎爐。”
15. 藏神於氣穴曰胎，氣至氣穴為息，胎其神息其氣，功夫進至胎息，則不出不入，永無凡息矣。

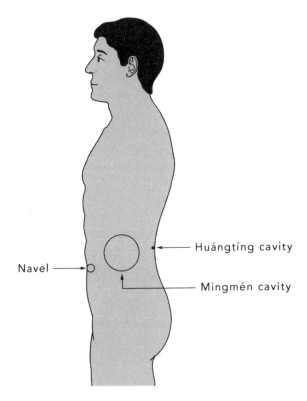

Figure 9-6. Huángtíng cavity

are called Yuánqiào (元竅), which means "original cavity," or "original key point." One of these places is called Huángtíng (黃庭) or "Yellow Yard." Daoists used to wear yellow robes, so naturally this name is used frequently in Daoist society. The Huángtíng cavity is behind the navel and in front of the Mìngmén (Gv-4) (命門) (Figure 9-6). It is at the center of gravity of your body. This is the place where the baby's cells start to multiply. In embryonic breathing, your Shén is able to reside at the Huángtíng and the Post-birth Qì is able to reach it. Then the Yáng Qì and Yīn Qì interact, and a new "baby" is born. The Daoist Lǐ, Qīng-Ān (李清庵) said: "Shén and Qì combine to originate the super spiritual quality, Xīn and breath are mutually dependent to generate the holy embryo."[16] Xīn here means mind and Shén.

The Daoist treatise *Wǔzhēnpiān* (*Treatise on Comprehending the Real*, 悟真篇) said: "There are three kinds of breathing. From coarse to fine, inhalation and exhalation through the nose is nose breathing. Keeping the center (Lower Dāntián) and ascending and descending, is Qì breathing. (When) extremely calm and return to its root is called 'Shén breathing.' Therefore, to number (means to evaluate) the breathing (meaning nose breathing) is not as high as regulating (abdominal real) breathing, and the regulating breathing is not as high as Shén breathing. When the Shén breathing becomes peaceful, then condense the Shén into

---

16. 李清庵詩云：〝神氣和合生靈質，心息相依結聖胎。〞

the Qì cavity (Huángtíng), then the breathing is really deep."[17] This saying explains the levels of breathing. First, you learn nose breathing from coarse to fine, until the breathing becomes relaxed, deep, smooth, and natural. Then you enter into abdominal breathing and eventually enter into real breathing. After you have reached the real breathing stage, you train Shén breathing until your Shén is able to reach the Huángtíng cavity and the Post-birth Qì is able to reach there also, so that the holy embryo will be generated and the elixir will be formed.

To conclude this section, it is important for a Qìgōng practitioner to learn the correct ways of regulating his breathing. There are many ways of regulating the breathing, which we have arranged from the most basic to the deepest and most difficult. To reach the final goal of embryonic breathing you must start with regulating the normal breathing. It is called Bíxí (鼻息), which means "nose breathing." From normal regular breathing, you will enter the abdominal breathing stage which enables you to build Qì at the Dāntián. It is this Qì that will lead you to the door of real Qìgōng practice. This training is called Qìxí (氣息), or "Qì breathing." When you have reached this level the Dāntiánqì is able to move up and down following your breathing. You have now reached the target of "real breathing" (Zhēnxí, 真息). Finally, you will lead the Post-birth Qì to the "Huángtíng Cavity" to interact with the Pre-birth Qì and generate the "holy embryo" (Shèngtāi, 聖胎). When you have completed this stage, you will have formed the "Elixir." This stage of breathing is called "Tāixí" (胎息), which means "embryonic breathing."

Reaching the final goal of embryonic breathing is very difficult. When you have reached this stage, you will have built the foundation of enlightenment. It is almost impossible to reach this stage without becoming a hermit. Very few Qìgōng practitioners have really done it. It is probably more feasible for the average person who is seeking good health and a long life to reach the stage of "real breathing."

9-4. GENERAL KEYS TO REGULATING NORMAL BREATHING (TIÁO PÍNGCHÁNG HŪXĪ DE YĪBĀN YÀOLǏNG, 調平常呼吸的一般要領)

If you are a Qìgōng beginner, you should start with regulating your normal breathing, and not worry about any other Qì regulating breath training. This will gradually lead you into Qì breathing.

There are eight key words for air breathing which a beginning Qìgōng practitioner should remember during normal breathing exercise. Once you understand them you will be able to substantially shorten the time needed to reach your Qìgōng goals. These eight key words are:

1. **Calm and Silent (Jìng, 靜).** The mind is calm and the breathing is silent. When your mind is calm and peaceful, you will be able to judge what is going on correctly and will be able to regulate your breathing more efficiently. Unless you are engaged

---

17. 悟真篇曰：〝息有三種：從粗入細，呼吸出入者鼻息也；規中升降者氣息也；靜極歸根者神息也。故數息不如調息，調息不如安息。神息既安，則凝神入氣穴，其息深矣。〞

in special training for some specific purpose, keep your breathing silent so that it is relaxed and peaceful.

2. **Slender (Xì, 細).** When you breathe, it is like a tiny stream—it should be smooth, natural, and slender. This key will lead you into deeper levels of meditation and relaxation.

3. **Deep (Shén, 深).** When you breathe deeply, draw the air down into your abdomen. Draw the air in by moving your diaphragm down, rather than by expanding your chest. Only expand your chest if you are doing a chest expanding exercise. Deep breathing will lead you to abdominal breathing and build the foundation for your Qìgōng practice.

    Deep and complete breathing does not mean that you inhale and exhale to the maximum. This would cause the lungs and the surrounding muscles to tense up, which in turn would keep the air from circulating freely, and hinder the absorption of oxygen. Without enough oxygen, your mind becomes scattered, and the rest of your body tenses up. In correct breathing, you inhale and exhale to about 70 percent or 80 percent of your maximum capacity, so that your lungs stay relaxed.

    You can conduct an easy experiment. Inhale deeply so that your lungs are completely full, and time how long you can hold your breath. Then try inhaling to only about 70 percent of your capacity, and see how long you can hold your breath. You will find that with the latter method you can last much longer than with the first one. This is simply because the lungs and the surrounding muscles are relaxed. When they are relaxed, the rest of your body and your mind can also relax, which decreases significantly your need for oxygen. Therefore, when you regulate your breathing, the first priority is to keep your lungs relaxed and calm.

4. **Long (Cháng, 長).** When you breathe, you should keep the breath as long as possible. However, you should remember that breathing long does not mean holding your breath. In order to breathe long, your lungs must be very relaxed and your meditative mind must have reached a deep level. In this case, your heartbeat will slow down, and you will require less oxygen. Only under these conditions can your breathing be long.

5. **Continuous (Yōu, 悠).** Your breathing must be smooth, natural, and most important of all, continuous. Unless it is for a specialized training, your breath should be continuous and without stagnation. When you stop or hold your breath, your body will tense. Continuous breathing will help you relax and lead you to a deeper meditative mind.

6. **Uniform (Yún, 勻).** Your breathing should be uniform. As we mentioned previously, your breathing is affected by your emotions. In order to attain uniformity in your breathing, you must regulate your emotional mind. Only this will allow you to keep your breath uniform and smooth.

7. **Slow (Huǎn, 緩).** Unless you are practicing a special training, your mind must be slowed down and you must take your time with your breathing. Take it easy and be natural. Do not rush your inhalation and exhalation.

8. **Soft (Mián, 綿).** When you breathe, your breathing should be easy and soft. Soft breathing makes you relaxed and leads you to a deeper meditative mind.

9-5. Six Stages of Regulating the Breath (Tiáoxí Liùjiē, 調息六階)

In Qìgōng society, there are six common words used in conjunction with regulating the breathing. They represent six stages in the practice. These words are:

1. **Count (Shǔ, 數).** Count means to count the breaths (Shǔxí, 數息). Counting is the first and most basic way to regulate the breathing. First, calm your mind and breath, following the eight keys to regulating explained above. Then, start to count your breaths slowly from one to ten and from ten to one. Alternatively, you may count only inhalations or exhalations. Paying attention to the counting keeps your mind from concentrating on your breathing and becoming tense. This helps you to lead your mind into a state of meditation. This is similar to the idea of counting sheep when you want to fall asleep.

2. **Follow (Suí, 隨).** Follow means to follow the breathing (Suíxí, 隨息). Once you can regulate your breathing with the counting method, you move on to this method. Be conscious of your breathing and follow the inhalation and exhalation. When you can do this without tensing up, your mind and breathing will unite and become one. The mind here means emotional mind, because it is the emotional mind which disturbs your calmness and peaceful thinking. It is said: "Xīnxī Xiāngyī" (心息相依), meaning "Heart (mind) and breathing (are) mutually dependent." When your mind is able to follow the breathing, the mind will enter a deeper meditative state and the breathing will slow down further. Following is an important technique in using the breathing and mind to help each other enter the deeper states of meditation.

3. **Stop (Zhǐ, 止).** Stop means to stop thinking about your breathing (Zhǐxí, 止息). An ancient Daoist named Lǐ, Qīng-Ān (李清庵) said: "Regulating breathing means to regulate the breathing until (you) stop."[18] This means that correct regulating means not having to consciously regulate. In other words, although you start by regulating your breath consciously, you must get to the point where the regulation happens naturally, and you no longer have to think about it. When you breathe, if you concentrate your mind on breathing, it is not true regulating, because the Qì in your lungs will become stagnant. When you reach the level of true regulating, no regulating is necessary, and you can use your mind efficiently to lead the Qì. Remember wherever the Yì is, there is Qì. If the Yì stops in one spot, the Qì will be stagnant. It

---

18. 調息要調無息息。

is the Yì which leads the Qì and makes it move. Therefore, when you are in a state of correct breath regulation, your mind is free. There is no sound, stagnation, urgency, or hesitation, and you can be calm and peaceful. When you reach this stage, you have obtained the real key to meditation.

4. **Look (Guān, 觀).** Look means to feel and to sense the breathing (Guānxí, 觀息). It is also commonly called Tīngxí (聽息), or "listening to the breathing." The words looking and listening here do not mean actually looking with your eyes and listening with your ears. They refer to using your mind to feel and sense what is happening. In meditation this is called Nèishì Fǎntīng (內視反聽), meaning "to see internally and to listen inwardly." Therefore, in Qìgōng meditation you do not pay attention to anything outside of your body. You use your mind to feel and sense (look and listen) internally. When you have reached the stage of regulating the breathing without regulating, your mind will be free. Then you are able to concentrate your mind on the movement of the Qì, and you may lead the Qì wherever you wish. You will be able to lead the Qì to every cell of your body and feel that your body is transparent.

5. **Return (Fǎn, 返).** Fǎnxí (return breathing, 返息) means to return your breathing to its natural way. That also implies that in this stage you will have reached the level of regulating the breathing without regulating. That means when you have mastered this stage you will have not only returned your breathing to the natural way, but have also reached the stage where your breathing combines with your mind and they become one. The breathing reflects the mind, and the mind reflects the breathing. Your breathing is now automatically regulated, and you no longer have to pay conscious attention to it, and your mind now regulates itself.

Regulating your mind requires that you understand the way (Dao) that Nature works. Your mind is now free and able to enter into a deep meditative state, and you can see beneath the surface of things and events and understand their real nature. The first step to this is understanding yourself. You need to comprehend the meaning of life. Breathing is the sign of life, and the dividing line of Yīn and Yáng. When you understand your breathing, you understand your life. This involves moving in your understanding from the poles of extreme Yīn and extreme Yáng to the middle, where all the fine gradations and shadings of existence are. When your mind is able to stay at the center, you are able to judge neutrally and see clearly. The two poles of Yīn and Yáng return back to their origin—"Wújí" (No Extremities, 無極). Natural breathing lets your mind be clear, so you can look at yourself and search out the real you. Only after you understand yourself are you able to understand real nature or the real "Dao."

Everything has its origin. In order to understand real nature, you must trace back to its origin. Fǎnxí is the process of returning yourself to your origin. This is a necessary step to becoming a "Buddha" or reaching "enlightenment." It is said: "Jiànxìng Liǎorán" (見性了然), which means "to see Nature and understand what it really is." When you have reached this stage, you have passed the stage of regulating your physical body and may concentrate on spiritual matters.

6. **Clean (Jìng, 淨).** "Clean" means "regulated," so in this method you use natural breathing to regulate your thoughts (Jìngxí, 淨息), although the term also refers to the stage when the breathing and the mind become one and the mind is regulated. Once you understand the real you and the real nature that lie beneath the surface appearances, you will use this breathing to regulate your mind into a state where you are free of emotions. Only then will you be able to reach the higher stages of spiritual cultivation. This cleaning process for the emotional mind is the final stage of religious Qìgōng. According to Buddhism, in order to become a Buddha, you must get rid of the seven emotions and six desires. Once you have reached this stage, your body is clean and your spirit is pure. When your mind and spirit has reached this stage, it is called "Jìng" (clean).

To conclude this subject, and hopefully to stimulate you to further thought, I would like to introduce more poetry related to regulating the breath. You should always remember that breath training gives you techniques and strategies which enable you to regulate your body and mind in Qìgōng practice. By regulating the body, mind, and breathing, you will be able to regulate your Qì and lead it smoothly and naturally. Qì and breathing are mutually related and cannot be separated. This idea is explained frequently in Daoist literature. The Daoist Guǎngchéngzi (廣成子) said: "One exhale, the Earth Qì rises; one inhale, the Heaven Qì descends; real man's (meaning one who has attained the real Dao) repeated breathing at the navel, then my real Qì is naturally connected."[19] This says that your abdomen should be the center of your breathing, almost as if you were breathing through your navel. The earth Qì is the negative (Yīn) energy from your kidneys, and the sky Qì is the positive (Yáng) energy which comes from the food you eat and the air you breathe. When you breathe from the navel, these two Qì's are able to connect and combine. Some people think that they know what Qì is, but they really don't. Once you connect the two Qì's, you will know what the "real" Qì is, and you may become a "real" man, which means one who has attained the Dao.

The Daoist book *Chàngdào Zhēnyán* (*Sing (of the) Dào (with) Real Words*, 唱道真言) says: "One exhale one inhale to communicate Qì's function, one movement one calmness is the same as (is the source of) creation and variation."[20] The first part of this statement implies again that the functioning of Qì is connected to breathing. The second part means that all creation and variation come from the interaction of movement (Yáng) and calmness (Yīn).

---

19. 廣成子曰：〝一呼則地氣上升，一吸則天氣下降，人之反覆呼吸於蒂，則我之真氣自然相接。〞
20. 唱道真言曰：〝一呼一吸通乎氣機，一動一靜同乎造化。〞

Huángtíngjīng (*Yellow Yard Classic*, 黃庭經) says: "Breathe Original Qì to seek immortality."[21] This means that in order to reach the goal of immortality, you must find and understand Original Qì, by means of correct breathing.

Moreover, the Daoist Wǔzhēnrén (伍真人) said: "Use post-birth breathing to look for the real person's (i.e., the immortal's) breathing place."[22] In this sentence, it is clear that in order to locate the immortal breathing place (the Dāntián), you must rely on and know how to regulate your Post-birth, or natural, breathing. Through regulating your Post-birth breathing, you will gradually be able to locate the residence of the Qì (the Dāntián), and eventually you will be able to use your Dāntián to breath like the immortal Daoists.

Finally, in the Daoist song "Língyuán Dàdàogē" ("The Great Daoist Song of the Spirit's Origin," 靈源大道歌) it is said: "The Originals (Original Jīng, Qì, and Shén) are internally transported peacefully, so that you can become real (immortal); (if you) depend (only) on external breathing (you) will not reach the end (goal)."[23] From this song, you can see that internal breathing (breathing at the Dāntián) is the key to training your three treasures and finally reaching immortality. However, you must first know how to regulate your external breathing correctly.

---

21. 黃庭經曰：〝呼吸元氣以求仙。〞
22. 伍真人曰：〝用後天之呼吸，尋真人呼吸處。〞
23. 靈源大道歌：〝元和內運即成真，呼吸外求終未了。〞

CHAPTER 10

Regulating the Emotional Mind

10-1. INTRODUCTION (JIÈSHÀO, 介紹)

The Daoists say: "(When) large Dao is taught, first stop thought; when thought is not stopped, (the lessons are) in vain."[1] This means that when you first practice Qìgōng, the most difficult training is to stop your thinking. The final goal for your mind is the "thought of no thought" (Wúniàn Zhīniàn, 無念之念). Your mind does not think of the past, the present, or the future, so you are independent of their influences. Your mind can be calm and steady, and you can gain peace. Only when you are in the state of "the thought of no thought" will you be relaxed and able to sense calmly and accurately.

You can see that regulating your mind is probably the second key to successful Qìgōng training. Regulating the mind is called "Tiáoxīn" (調心), which means "to regulate the (emotional) mind." In the third chapter we discussed the differences between the emotional mind (Xīn) and the wisdom mind (Yì). Before we discuss how to regulate your emotional mind, we would like to summarize the differences between Xīn and Yì.

1. Yì is the mind that is related to your wisdom and correct judgment. Yì is generated from clear thinking and is calm, peaceful, and clear. Xīn is the mind which expresses your feelings, emotions, and desires. Xīn can be excited, energized, and confused. When Xīn and Yì work together, your inner humanity and personality will be manifested.
2. Yì is considered the "Water Mind" and is nourished with the "Water Qì" (Original Qì) generated from Yuánjīng (Original Essence), while the Xīn is considered the "Fire Mind" and is nourished with "Fire Qì" converted from the food and air essences.

In Qìgōng training, regulating your mind means using your wisdom mind (Yì) to regulate your emotional mind (Xīn). After the emotional mind is under the control of wisdom

---

1. 大道教人先止念，念頭不住亦徒然。

mind, you will be calm and peaceful. Yì is the master of the Xīn. After your Yì has control of your Xīn, you will be able to regulate your Yì into a deeper meditative level and finally reach the stage of the "thought of no thought." This mind regulating practice is called Qínyuán Zhuōmǎ (擒猿捉馬), which means "Seize the ape and catch the horse." The ape represents the Xīn and the horse represents the Yì. Xīn, the emotional mind, is like an ape which is always running around. You have to put it on a leash and train it so that, although it is still emotional and excitable, it is now under your control. The Yì is like a horse which is strong and very useful, but which still has to be trained and harnessed before it can be used. Once the horse is tamed and trained, it can be calm, steady, and peaceful.

The Daoist Chóngyángzǔ (重陽祖) said: "Sleepy, then seize the ape and catch the horse, when you waken, again pluck 'Língzhī,' repeat the practice hundreds of days, only your heart (Xīn) knows. Conserve your real Qì, hide (it) at the Dāntián, the human will not die."[2] This saying means that if you feel sleepy while you are meditating, you should seize your Xīn (emotional mind) and catch the Yì (wisdom mind). The emotional mind makes you feel tired and sleepy. You should take control of your Yì and Xīn and wake yourself up by raising your spirit and keeping it at the center. Língzhī (*Fomes Japonica*, 靈芝) is a hard, dark brownish fungus which is supposed to possess supernatural powers. Here, Língzhī means the elixir which enables you to have a long life.

Once you have reached the stage of "no thought," your mind is clear enough to sense things accurately. You have to be able to sense things clearly inside your own body before you can direct the circulation of Qì and nourish your Shén. If your emotional mind (Xīn) is properly regulated, you can use it to sense what is going on inside you, and use your Yì to evaluate and correct the situation.

One of the most common processes of regulating the mind, which is especially popular with scholars, was originated by Confucius (Kǒngzǐ, 孔子). He said: "First you must be calm, then your mind can be steady. Once your mind is steady, then you are at peace. Only when you are at peace are you able to think and finally gain."[3] This procedure can also be applied to non-scholar meditation or Qìgōng exercises: First Calm, then Steady, Peace, Think, and finally Gain. So, when you practice Qìgōng, you must first learn to be emotionally calm. Once calm, you will be able to see what you want and firm your mind (steady). This firm and steady mind is your intention or Yì (it is how your Yì is generated). Only after you know what you really want will your mind gain peace and be able to relax emotionally and physically. After you have reached this stage, you must concentrate or think in order to execute your intention. When your mind is thoughtful and concentrated, your Qì will flow and you will be able to gain what you wish.

In this chapter we will first discuss the concepts of Xīn (emotional mind) and Niàn (thought). Once you understand these two concepts you will be able to learn how to control

---

2.　重陽祖日：“睡則擒猿捉馬，醒來復採瓊芝，每依時百日，只許心知，惜真氣，藏丹田，其人不死。”

3.　孔子日：“先靜爾后有定，定爾后能安，安爾后能慮，慮爾后能得。”

them and finally reach the goal of regulating the mind. One of the main purposes of regulating your mind is so that you can use it to lead or regulate the Qì. Therefore, we should review the relationship of Yì and Qì. Then we will discuss the concept of regulating the Qì in your organs. Finally, we will explain the relationship between Xīn, Yì, and Shén.

10-2. XīN, Yì, AND NiàN (XīN, Yì, NiàN, 心、意、念)

As discussed before, there are two concepts in Chinese which are both translated "mind." One is the emotional mind (Xīn, 心), and the other is the wisdom mind (Yì, 意). Both of these minds originate (generate) ideas. Most of these ideas last only a short time, and do not remain in your consciousness. However, many others remain, residing in your brain and affecting your thinking. When this happens, the idea generated from Xīn or Yì is matured, and become a "thought." A thought will continue to affect your thinking and decision-making, and oftentimes disturb your emotions. This matured thought is called Niàn (念) in Chinese. The Chinese frequently combine the two (idea and thought) and use the term "Xīnniàn" (心念) (emotional mind-thought) to distinguish the thoughts generated by Xīn from those generated by the wisdom mind, which would be called Yìniàn (wisdom mind-thought, 意念).

For example, when you hear something sad which upsets you, your emotional mind (Xīn) has grasped an idea which causes an emotional reaction in it. If this state of mind persists and continues to upset you emotionally, it has become a thought and is "Niàn" instead of "Xīn." When you see a beautiful car and wish you owned it, this idea is called "Xīn." If this idea continues to bother you, then it is "Niàn." Xīn is the cause of thought, and thought is the product of Xīn.

The Yì is also able to generate thoughts. They are usually calm, wise thoughts which do not disturb you emotionally or mentally. However, what usually happens with most people is that the idea which the Yì has generated is taken over by the Xīn. For example, from your Yì, you know you should get up at six o'clock in the morning for Qìgōng practice. This idea is an Yì. However, when morning comes around, your emotional laziness has conquered the idea which was originally generated from Yì, and you decide to turn over and go back to sleep. In this case, the new idea (of laziness) is generated from Xīn. Once you finally get up, you feel guilty and sorry for yourself. If this emotional, conscious feeling persists, then it is a "thought" (Xīnniàn).

In Qìgōng, thoughts which originate with the emotional mind (Xīn) are classified as fire thoughts, because they are able to disturb or raise your emotional feelings, while the thoughts which originated with the Yì are classified as water thoughts, because they can cool down your emotions. Generally speaking, in Qìgōng practice it is the emotional mind and thoughts which disturb and slow down your cultivation. Therefore, when regulating the mind is mentioned in Qìgōng society, they usually mean regulating the Xīn (emotional mind) and the thoughts it generates.

Regulating your Xīn means to cut down on the amount of ideas generated from your emotional feelings, and to disperse thoughts (Niàn) which formed from Xīn concerning the past, present, and future. If you want to stop thoughts from being produced, you must find the source of the Xīn and the Niàn. Only when you have traced them to their source will you be able to stop your thoughts at their root.

Buddhists believe that emotional feelings are generated by attachment to the seven emotions and the six sensory pleasures (Qīqíng Liùyù, 七情六慾). The seven emotions are: happiness, anger, sorrow, joy, love, hate, and desire; and the six sensory pleasures are the pleasures derived from the eyes, ears, nose, tongue, body, and mind.

The Buddhists believe that all human suffering comes from these roots. In order to be emotionally neutral and become a Buddha, you must first cultivate your Xīn and become detached from all emotional roots. They are aiming for the state of the "Four Emptinesses" (Sìdà Jiēkōng, 四大皆空), which means that the four elements (earth, water, fire, and air) are absent from the mind and one is indifferent to worldly temptations.

The first step toward reaching this goal of regulating the Xīn is "Guānxín" (觀心), which means "inspect or look at (your) Xīn." In other words, you must first investigate yourself, and come to understand yourself. Therefore you must first withdraw all of your attention from the outside world, and concentrate it wholly on your inner world. This training is called Nèishì Gōngfū (內視功夫), which means "the Gōngfū of internal vision."

After you have found the roots of your emotional disturbance, you will start to regulate your Xīn. Regulating your Xīn involves using your Yì and conscious feeling to stop the activity in your Xīn, setting it free from the bondage of ideas, emotions, and conscious thoughts. When you reach this level, your mind will be calm, peaceful, empty, and light.

Naturally, most Qìgōng practitioners are not aiming at the goal of enlightenment or Buddhahood. Their major priorities are health, happiness, and longevity. Buddhist monks will generally retreat into the mountains and separate themselves from the normal human world to avoid emotional disturbance during their cultivation. As a general Qìgōng practitioner, you are aiming to regulate your Xīn with your Yì. You do not want to get rid of your emotional mind, but you want it to be controlled by your Yì. Through this training, you will be able to put your mind in neutral when necessary and attain your goal of a calm and peaceful life.

In Qìgōng practice, only if your mind has reached the stage of real calmness and peace will you be able to relax deep into your marrow and internal organs. Then your mind will be clear enough to see (feel) the internal Qì circulation, and communicate with your Qì and organs. Finally, your Yì will be able to regulate your Qì and lead it to a state of balance.

Although this theory is simple and easy to understand, in practice it is very difficult to regulate your mind. In the last several thousand years, meditators have developed several ways of doing it. In the next section we will list some of them for your reference.

10-3. Methods of Stopping Thought (Zhǐniànfǎ, 止念法)

Before you start, you should understand that there are no techniques which are absolutely effective for everybody. It depends on the individual. It may also depend on the situation and timing. Remember that the final goal of regulating your thoughts is to reach "the thought of no thought." In other words, to regulate your thoughts without thinking of regulating. Therefore, you must continue practicing until the regulating happens naturally and you do not need to consciously regulate your thoughts. Only when you reach this stage will your mind be free and neutral.

Stop and Look Method (Zhǐguānfǎ, 止觀法)

"Zhǐ" means "to stop" and "Guān" means "to look after," "to investigate," and "to take care of." This means that after your Yì has controlled your Xīn, you should concentrate on watching the thoughts as they appear. When one comes, you should stop it immediately, not allowing it to grow. You should keep your consciousness aware of what is happening and use your Yì to stop each new thought. This process is called Zhǐniànfǎ ("stopping thought method," 止念法).

You will often find that, once you have stopped one thought, another one appears immediately. You stop that one, but another one pops up as if there is no end to the cycle. In order to stop this negative cycle, you must wait until your mind is clear, calm, and peaceful, and then put your Yì there before any more thoughts come up from the Xīn. If you can keep your mind in this neutral state, further thoughts will be stopped. The following are methods commonly used by meditators to stop the new thoughts from appearing.

Generally, there are three steps to stopping the Xīn and Niàn:

1. **Tie to the Origin and Stop Method (Xìyuánzhǐ, 繫緣止).** "Xì" means "to tie," "to bind," "Yuán" means "relationship, origin, and cause," and "Zhǐ" means "to stop." In this training you bind your Xīn and Niàn to one place in the same way that you would tie an ape to a post. If you can keep your Yì centered in a particular spot, you can control your Xīn and Niàn, but if your Yì is weak, your Xīn and Niàn will run wild.

   There are two places which are commonly used to center your Yì. The first place is your nose. Place your Yì on your nose and pay attention to your breathing. Gradually, the generation of new Xīn and Niàn will stop. The second common place is the Lower Dāntián. Concentrate your Yì at the Dāntián and feel and sense the generation and movement of Qì. Gradually your Xīn and Niàn will become quiet.

2. **Restrain the Xīn and Stop Method (Zhìxīnzhǐ, 制心止).** Once you have tied up the ape, you still have to calm it down, or it will continue to run around the post. This is the taming process. Once you are able to bind your Xīn and Niàn in one place, you must stop the thoughts from being generated by the Xīn. You need to understand the reason why the ape is still running wild, whether it is due to hunger

or some disturbance, and you need to understand why your Xīn is still generating distracting thoughts. If you are taming an ape, in order to keep the ape in the cage without running wild, you must understand the feelings of the ape and try to solve the problem in order to calm it down. Once the ape realizes that he will not be able to escape and will not be harmed, and furthermore, that he will be taken good care of by the master, he will gradually get used to it and calm down.

3. **To Comprehend the Real and Stop Method (Tǐzhēnzhǐ, 體真止).** This is the last step in stopping thought. In this step you analyze how Xīn and Niàn are being continually generated. Like dealing with an ape, once you understand the cause of its wildness, you can determine how to calm it down. Only after you have calmed it down are you able to lead the Xīn to understand and comprehend the nature of reality. Finally, the new disturbances of your Xīn will be stopped. It is like educating the ape so that he understands that when he is staying with the master, he will have plenty of food and a nice place to stay. At this point you will not need to keep the ape tied up. Only when you are able to untie the ape (your mind) and have it stay calm and peaceful have you reached real regulation. Then the Xīn and Niàn which are generated will not run wild, and the Yì will be able to direct them effortlessly.

There are also three ways of looking at or investigating your thoughts. They are called "The Three Looks" (Sānguān, 三觀). When your mind is calm and peaceful, pay attention to your thoughts and learn how to analyze them.

1. **The Empty Look (Kōngguān, 空觀).** When you use the Empty Look you look at and investigate everything in this universe: how it is generated, and how it grows, changes, and finally dies. As you look at things, you discover why they happen and what their causes are, and you learn the effects they cause. Everything that happens is ultimately empty. Your experiences are vain, illusory, they gain you nothing but a feeling which is false and temporary in comparison with the existence of the universe. When your Xīn understands this principle, it will not continue to think. Buddhists believe that all motivations and desires generated from the emotional mind do not last long, and ultimately accomplish nothing. If you can see this, you will be able to stop the generation of new Xīn and Niàn.

2. **The False Look (Jiǎguān, 假觀).** "Jiǎ" in Chinese means "false, imaginary, not real." In this method, when you find yourself in a bad situation, perhaps stuck in traffic, you look into the past to see how the traffic jam may have come about, and you look into the future to see how it will surely clear up. You look into the past and future to help you control your Xīn in the present. However, since the past and future are not the now, they are false. In this method, you are looking at false things and using them to help yourself let go of unsettling feelings and control your Xīn.

3. **The Centered Look (Zhōngguān, 中觀).** After you have used the other two Looks and your Xīn comprehends the nature of emotional disturbances, you will have seen

through every emotional feeling and desire, and you will understand that they are all only temporary. Since your physical life is so short, you should not be bothered by empty emotional feelings. Once you have realized this, you will keep your attention on (look at) only the here and now. Your mind will now be centered and neutral. All of these Looks use your Yì to lead the Xīn to understand the truth about emotional feelings. Then Xīn will not bother the Yì again.

For example, if you are driving somewhere and suddenly get caught in a traffic jam, do you get upset? Most people would, but if you stop to think about it, what do you gain from getting upset? Will the jam disappear or will the cars start moving faster? What do you gain from getting upset, and what do you lose? If you understand all of this, you will see that there is no benefit derived from getting upset, and you will use the time more gainfully, perhaps by just enjoying the music on the radio. If you can do this, then your mind is centered and regulated.

The Behold and Think Method (Guānxiǎngfǎ, 觀想法)

"Guān" in Chinese means "to admire, to look up to, or to view someone or something" as an example. "Xiǎng" means "to imagine, to think, or to meditate." In this method, when you meditate to regulate your Xīn you hold an image or idea in your mind of a person, such as Buddha, or something, such as moonlight, which occupies your attention. If you concentrate on this image, your Xīn will be steady and calm, and, consequently, your mind will be regulated. The person or thing upon which you concentrate is the source of the power which encourages and enables you to conquer your emotional mind.

The Guānxiáng method is widely used by Buddhists. When Christians meditate on the image of Christ to lead their minds into a steady, calm state and finally regulate their minds, they too are using the Guānxiáng method. In Daoist and Buddhist meditations, a Buddha is usually used as an image, and a poem or verse written by the Buddha will be read to help the Xīn be steady and peaceful. People use other things as images too. Sometimes people will use the moon, because it is peaceful, gentle, and calm, and can help you to lead your mind into a deep meditative state.

The One Point Spiritual Enlightenment Method (Yīdiǎn Língmíngfǎ, 一點靈明法)

"Yīdiǎn" means "a point." "Líng" is "the supernatural part of the Shén." "Míng" means "enlightenment." In this technique you focus on the highest, most refined level of your Shén. You are looking to enlighten the supernatural Shén, or Líng, and focus it on a tiny point in your Upper Dāntián (i.e., the third eye). When you are doing this, your thought will have a target. This effort will regulate your Xīn and redirect it into a peaceful and calm state.

The Large Hand Stamp Method (Dàshǒuyìn, 大手印)

"Dàshǒuyìn" literally means the "Large Hand Stamp." Large Hand means the fingers, and Stamp means pressing the fingers together. The Large Hand Stamp meditation method originated with the Indian Buddhists, and was later widely adopted by the Tibetan

Buddhists. After a thousand years of study and practice, this method has become a major meditation technique in Tibetan Qìgōng practice.

In this practice, you press your fingers together in specific ways. The fingers of one hand may press fingers on the other hand, or on the same hand, or the fingers may be interlocked in certain ways. Your mind concentrates on where you are pressing, and at the same time your concentrated mind leads your Shén to a higher state.

Leading your Shén to a higher state is the key to success in regulating. When your Shén is raised, your Yì is strong and the Xīn will be controlled. Frequently people will generate a sound or else shout to awaken and raise the Shén and stop the generation of distracting thoughts. For example, when you meditate you may discover that your emotional mind bothers you and you cannot stop it. If you open your eyes and look fiercely and utter the sound "Hā" (哈), you will stop the emotional thought and lead yourself to a new stage of meditation.

Religious meditators will often regulate their minds by raising their Shén. Another method is to concentrate the Shén, rather than raise it. When the Shén is focused, the Yì will naturally also be focused, and the Xīn will be controlled. Often a gong is used to help the meditator focus his Yì and Shén.

10-4. Yì AND Qì (Yì Yǔ Qì, 意與氣)

All of the above discussion focused on how to regulate your Xīn. Once your Xīn is regulated, your mind will be peaceful and calm, and your Yì will be able to direct and regulate the Qì.

However, in order to regulate your Qì effectively, you must train your Yì. The first step in this process involves understanding how the Yì communicates with your Qì. Communicate means to feel, to sense, and to correspond to. Your Yì must be able to sense and feel the Qì flow, and understand how strong and smooth it is. In Tàijí Qìgōng it is said that your Yì must "listen" (Tīng, 聽) to your Qì and "understand" (Dǒng, 懂) it. "Listen" means to pay careful attention to what you sense and feel. The more you pay attention, the better you will be able to understand. It is important to understand that paying attention to your Qì does not mean that your Yì is right with the Qì. It means that your Yì is aware of what is going on with the Qì, but it does not directly interfere with it. Only when you understand what is going on with the Qì can you set up an effective strategy which allows you to accomplish your goals. In Qìgōng, when you want your Qì to do a certain thing, your mind (Yì) must first generate an idea. In other words, you form a clear idea or visualize what you want your Qì to do. When a general wants his troops to do something, he must first know where they are, and then communicate to them where he wants them to go. In the same way, when you want your Qì to do something, you must understand how and where your Qì presently is, and form a clear idea or image of where you want it to go.

Next, you should know how to direct your soldiers. In Qìgōng training it is said: "Use your Yì (mind) to lead your Qì" (Yǐyì Yǐnqì, 以意引氣). Notice the word lead. Qì behaves like water—it cannot be pushed, but it can be led or guided. When Qì is led, it will flow smoothly and without stagnation. When it is pushed, it will flood and enter the wrong paths. Since Qì follows wherever the Yì goes, you lead the Qì simply by placing your Yì wherever you want the Qì to go. For example, if you intend to lift an object, this intention is your Yì. Your Yì goes to the object, the Qì moves out into your arms, and the arms go to the object. The Yì moves upward and the Qì follows, and the arms lift the object. You should also remember: when the Yì is strong, the Qì is strong, and when the Yì is weak, the Qì is weak.

You can see that in order to regulate your Qì, you must first train your Yì. You have to learn to concentrate it more than you normally do in your everyday life. It also means that you must train your Yì to understand and lead the Qì in your body. Your Yì is like a general on a battlefield, and the Qì is like the soldiers. As a general, you must be calm and know what you are doing. You must know the condition of your soldiers and how they can be arranged for battle.

It is said: "Your Yì is on your refined spirit (i.e., Jīngshén or spirit of vitality, 精神), not on your Qì. Once your Yì is on your Qì, the Qì is stagnant."[4] When you want to walk from one spot to another, you must first mobilize your intention and direct it toward the goal, then your body will follow. The mind must always be ahead of the body. If your mind stays on your body, you will not be able to move. It is as if you are a general conducting a battle. Although you should be aware of the situation of the soldiers, your mind cannot be on the soldiers. Your mind should be on strategy and where you should move your troops. If your mind is only on where the soldiers are now, you will not be able to lead your army to victory.

10-5. Yì and the Five Organs (Yì Yǔ Wǔzàng, 意與五臟)

One of the final goals in Qìgōng health training is to regulate the Qì in your five Yīn organs. As mentioned several times, these five organs are the lungs, heart, kidneys, liver, and spleen. It is believed in Chinese Qìgōng society that these organs are the most vital organs and that they directly affect your health. If you want to have good health and slow down the degeneration of your body, you must regulate the Qì in these five organs so that it is neither too Yáng nor too Yīn. This process is called Wǔqì Cháoyuán (五氣朝元), or "The five Qì's toward their origins."

However, this is a very profound subject, and it is sometimes interpreted differently by Oriental physicians and by Qìgōng practitioners. In order to reach this target, your Yì must be able to sense the situation in these five organs. To do this, you must be able to relax deep into the organs, and then your Yì must be directed to a deep, sensitive level through meditation. If you are able to regulate your body and your Yì, you may be able to sense the different elements which make up your body: solid matter, liquids, gases, energy, and spirit. You may even be able to see or feel the different colors that are associated with the five organs—green (liver), white (lungs), black (kidneys), yellow (spleen), and red (heart). When understood

---

4.   意在精神，不在氣，在氣則滯。

properly, it can give you a method of analyzing the interrelationship of your organs, and help you devise ways to correct imbalances.

Another method of regulating the five organs involves using the principle of the five elements (Wǔxíng, 五行). Each of the five elements relates to one of the Yīn organs: Metal to the lungs, Fire to the heart, Water to the kidneys, Wood to the liver, and Earth to the spleen. The way the organs relate to one another is similar to how the elements relate to each other. You can use this concept to regulate your organs. For example, Metal (the lungs) can be used to adjust the heat of the Fire (the heart), because metal can take a large quantity of heat away from fire (and thus cool down the heart). When you feel uneasy or have heartburn (excess fire in the heart), you may use deep breathing to calm down the uneasy emotions or cool down the heartburn.

Naturally, it will take a lot of practice to reach this level. In the beginning, you should not have any ideas or intentions, because they will make it harder for your mind to relax and empty itself of thoughts. Once you are in a state of "no thought," place your Yì on your Dāntián. It is said "Yìshǒu Dāntián" (意守丹田), which means "The Yì is kept on the Dāntián." The Dāntián is the origin and residence of your Qì. Your mind can build up the Qì here (start the fire, Qǐhuǒ, 起火), then lead the Qì anywhere you wish, and, finally, lead the Qì back to its residence in the Dāntián. When your Yì is on the Dāntián, your Qì will always have a root. When you keep this root, your Qì will be strong and full, and it will go where you want it to. You can see that, when you practice Qìgōng, your mind cannot be completely empty and relaxed. You must find firmness within relaxation, then you can reach your goal.

10-6. XĪN, YÌ, AND SHÉN (XĪN, YÌ, SHÉN, 心、意、神)

In order to regulate your mind (Xīn and Yì) effectively, you must also know the relationship of your Xīn, Yì, and Shén. Xīn, Yì, and Shén are mutually related and cannot be separated. First, you should understand that in Qìgōng training your Yì is the origin of your being and the control tower, and Xīn is the energy source of your Shén. In order to raise your Shén, your Yì must first generate an idea of raising your Shén. From this idea, under the control of your Yì, your Xīn will raise the Shén to a higher energy state. For example, a common way of traiNíngshén is to image that the Upper Dāntián is on fire. This is the step of raising the Shén to an energized state. Then you use your Yì to lead or to focus the fire spreading around the Upper Dāntián to a tiny point. In this case, you have raised your Shén with your Xīn, yet controlled it with your Yì.

Although the Xīn is able to raise your Shén, it can also make you excited, which will lead your Shén away from its residence in the Upper Dāntián. For example, if you receive surprising news, you may become excited and your Shén may be raised. Usually, when this happens your Yì loses its control of the Xīn, and you lose your calmness and clear judgment. In Qìgōng practice, your goal is to raise your Shén as high as possible and still have it controlled at its center by your Yì (Figure 10-1). Many Qìgōng practitioners, especially monks, believe that once they have reached a high level of Qìgōng and can regulate their Xīn completely, they should be able to raise their Shén solely with their Yì, instead of with their Xīn.

You can see that when you regulate your Xīn and Yì you are regulating your Shén as well. There are many steps in using your Yì to regulate your Shén. They are: 1. Shǒushén (to keep and protect the Shén, 守神); 2. Gùshén (to firm and solidify the Shén, 固神); 3. Dìngshén (to stabilize and to calm the Shén, 定神); 4. Níngshén (to condense or to focus the Shén, 凝神); 5. Yǎngshén (to nourish, to raise, or to nurse the Shén, 養神); and 6. Liànshén (to refine, to train, or to discipline the Shén, 煉神). We have discussed these briefly in the third chapter, and we will cover them again when we discuss regulating the Shén.

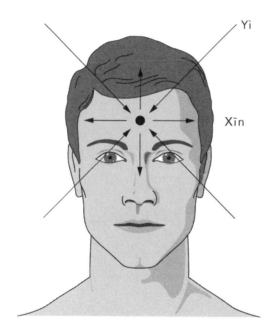

Figure 10-1. Use Yì to control Xīn at the Upper Dāntián

CHAPTER 11

Regulating the Essence

11-1. INTRODUCTION (JIÈSHÀO, 介紹)

Of the three roots—Jīng, Qì, and Shén—essence (Jīng) is probably the most important element in successful Qìgōng practice. To regulate your essence means to conserve it and convert it into Qì without any waste. You must learn how to keep your Original Essence in the kidneys, its residence, by strengthening the kidneys. You must also learn how to conserve the essence by not abusing it, and by learning how to convert it into Qì efficiently.

As mentioned, the essences which are converted into Qì can be classified as Fire Essence, which is obtained from food and air, and Water Essence, which you inherit from your parents. In order to reduce the Fire Qì, you must reduce the Fire Essence by taking in high quality food and air. There are many texts available which discuss this idea.

When Qìgōng practitioners refer to essence, they are usually referring to Original Essence, which is also called "Water Essence." It is usually of more importance in Qìgōng training than the Fire Essence. It is easy to regulate Fire Essence, but you need a lot of understanding and training to regulate the Water Essence.

As mentioned in the third chapter, Chinese medical society calls two pairs of your body's organs kidneys: your real kidneys (also called "the internal Kidneys"; Nèishèn, 內腎), and the testicles or ovaries (also referred to as the external kidneys; Wàishèn, 外腎). It is believed that after your birth, your Original Essence stays in your internal kidneys. The internal kidneys are closely related to the external kidneys. When the Original Essence in the kidneys is converted into Original Qì, part of it is used to nourish the external kidneys and enliven the production of sexual essence or hormones. Clearly, if your internal kidneys are weak and the Original Qì cannot be converted efficiently from the Original Essence, the production of hormones or essence by the testicles will also be reduced. Therefore, if you wish to regulate your essence, you must first learn how to regulate the Original Essence in the internal kidneys.

In Marrow/Brain Washing Qìgōng, the sexual essence is the main source that is converted into Qì to fill up the four Qì vessels (reservoirs) in your legs. It is also believed that part of this Qì is led through the Thrusting Vessel (Chōngmài, 衝脈) through the spinal cord to the brain to nourish it. When people get old and start to lose their sexual vitality, they often lose their memory and their legs become weak. This is simply because there is an insufficient amount of sexual essence to supply Qì to the brain and the four vessels in the legs. For this reason, the main task in Marrow/Brain Washing Qìgōng is to increase the production of sexual essence and convert it efficiently into Qì. If you are interested in knowing more about this subject, please refer to the book: *Qìgōng—The Secret of Youth*, from YMAA Publication Center. Here we will discuss regulating the essence in the internal kidneys.

11-2. STRENGTHENING YOUR KIDNEYS (QIÁNGSHÈN, 強腎)

In order to regulate your Original Essence, you must first take care of its residence, the kidneys, so that the essence will be protected. The first step to strengthening the kidneys is to keep them healthy. This is called Gùshèn (固腎), which means "to firm and to solidify the kidneys." To strengthen the kidneys is called Qiángshèn (強腎).

To Firm and to Strengthen the Kidneys (Gùshèn and Qiángshèn, 固腎，強腎)

Several thousand years of study and experimentation have yielded many ways to maintain the health of and strengthen the kidneys. All of them work by maintaining the Qì in the kidneys at the proper level. In order to do this you need to know how the kidneys are affected by weather, food, and emotions (Table 11-1).

Kidneys and the Weather

Your kidneys are Yīn organs. When the weather is cold, especially during the winter, the surrounding air is also Yīn, and the Qì level of the kidneys is diminished. When this happens, the Qì flow will be sluggish and the back will become sore and ache, especially the lower back. It is therefore important that the kidney area be protected so that Qì will not be lost out of your body. The best method is to wear warm clothes, especially around your waist. In addition, you should learn a few massage techniques to improve Qì circulation in the kidney area and to use the Qì in your hands to nourish the kidneys. We will now discuss a few massage techniques which are commonly used in Qìgōng.

Massaging the Kidneys Directly. This is the most common technique. Use the center of your palms to rub the back over the kidneys with a circular motion. The tops of both circles should move inward toward each other. There is a Qì gate or cavity called Láogōng (P-8) 勞宮) in the center of your palm (Figure 11-1). This cavity belongs to the Pericardium. The Pericardium includes the blood vessel which enters into the heart and the membranous sac which encloses the heart. In the Chinese medical theory of the five elements, the heart is classified as Fire and the kidneys are classified as Water.

Therefore, when you use the center of your palms to massage the kidneys, you are using fire to warm up the water, and are therefore nourishing the kidneys. When you massage the kidneys with a circular motion, the top of the motion should be inward (Figure 11-2) in order to nourish the kidneys. If you rub in the opposite direction, you are spreading the Qì away. When you rub the kidneys, you do not have to press heavily. Place your hands on the skin firmly and circle. In just a few minutes or so, you will feel the Qì inside near the kidneys circulating in the same direction. This means that you have improved the Qì circulation there. Naturally, you will be more relaxed and the massage will be more effective if someone

	WOOD 木	FIRE 火	EARTH 土	METAL 金	WATER 水
Direction	East	South	Center	West	North
Season	Spring	Summer	Long Summer	Autumn	Winter
Climactic Condition	Wind	Summer Heat	Dampness	Dryness	Cold
Process	Birth	Growth	Transformation	Harvest	Storage
Color	Green	Red	Yellow	White	Black
Taste	Sour	Bitter	Sweet	Pungent	Salty
Smell	Goatish	Burning	Fragrant	Rank	Rotten
Yin Organ	Liver	Heart	Spleen	Lungs	Kidneys
Yáng Organ	Gall Bladder	Small Intestine	Stomach	Large Intestine	Bladder
Opening	Eyes	Tongue	Mouth	Nose	Ears
Tissue	Sinews	Blood Vessels	Flesh	Skin/Hair	Bones
Emotion	Anger	Happiness	Pensiveness	Sadness	Fear
Human Sound	Shout	Laughter	Song	Weeping	Groan

Table 11-1. Table of Correspondences associated with the Five Phases

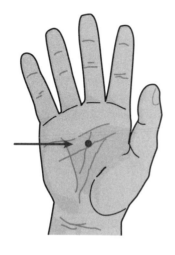

Figure 11-1. The Láogōng
cavity (P-8)

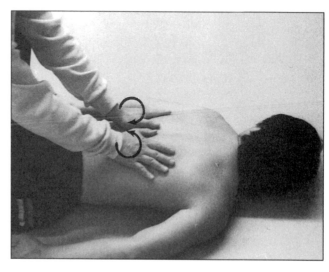

Figure 11-2. Massaging the kidneys

else can massage you. This direct massage is very effective and useful in winter time. Please remember that you should warm up your hands first; cold hands will drain Qì from the kidneys.

Massaging the Bubbling Wells. Massaging the Bubbling Well cavities (Yǒngquán, K-1, 湧泉) (Figure 11-3) is probably the second best techniques in nourishing the Qì and improving the Qì circulation around the kidneys. The Bubbling Well cavities belong to the Kidney Qì Channel. Usually the thumb is used to massage these two cavities with a circular motion (Figure 11-4). You may also use the center of your palm to rub the bottom of your feet (Figure 11-5). Alternatively, you may rub your palms against each other first until they are very warm, then place the centers of your palms (Láogōng cavities) on the top of the Bubbling Well cavities. In this case, you are using the Heart Fire to nourish the kidney water.

Massaging with Movement. Massaging the kidneys with movement is a common Wàidān Qìgōng practice, and is used in such exercises as the Eight Pieces of Brocade (Bāduànjǐn, 八段錦). The method is simple and very effective. Generally, there are two major movements which are able to massage the kidneys and improve the kidneys' Qì circulation. The first movement is bending forward (Figure 11-6). This stretches and tenses the two major sets of muscles on the sides of the spine, and presses down on the kidneys which are beneath them. You should stay there for about five seconds and then straighten your body. This releases the pressure on the kidneys and lets them return to their original state. Doing these movements repeatedly massages the kidneys.

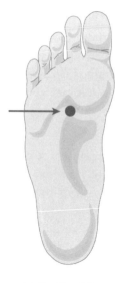

Figure 11-3. The Yŏngquán
cavity (K-1)

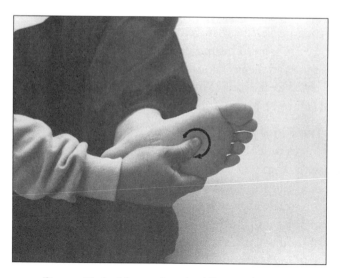

Figure 11-4. Massaging the Yŏngquán cavity
with the thumb

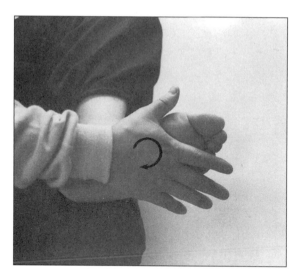

Figure 11-5. Massaging the Yŏngquán
cavity with the hand

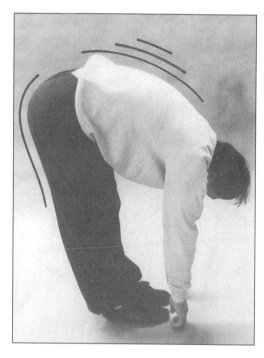

Figure 11-6. Bend forward to
massage the kidney

The second movement is twisting your upper body to the sides (Figure 11-7). Though the muscles are stretched differently than in the preceding exercise, the principle and effect are the same. This movement, in addition to massaging the kidneys, also loosens the entire spine and the back muscles, and increases Qì circulation in the Governing Qì Vessel (Dūmài, 督脈) in the back. You may also combine the last two movements to massage your kidneys (Figure 11-8).

The Kidneys and Food

In order to maintain your health and lengthen your life, you must always be concerned with what you eat. Everything you eat will be converted into Qì and nourish your body. According to Chinese medicine, too much acidic food can make your body too Yáng, and too much alkaline food can make it too Yīn. For example, eating too much acidic food will increase heartburn, and soft drinks will cool down the fire and body heat. Different kinds of food will place stress on different organs. For example, too much alcohol will increase the working load and stress on your liver.

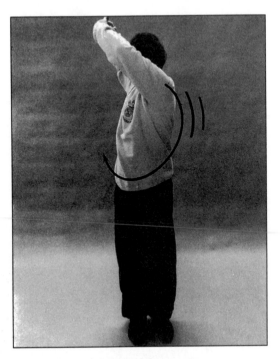

Figure 11-7. Twist sideways to massage the kidneys

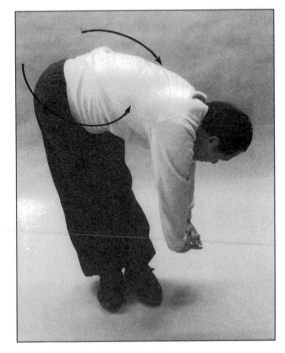

Figure 11-8. Twist and bend to massage the kidneys

There are also several foods which, when eaten to excess, will affect the condition of your kidneys. For example, too much salt will weaken your kidneys, so you should moderate the amount of salt you eat, especially as you get older. Experience has also shown that eating too much eggplant will weaken your kidneys. Ginseng is good for the kidneys in the wintertime, but it is not as good in the summer since you always have enough Qì to nourish the kidneys then. Many Chinese herbalists have studied and experimented with different prescriptions of herbs for different organs. We will leave this subject to a more qualified author.

The Kidneys and Emotions

From Table 11-1 you can also see that your emotions are closely related to the condition of your organs. In order to protect your kidneys, you should avoid fear. Fear originates in your mind. You should understand that fear will not solve any problems. You must face your problems and find the solutions. Once your mind is clear, you will know how to avoid situations which cause you fear. This is the process of regulating your mind, and is the way to maintain your kidneys in good condition.

11-3. REGULATING THE ESSENCE (TIÁOJĪNG, 調精)

The above discussion concentrated on how to protect the residence of your essence. Now we must discuss how to regulate the essence itself. To regulate the essence is to convert it into Qì in the most efficient way, and to conserve the use of the essence. This is a very broad subject, and it is difficult to say which is the best way to conserve your essence, since it depends on individual lifestyles and habits. However, we will discuss some of the most common methods which might give you a deeper understanding of regulating your essence.

Increasing the Efficiency of the Conversion of Essence into Qì

Abdominal Exercises. It is very important in Qìgōng training to know how to lead the Qì which was converted from Original Essence to its residence, the Lower Dāntián. The trick to this is abdominal exercises. When you move your lower abdomen in and out in coordination with your breathing, the muscles need more Qì than they normally do. The muscles therefore draw in both the Post-birth Qì which was converted from the essence of food and air, and the Pre-birth Qì which was converted from your Original Essence in the kidneys. The Qì which the muscles don't need is stored in the Dāntián for future use.

According to Chinese acupuncture, there are two cavities called Shènshū (Kidney Doors, B-23, 腎俞) or Jīngmén (Essence Doors, 精門) located on your back (Figure 11-9). They are the gates used to regulate the Qì level of the kidneys. Whenever the Qì level is too Yáng in the kidneys, Qì will leak out of your body through these two doors. Normally, when you are young, your essence is strong, fresh, and vigorous, and you have an abundant supply of Qì. Some of this Qì will leak out through these two gates and be wasted. One way to reduce this Qì leakage is to lead it to the front with abdominal exercises and store it in the Dāntián.

After you have practiced a lot of Qìgōng you will develop the ability to lead the Qì from the kidneys to the Lower Dāntián simply by thinking or meditating about it. At this time, the physical abdominal exercises will no longer be necessary.

Protecting the Essence Doors. Not only should you know how to lead Qì to the Dāntián, you should also know how to protect the Essence Doors, especially during the winter. As mentioned earlier, Chinese medicine classifies the kidneys as Yīn. In the winter the surrounding air is also Yīn, in fact it is more Yīn than the kidneys. Because of this, the Qì in the kidneys will leak out into the air. If you want to prevent this, you must dress warmly, and be especially careful to keep the kidney area warm. Often Qìgōng practitioners will massage the kidney doors to warm the kidneys and increase the conversion of Qì, and at the same time use abdominal exercises or concentration to lead the Qì forward to be stored in the Dāntián. You should remember that you will be strong and healthy only when your Dāntián and Qì reservoirs are full.

Massaging the Kidneys and the Bubbling Well Cavities. Massaging the kidneys and the Bubbling Well cavities improves and smoothes the Qì circulation in the kidneys, and keeps them functioning at high efficiency. It also improves the efficiency of the Jīng and Qì conversion. This has been covered in the previous section.

Marrow/Brain Washing Training. In Marrow/Brain Washing Qìgōng, the essence of the testicles or ovaries is converted into Qì. Although the testicles or ovaries are not the internal kidneys themselves, they are closely related to them. Normally, you may increase the Jīng to Qì conversion of the internal kidneys through Marrow/Brain Washing practices which work with the testicles and ovaries. Many techniques are used to stimulate the sexual organs and increase the production of essence. Once the essence is full, it is converted into Qì and used to fill up the Qì reservoirs in the legs. This Qì is then led up through the spinal cord to nourish the brain. This has been discussed in more detail in the second volume of the YMAA Qìgōng book series: *Qìgōng—The Secret of Youth*.

Conserving Your Essence (or Qì)

Conserving your essence means abusing neither it nor the Qì which was converted from it. If you waste an excessive amount of Qì, the Qì in your body will be deficient because the conversion process of essence into Qì is very slow. One of the most serious ways that a man can abuse his Qì and essence is through too much sexual activity. Too much sex drains Qì out of your Qì reservoirs and lowers the level of Qì in the whole body. Since essence must be converted into Qì to replace the loss, you also decrease your supply of essence.

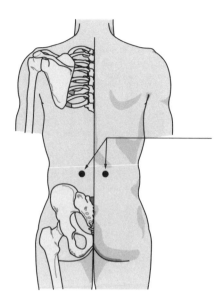

Figure 11-9. The Shènshū cavities

In Chinese medical science, it is believed that sperm is a product of the essence which is stored in the testicles (sperm is called "Jīngzǐ," which means "the sons of essence," 精子). Qì is required to produce sperm and hormones from your essence. After you have sex, it takes at least three days for the Qì nourishment of the groin to reach its normal level. This is why, in traditional training, it is urged that the practitioners not practice Qìgōng (especially Nèidān, which involves the lower abdominal area) for at least three to four days after sexual activity. After the Qì has recovered its normal level, conservatively speaking, it will take about one week for the normal male to replenish his supply of sperm essence. In ejaculation, Qì is drained out of the man's reservoirs, especially in the legs, and is passed into the woman's body. Roughly estimated, a man might lose about 40 percent of his Qì with one ejaculation, and if he has another ejaculation soon after, he will lose 40 percent of the remaining Qì. Naturally, this figure varies from person to person.

Women do not have to worry about losing Qì. As a matter of fact, they receive the man's Qì and use it to nourish their body. However, there are some Qìgōng techniques whereby the man retains his Qì and makes his body's Qì level lower than the woman's. In this case, the man is the one who benefits. There are a number of books available on Daoist sexual practices which can be consulted for further information.

CHAPTER 12

Regulating the Qì

12-1. Introduction (Jièshào, 介紹)

If you take a look at your whole being, you will see how your body is made up of a number of parts: 1. Physical body (including water); 2. Air (mainly oxygen); 3. Mind (Xīn and Yì); 4. Qì; and 5. Shén. All of these five elements are closely related and cannot be separated. Among these five, Qì is the energy which makes the other four function. Whenever the Qì flow is stagnant or stops, you will sicken and die. For this reason, one of the major goals of Qìgōng training is to regulate the Qì in your body. When Qì flows normally and smoothly, all the other elements will be well-nourished and will retain their normal, healthy condition, and you can expect to live a long time.

In Qìgōng practice, before you can regulate your Qì you must first regulate your body, breath, and mind. If you compare your body to a battlefield, then your mind is like the general who generates ideas and controls the situation, and your breathing is his strategy. Your Qì is like the soldiers who are led to various places on the battlefield. Your essence is like the qualitative background of your soldiers. For example, if your soldiers are well educated, highly disciplined, and strong of body, you will have a strong army. In addition to this, in order to win a battle, you and your soldiers must also have high morale. This morale is your Shén. All of these elements are necessary, and all must be coordinated with each other if you are to win the war against sickness and aging.

If you want to arrange your soldiers most effectively for battle, you must know which area of the battlefield is most important, and the points at which you are vulnerable (where your Qì is deficient) and need to send reinforcements. If you have more soldiers than you need in one area (excessive Qì), then you can send them somewhere else where the ranks are thin. As a general, you must also know how many soldiers are available for the battle, and how many you will need for protecting yourself and your headquarters. To be successful, not only do you need good strategy (breathing), but you also need to communicate effectively with your troops, or all of your strategy will be in vain. When your Yì (the general) knows how to regulate the body (knows the battlefield), how to regulate the breathing (set up the strategy), and how to effectively regulate the Qì (direct your soldiers), you will be able to reach the final goal of Qìgōng training.

12-2. WHAT QÌ SHOULD BE REGULATED? (SHÉNMEQÌ XŪYÀOTIÁO? 什麼氣 需要調?)

As discussed in the third chapter, Qì can be classified into many different categories according to their origins or according to the roles they play in the body. According to the origin of the Qì, the Qì can be identified as Pre-birth (or Original) Qì, or Post-birth Qì. Pre-birth Qì is converted from the Original Essence you inherited from your parents, while the Post-birth Qì is converted from the food and air you take in. The first step in regulating the quality of your Qì is regulating your essence, which was discussed in a previous chapter. The next step is regulating the Qì according to its function. From this point of view, you have both "Managing Qì" and "Guardian Qì."

Managing Qì (Yíngqì, 營氣)

Regulating the Qì in the Eight Vessels and Twelve Qì Channels. The first task in regulating the Managing Qì is to regulate the Qì supply to the twelve internal organs through the twelve primary Qì channels. In order to reach this goal, you must also learn to regulate the Qì in your eight Qì vessels. To continue with the battlefield analogy, the twelve internal organs are like a line of twelve forts, and your eight vessels are like the eight training camps behind the lines which supply soldiers to the front line. In the front line, if any one of the forts is lost, the others are placed in jeopardy, and the whole line may be lost. It is therefore important to keep the right number of troops in each fort so that the whole arrangement can function efficiently. Both quality and quantity are important in this.

Among these twelve forts are six which are considered positive (Yáng). These are the nourishing and absorbing systems, and handle the digestive and absorptive functions. These six Yáng organs are the Stomach, Large Intestine, Small Intestine, Urinary Bladder, Gall Bladder, and Triple Burner. The other six organs are considered negative (Yīn), and are responsible for storing the body's essence and maintaining life. These organs are the Lungs, Heart, Kidneys, Liver, Spleen, and Pericardium (although the Lungs absorb oxygen, Chinese medicine considers them to be one of the life managing organs).

Normally, the Yáng organs have more Qì than the Yīn organs. Five of the Yīn organs (excluding the Pericardium) are considered the most important organs, and determine whether you win or lose the battle for your health. They decide your life and death. You must regulate their Qì first. In Qìgōng it is said "Wǔqì Cháoyuán" (五氣朝元), which means to lead the "Five Qì's to their Origins." This means that in order to reach the goal of health, you must regulate the Qì in these five organs to its original levels. Only then will they function properly, and degeneration be kept to a minimum.

Nourishing the Brain and Shén with Qì. The second task in regulating the Managing Qì is regulating the Qì supply to the top of your head to nourish your brain and Shén. In Qìgōng practice, your brain and the Shén are considered to be the headquarters of your thinking and Qì. If you do not have the best personnel and facilities in your headquarters, it will not function well, and the whole body will be unhealthy. Your brain generates the Yì, which is like a general, and your Shén is like the morale which is able to raise the soldiers' fighting spirit. It is this Shén which enables the entire fighting unit to work and communicate in the most efficient way.

In Marrow/Brain Washing Qìgōng, it is believed that the brain and the Shén are the most important factors in maintaining health and lengthening life. If you are able to nourish your brain and Shén with Qì constantly, you will be able to direct your Qì to regulate the entire body, and will have won most of the battle.

Guardian Qì (Wèiqì, 衛氣). Regulating the Guardian Qì is different from regulating the Qì which circulates in the twelve channels and the Qì which nourishes the brain. When you regulate your Guardian Qì, you are regulating the Qì out from the Qì channels to the surface of the skin. This means you lead the Qì outward to the surface of your skin and inward to the bones.

The function of your Guardian Qì is to generate a Qì shield around you to prevent any negative influences from invading your body. The size of your Qì shield is adjusted according to the weather and the environment around you. If you are able to keep this Qì shield strong, the Qì will smoothly reach out to your hair and beyond, and your hair and skin will stay healthy.

The Qì should also be led inside so that it penetrates even the bone marrow. The marrow manufactures blood cells. When your marrow has plenty of Qì, it will produce fresh and healthy blood cells which will keep your whole body functioning optimally and protect it internally.

12-3. REGULATING THE Qì (Tiáoqì, 調氣)

Regulating the Qì is one of the main goals of Qìgōng training. Regulating includes adjusting, protecting, keeping, and raising. You can see that the definition of regulating the Qì is very wide and the purposes are varied. Many Qìgōng styles have been created and developed to reach the different goals of Qì cultivation. To scholars, regulating means keeping and protecting the Qì circulation in the body. To medical doctors, regulating means adjusting and correcting the Qì level. To martial artists, regulating means concentrating, and leading the Qì to energize the muscles more efficiently. To Buddhists, regulating means protecting, nourishing, and cultivating. To Daoists, regulating means building up, raising, training, and disciplining.

Although when you practice one category of Qìgōng you also cover some of the training done by other categories, the emphasis is different. For example, if you learn to regulate the Qì from a medical Qìgōng style, although you also reach the goal of maintaining health and training to build up your Qì, you will be using methods designed mainly for curing illnesses. Therefore, in order to learn how to regulate Qì, you should know what your goal is, and how deeply you would like to enter. Then, you will be able to decide which category you want to learn.

Nobody knows your body and its inner workings better than you do. After all, you live in it, and you are the only one who is able to feel it directly. Therefore, you are the one who is best qualified to judge which Qìgōng style is the most beneficial for you. If you are a Qìgōng beginner, I suggest that you start with one of the easier systems developed by scholars and medical doctors, such as the "Eight Pieces of Brocade" or "Five Animal Sports." They are easier to understand, learn, and experience without incurring any potential of serious danger. Training in these systems will teach you the "why," "what," and "how." For example, by studying scholarly Qìgōng you may grasp the idea of regulating the mind, and from practicing medical Qìgōng you may come to understand more clearly how to regulate your body. It does not matter which Qìgōng style you have decided to train deeply. Before you regulate your Qì, you must always regulate your body, breathing, and mind. Once you have gained the experience and understood the theory, you will be able to understand the deeper martial or religious Qìgōng such as "Small Circulation," "Grand Circulation," or "Marrow/Brain Washing Qìgōng" more easily.

In this section, I believe that we should first discuss two major subjects before going on to the general concepts of regulating the Qì. These two subjects are: A. The communication between your Yì and Qì; and B. Two general attitudes toward regulating the Qì.

Communication Between Yì and Qì. Learning how to open communications between your Yì and Qì is probably the most crucial factor in successful Qìgōng training. There are two ways that Qì flows in your body. One of them is the natural, automatic circulation which is responsible for the internal functioning of the body. This circulation does not need your conscious attention. For example, you do not need your Yì to lead the Qì to the organs to keep them functioning. This happens naturally and automatically. However, if you desire to lift an object, first your Yì must generate the idea of lifting, and this idea or intention will lead Qì to the arms to energize the muscles. You understand already that the muscles do not function without Qì, any more than an electric fan will run without electric current.

Regardless of which purpose a Qìgōng practitioner is training for, first he must learn how to increase the communication between his Yì and Qì. Communication means not only that your Yì is leading the Qì—your Yì must also feel or sense what is going on with the Qì. This mutual interaction allows you to understand the Qì situation. It is commonly said in internal arts society that "First, you must listen carefully, then you will be able to understand." "Listen" here means to "feel" or to "sense." Only if your Yì is able to communicate and understand the situation, will you be able to regulate the Qì. It is just like in a battle; the general in his headquarters must be able to communicate efficiently with his soldiers, otherwise he will not be able to apply his strategy.

In Qìgōng, in order for your Yì to communicate with your Qì, you must first regulate your body, your breathing, and your mind. These three prerequisites are the major paths to regulating your Qì. After you have regulated these three elements, the communication between your mind and Qì will happen automatically and naturally. At first, your mind is able to feel or even sense the Qì flow. After you have been doing this for a while, you start to understand the Qì. It is as if you are learning a new language. The more you practice and experience it, the more you will be familiar with it and understand it. Only then is your mind able to direct and lead it.

Two Attitudes toward Regulating the Qì. In order to regulate your Qì so that it moves smoothly and in the correct paths, you need more than just efficient Yì-Qì communication. You also need to know how to generate Qì. If you do not have enough Qì in your body, how can you regulate it? In a battle, if you do not have enough soldiers to carry out your strategy, you have already lost.

In Chinese Qìgōng society, there are two major attitudes in regulating the Qì. Both of them have their own theories, disadvantages, and advantages. From these two different viewpoints were developed two major approaches to regulating the Qì. One is called Yǎngqì (養氣) and the other is called Liànqì (煉氣). Yǎng means to gradually raise, nourish, keep, and protect; while Liàn means to refine, train, build, and strengthen. According to analysis of the available documents, it seems that the Scholars and the Buddhists favor Yǎng Qì, with the Buddhists becoming the authorities in both theory and training, while the Daoists and martial artists train more Liàn Qì which, in regard to health, is considered more advanced. It is not surprising that medical Qìgōng exercises include both, and vary according to training purposes.

In practicing regulating the Qì, it is crucial to increase the quantity of Qì while maintaining a neutral state in the body. As you know, excess (Yáng) or deficient (Yīn) Qì will cause health problems and speed up aging. It is important, therefore, to learn how to fill up the Qì reservoirs (eight Qì vessels) without letting this abundant Qì overflow into the twelve Qì channels. In the Yǎng Qì training, the scholars and Buddhists practice the ways of nursing and protecting the Qì first. Then they learn to gradually raise or cultivate the Qì to a healthier level. This gentle and conservative method is meant to maintain a healthy Qì flow without significantly affecting the Qì level and the natural circulation. This training is especially important when the practitioners are getting old and the Qì level in the reservoirs is lower.

In Liàn Qì training, the Daoists work on training and refining their Qì, and also on strengthening or increasing the Qì level in the Qì reservoirs. Daoist Qìgōng practitioners believe that in order to obtain the goal of longevity, not only must you maintain smooth Qì flow, but you must also increase the Qì level to strengthen the physical organs. They believe that the quality and strength of your physical body can be improved by nourishing the Qì correctly.

Your body is like an electrically powered machine in that it needs current to run, and if you continually run an inadequate current through it, it will deteriorate quickly. However, your body is different from a machine in that if you gradually increase the amount of current, your body will adjust to the current, and will become stronger and start to function better. It is just like if you are able to run five miles a day and do so on a regular basis, you will maintain your health and a certain amount of strength. This is the scholarly and Buddhist way. However, if you gradually increase the distance as time goes on, your body will readjust itself to fit the new requirement, and your conditioning will improve. This is the Daoist way.

You can see that the Scholarly and Buddhist way is gentle and more conservative, while the Daoist way is more active. Sometimes the Daoist training methods are more difficult and dangerous than those of the Buddhists. They always need to keep track of what is happening in their physical bodies as they train, and be careful that the Qì they have built up is not mishandled and does not move the wrong way.

Beginners in Qìgōng should first learn how to keep their Qì flowing smoothly. Only after you understand yourself and Qìgōng theory should you start training gradually to refine and train your Qì to a higher level. This normally takes at least ten years of correct practice under the instruction of a qualified master.

How to Regulate the Qì

Every Qìgōng style has its own unique methods for regulating the Qì. Because regulating the Qì is one of the final goals of Qìgōng, methodology will be the major subject when we introduce the different Qìgōng styles in the future. In order to help you grasp the general theory of how to regulate Qì, we will introduce the general concepts of regulating your Managing Qì, Guardian Qì, and the five organs' Qì.

REGULATING THE MANAGING QÌ

1. **Qì Vessels and Channels.** One of the goals of regulating the Managing Qì involves regulating the Qì in the eight vessels and twelve primary Qì channels. The key targets of the regulating are keeping the Qì vessels full, and keeping the Qì circulating in the twelve channels smoothly with the right Qì level.

   Though many scholarly and medical Qìgōng styles studied this subject, it was probably not until about 500 CE that specific and deep training was introduced. This was done by Dámó in his *Yìjīnjīng* (*Muscle/Tendon Changing Classic*). He was most concerned with two of the eight vessels, the Conception and Governing Vessels. It is believed that these two vessels govern the twelve Qì channels, and so the "Small Circulation" (Xiǎozhōutiān, 小周天) was developed to train them. Once you have completed the training of the small circulation, you will then train the "Grand Circulation" (Dàzhōutiān, 大周天). which will help you to open up all of the blockages along the twelve channels. This will improve the smooth circulation of the Qì significantly and, therefore, help you to reach the goal of strengthening your physical body.

   Although after Dámó numerous styles were created to achieve the same purpose, they still follow the same training theory and principles.

2. **Brain and Shén.** The brain is the headquarters and the Shén (spirit) is the Qì control center of your whole being. Therefore, keeping them functioning normally is the key to health and the door to increasing your longevity. In order to regulate your Managing Qì, you must first regulate its headquarters. For this reason, Dámó passed down a training methods in *Xǐsuǐjīng* (*Marrow/Brain Washing Classic*).

In Marrow/Brain Washing Qìgōng training, you learn how to fill up the Qì in the other six vessels. It also teaches you how to lead Qì to your head to nourish your brain and Shén. We discussed Marrow/Brain Washing training briefly in chapter 6. For a detailed discussion, see the book: *Qìgōng—The Secret of Youth*.

REGULATING THE GUARDIAN QÌ

Though regulating the Guardian Qì is not considered as critical as regulating the Managing Qì, it still plays an important role in Qìgōng training. The target of regulating the Guardian Qì is to strengthen the Qì circulation to your skin to generate a Qì shield against negative influences and to maintain healthy growth of your hair and nails.

Guardian Qì training is found in both Wàidān and Nèidān. There are several common methods:

1. **Massage.** Massage is the easiest way. It increases Qì circulation near the skin and therefore leads Qì to the skin.

2. **Slapping.** Though slapping is part of massage, there are several exercises which particularly emphasize the effectiveness of slapping or lightly beating the skin, which stimulates and leads Qì to the skin.

3. **Physical Exercise.** Physical exercise is probably the most common method. When you move or exercise, an abundance of Qì is led to the extremities to energize the muscles. Afterwards, the excess Qì moves out through the skin, increasing the Qì circulation there, and finally dissipates into the surrounding air. When you do this, you normally exercise until you start sweating, which indicates that Qì has been led to the skin and is energizing the pores.

4. **Internal Qì Expansion.** Internal Qì expansion is the hardest, but probably the most effective way to lead Qì to the skin to generate a Qì shield. This is the method which Qìgōng practitioners use. There are many ways to do it. For example, when you have achieved a certain degree of mental concentration, you may imagine that your body is on fire. You will begin to feel warm, and this feeling and the idea of strengthening your Qì shield will lead Qì to the skin. Another way is to imagine that you are a beach ball. As you inhale and exhale, imagine that the ball is shrinking and expanding. After training for a while, you will feel that when you exhale your body expands and all of the pores open. This training will be discussed more thoroughly in a later volume.

REGULATING THE QÌ OF THE FIVE ORGANS

Regardless of which style of Qìgōng you use to reach the goal of health and longevity, they all teach how to regulate the organ Qì, especially of the five Yīn organs (lungs, heart, liver, kidneys, and spleen).

When you regulate your organ Qì, your mind must be able to understand the condition of each organ. In order to do this, your body must be able to relax deep into the organs so that the Qì can flow smoothly there. Also, your meditative mind must be able to sense and communicate with the organs.

There are many ways to regulate the organ Qì. Wàidān uses certain movements to affect specific organs. For example, you can bend forward so that the back muscles press down on the kidneys, and then straighten up so that the pressure is released. This massages the kidneys and increases the Qì circulation.

In Nèidān, you use your mind to lead Qì to the organs. You need to be able to feel and sense the condition of the organs, and you also have to understand the relationships between the five organs, the five elements, and the emotions. For example, the liver belongs to the element Wood and is related to the emotion anger. Whenever you are angry, the liver becomes tense and the normal Qì circulation is upset. Your heart belongs to the element Fire and is related to the emotion happiness. When you are too happy you become very excited. This brings an excess of Qì to the heart and may cause problems. You can see that you have to regulate your emotional mind before you can use your Yì to regulate the Qì in your organs. For example, if you are very excited and your heart is beating too rapidly, put your mind on your lungs and breathe deeply. This will draw the excess Qì from the heart and cool it down. You can see that Nèidān is much harder than Wàidān.

Diet is also useful in regulating the organ Qì. For example, too much alcohol will make your liver, heart, and lungs too Yáng. Tobacco and drugs will make the Qì circulation in your lungs stagnant. Table 11-1 explains the relationship between the properties of food and your organs. The easiest way to regulate your Qì is by controlling your diet.

CHAPTER 13

Regulating the Spirit

13-1. Introduction (Jièshào, 介紹)

There is one thing which is supremely important in battle, and that is fighting spirit. You may have the best general who knows the battlefield well and is also an expert strategist, but if his soldiers do not have high fighting spirit (morale), he may still lose. Remember, spirit is the center and the root of a fight. When you keep this center, one soldier can be equal to ten soldiers. When his spirit is high, a soldier will obey his orders accurately and willingly, and his general will be able to control the situation efficiently. In a battle, in order for a soldier to have this kind of morale, he must know how to fight, why he is fighting, and what he can expect after the fight. Knowing what he is doing and why will raise his spirit, strengthen his will, and increase his patience and endurance.

It is the same with Qìgōng training. In order to reach the final goal, you must have three basic moral virtues: will, patience, and endurance. You must also know what, why, and how. Only then will you be able to be sure of your target and know what you are doing.

Shén, which is the Chinese term for spirit, originates from Yì (the wisdom mind). When the Yì is firm, Shén will be steady and calm. When Shén is strong, the Yì is firm. Shén is the mental part of a soldier. When Shén is high, the Qì is strong and easily directed. When the Qì is strong, Shén is also strong.

In Qìgōng training, it is said: "Yǐshén Yùqì" (以神馭氣), which means to use your Shén to govern the Qì. Shén is thought of as the headquarters that controls the movement of Qì, and it is able to raise or calm the Qì and move it wherever you desire. You may have noticed that when your spirit is high, you can somehow find enough energy to do just about anything. If your Yì is also concentrated and is able to control your Shén at its residence, your judgment will be clear and calm. It is believed in Qìgōng training that when your Shén is properly trained it can lead your mind to supernatural states.

It is also believed that when your Shén is high it is able to lead the Qì smoothly and fluidly to an injured place to speed healing. We have all heard of cases where the doctor felt that a patient was so sick that he would not be able to last for a month. The patient, however, felt differently, and was determined to survive. His spirit was so high that, through sheer force of will, he was able to far outlast the doctor's prognosis. In such cases, some patients even experience miraculous cures. According to Qìgōng theory, this patient's spirit led Qì to the damaged place and overcame the physical damage.

Many people have experienced another phenomenon. A man's boss tells him that if he completes a big project in a very limited time, he will get a week's vacation. The man concentrates totally on the project, working day and night with very little sleep. He is very enthusiastic about the job, finding it challenging and exciting, and is surprised at how healthy and energetic he feels. Finally the job is done. When the man finally gets to relax on his vacation, suddenly he becomes sick. According to Qìgōng theory, this is easy to explain. When you are deeply involved in something for which you are responsible, your spirit is high. This high spirit energizes the Qì in your body so that it flows strongly and smoothly and your Guardian Qì is strong. This keeps you from getting sick. Once you relax, your spirit is lowered and your Qì is not energized any more. Sickness will then be able to break through the shield of your Guardian Qì. Most often you catch a cold.

These two examples should give you an idea of how the Shén is able to affect your health and longevity. Because it plays such an important role, Shén training is considered one of the final stages of Qìgōng. Training and refining your Shén into a supernatural state is a necessary step in achieving Daoist enlightenment and Buddhahood.

13-2. Regulating the Spirit (Tiáoshén, 調神)

In general, there are four major tasks in regulating your Shén: 1. learning how to raise your Shén; 2. how to keep it at its residence and strengthen it; 3. how to coordinate it with your breathing; and finally, 4. how to use your Shén to direct your Qì effectively. All of these are called Liànshén (煉神) by Daoist Qìgōng practitioners. Lian means to refine, to train, or to discipline. In religious Qìgōng, there is another ultimate goal in regulating the Shén, and that is to train it to be independent enough to leave the physical body. This final goal will be discussed in books discussing religious Qìgōng.

Raising the Shén (Yǎngshén, 養神)

Yǎng means to nourish, to raise, or to nurse. Yǎngshén has been the main task for Scholars and Buddhists in their training to regulate the Shén. Shén needs to be nourished by Qì. Normally, the Fire Qì which comes from food and air is able to raise the Shén easily, however, this Fire Qì also increases emotional disturbance and therefore leads the Shén away from its residence. Using your Yì, which is nourished by the Water Qì, to raise your Shén is harder. However, if you are able to do it, this Shén can be stronger and more concentrated than when you use the Fire Qì. In Qìgōng practice, you are learning how to adjust your Xīn and Yì to raise your Shén. If you are able to use your Xīn and Yì properly, your Shén will be raised but not excited, and it will be able to remain at its residence.

Learning how to raise the Shén the right way is almost like raising a child. You need a great amount of patience and perseverance. One way to raise a child is to help him restrain his attraction to the seven emotions and six desires. Another way is to let him keep this contact with his human nature, yet educate him and help him to develop his wisdom so that he can make clear judgments. It is a long process, and demands a lot of understanding and patience. In Qìgōng, raising the Shén is not a question of increasing your emotional excitement. This would scatter the Yì, and your Shén would become confused and lose its center. Yǎngshén training builds a strong center for your spirit, and helps the spirit take control over a larger part of your life.

Keeping the Shén in Its Residence and Training It

After raising your Shén, you must learn how to keep it at its residence and train it. As with a child of a certain age, you must be able to keep his mind in the family instead of straying outside and running wild. Then you will be able to educate him. In Qìgōng training, to keep and train the Shén includes four major steps:

To Protect the Shén (Shǒushén, 守神). "Shǒu" means "to keep and to protect." The very beginning of the training involves learning how to keep your Shén at its residence. While it is relatively easy to raise your spirit, it is much harder to keep it in its residence. In Shǒushén training, in order to keep the Shén in its residence you must use your regulated mind to direct, to nurse, to watch, and to keep the Shén there. It is just like keeping your child at home instead of letting him leave home and run wild. You must be patient and control your temper (regulate your mind). You can see, therefore, that the first step in regulating your Shén is to regulate your Xīn and Yì. If you lose your patience and temper, you will only make the child want to leave home again. Only when you have regulated your Xīn and Yì will you be able to watch and to keep your Shén effectively.

To Firm the Shén (Gùshén, 固神). "Gù" means "to solidify and to firm." After you can keep your Shén in its residence, you then learn how to firm and solidify it (Gùshén). Gùshén means to train your Shén to stay at its residence willingly. After you are able to control your child in the house, you must make him want from his heart to stay. Only then will his mind be steady and calm. Naturally, in order to reach this stage, you will need a lot of love and patience to educate him until he understands how important it is for him to stay home and grow up normally and healthily. Qìgōng training operates on the same principle. The second step of Shén training is to make the Shén willing to stay in its residence. In order to do this, your mind must be able to regulate all emotional thoughts. Only then will your Shén be able to stay in its residence in peace.

To Stabilize the Shén (Dìngshén, 定神). "Dìngshén" means "to stabilize and to calm the Shén." When you have brought your child into the stage of peace, he will not be as excited by and attracted to outside emotional distractions. In regulating your Shén you must learn to calm down the Shén so that it is energized but not excited. Then the mind will be peaceful and steady.

To Focus the Shén (Níngshén, 凝神). "Níng" means "to concentrate, to refine, to focus, and to strengthen." You can see from the above three processes that keeping, firming, and stabilizing are the foundation of the cultivation of your Shén. It is like a child who is able to stay at home willingly with a calm and steady mind. Only then will you be able to teach and train him. In Qìgōng, once you have passed these three initial steps, you will learn to condense and to focus your Shén in a tiny spot. The Condensing the Shén stage is where you can train the Shén to a higher spiritual state. When the Shén is focused in a tiny point, it is like a sunbeam which is focused through a lens. The smaller the point, the stronger its beam.

Combining Shén with the Breathing

After the Shén has been trained to a high degree, you can put it to work. The first assignment for your Shén is coordination with your breathing. Remember, in Qìgōng training your breathing carries out your strategy. When this strategy is directed by your Shén, it will be able to obtain maximum results. This is called "Shénxí Xiāngyī" (神息相依), which means "the Shén and the breathing are mutually dependent." In Qìgōng training, this is called Shénxí (神息) which means "Shén breathing." At this stage, your Shén and breathing have united into one. When you have accomplished this, your Qì will be led most efficiently. Naturally, this is not an easy task. In order to reach this stage, you must have regulated your body, breathing, and mind.

Combining Shén with Qì

The last stage of regulating Shén for health involves learning to use the Shén to direct the circulation and distribution of Qì in the most efficient way. In Qìgōng society, this stage is called Shénqì Xiànghé (神氣相合), which means "the Shén and Qì combine together." In a battle, if the spirit of the soldiers is kept high, their fighting ability and efficiency will be increased, and the strategy will be carried out more thoroughly.

Obviously, cultivating your Shén is a long and painstaking process. There is no limit to Shén cultivation. The more you refine it, the higher it is able to go. In religious Qìgōng training, the final stage of regulating the Shén is to train the Shén to separate from the physical body. In order to reach this goal, you must first accomplish the preceding four phases of training. Only when your Shén and Qì are combined will the Qì nourish the Shén so that it grows and matures. We will discuss this subject in a later volume.

CHAPTER 14

Important Points in Qìgōng Practice

14-1. INTRODUCTION (JIÈSHÀO, 介紹)

Qìgōng is the science of working with the body's energy field. This is something completely new for most people, and so you will encounter many new experiences, have many questions, and even experience difficulties or unusual phenomena which may lead you away from correct practice. If you are a beginner and have not built up a strong Qì field in your body, straying from correct practice may not significantly harm your health. However, if you have reached a level where you have built up strong Qì circulation, incorrect practice may be harmful and dangerous. You will not just stop making progress in your training, but you will probably also disturb your normal Qì circulation. Therefore, before you start training you should study the common phenomena and deviations (which means entering the wrong path) which many Qìgōng practitioners have experienced before. You should also study the cause of deviation and understand how to correct the mistakes. However, it is important for you to remember that you shouldn't expect these things to happen. Expectation is the worst emotional disturbance. What will happen will happen, what won't happen, won't.

In this chapter, we will first discuss the common phenomena which may be experienced by the Qìgōng beginner. This section will help the beginner to avoid confusion and to stop his mind from wandering. As you advance in the training, you will have many different sensations. Usually this is a sign that you are progressing. We will discuss some of the common sensations in the third section. Then we will discuss the most important subject in Qìgōng practice: the causes of the deviations and how to correct them. Finally, in the last section we will list twenty-four rules for Qìgōng practice.

14-2. COMMON EXPERIENCES FOR QÌGŌNG BEGINNERS (QÌGŌNG CHŪXUÉZHĚ DE YĪBĀN JĪNGYÀN, 氣功初學者的一般經驗)

In this section we will discuss many of the phenomena Qìgōng beginners often experience in practice. Some of these phenomena are common, and normally caused by improper posture, timing, training methods, or other reasons. Since most beginners cannot generate a significant amount of Qì, these phenomena are usually harmless. However, if you ignore these clues and continue to train incorrectly, you will build bad habits which may eventually bring you harm. It is therefore important that you pay attention to them, understand them, and study their causes.

The Mind is Scattered and Sleepy

The Daoist Níwánzǔ (泥丸祖) said: "For one hundred days (of Qìgōng practice), prohibit sleepiness. Sleepiness and confusion (make the mind) scattered and disordered, and (you will finally) lose the real."[1] This sentence says that when the beginner practices Qìgōng, he will frequently be sleepy and his mind will be scattered. If you do not keep this from happening, you will have lost the real way (Dào) of training. Having a scattered and disordered mind is one of the most common experiences of beginners. This happens because your Yì is not able to control your emotional Xīn. Though your Yì is strong, your Xīn is even stronger. In this case, you must first regulate your Xīn and analyze the causes and the possible results of this disturbance. After you completely comprehend the nature and cause of your emotional disturbance, you will know the why, how, and what, and it will be easier for your Yì to control your Xīn and bring you peace. Only when you do this will you be able to keep your mind from being confused and scattered.

It is also common for beginners to fall asleep, especially in still meditation. One reason this happens is because of physical and mental fatigue. When you are tired, your spirit is low and your mind is disordered. If you find this happening, the best thing is to stop trying to practice, and either relax or take a nap. If you try to force yourself to continue, you will only do more harm than good. A good way to relax is to lie down comfortably and pay attention to your breathing. Every time you exhale, bring your relaxation to a deeper level. Pretty soon your breathing and heart beat will slow down, and you will feel nicely rested. After the rest, your mind will be clear and your spirit will be fresh. Now you will be able to raise your Shén and keep it at its residence. When you have reached this stage, you will find your spirit and mind centered and balanced.

Feeling Cold

This usually happens during still meditation. In moving Qìgōng exercises you are usually energizing your physical body, so you tend to feel warm and your body is more Yáng. However, in still meditation you are calming your mind, slowing down your breathing, and reducing your pulse rate. This causes your body to be more Yīn. Especially in winter, when you are in a relaxed meditative state your body releases energy into the surrounding air and

---

1.　泥丸祖曰：〝百日之中功忌昏，昏迷散亂失卻真。〞

becomes even more Yīn. It is therefore advisable, when you meditate in the early morning or in the winter, to wear warm clothes and to cover your legs, especially your knees, with a blanket.

However, sometimes you will feel cold even when you are dressed warmly and the room is a comfortable temperature. This is most likely caused by your mind. Your mind has a very significant influence on the circulation and distribution of Qì in your body. Sometimes you can feel cold because of nervous tension, emotional upset, or fear. Have you ever had the experience, during a hot summer day, of something happening which makes you suddenly afraid, and you feel a chill run through your body? Since your mind has such an effect on you, it is important to regulate your mind before you meditate, so that you are calm and steady.

Numbness

Numbness is very common in Qìgōng training. For example, when you sit for a long time in meditation, your blood and Qì circulation slow down, reducing the supply of oxygen and nutrition to your legs. This is very common with beginners. When this happens, you should not continue your meditation, because your concentration and relaxation will be affected. Stretch your legs and massage the bottoms of your feet, especially the Bubbling Well (K-1) (Yǒngquán, 湧泉) cavities. This will speed up the recovery of the circulation. If you meditate regularly and consistently, you will find that you can sit longer and longer without your legs becoming numb. This is because your body has a natural instinct to readjust the oxygen and nutrition supply system to fit the new situation. Normally, after six months of regular practice, you will be able to sit at least thirty minutes without any problem.

Numbness will sometimes also happen in moving Qìgōng training while you are standing. This is most common when you are standing stationary for a long period of time, such as when you are doing Dámó's *Yìjīnjīng*. The numbness occurs most frequently in the ankles and heels, because your body's weight presses down on them and cuts down the circulation. In this case, after you have finished your practice, simply walk for a few minutes or rock back and forth on your heels and toes a few times. This will restore the circulation in a few seconds.

There are certain Qìgōng styles which use stationary postures to build up Qì in specific areas, and later let this accumulated Qì circulate in the body. In this case, numbness and soreness are expected and normal.

Soreness and Pain

Soreness and pain are frequently caused by incorrect posture. If you do not understand the theory of the exercise, you may cause yourself serious injury. The joints are particularly susceptible. For example, the wrong posture in sitting meditation can cause back pain. If you do not correct it, you may even injure your spine. Another common example is the horse stance. When done incorrectly, the knees can be injured seriously. Therefore, before you practice you must first accurately understand the theory and the training methods.

In martial Qìgōng training, certain parts of the body or the joints will be trained in order to increase their strength. In this case, soreness and pain are expected. In this type of training you must build your strength gradually. Normally, it will take at least six months for your muscles to grow and adapt to the new situation. If you are impatient and speed up the training, the weak muscles will lose their capacity to function normally and the ligaments around the joints will be injured.

Half of the Body Feels Hot

Sometimes in Qìgōng practice, half of your body will feel hot. It may be the left, right, upper, or lower half, or just one portion of your body will feel cold while the rest feels hot. This usually happens when you are emotionally upset, when you are sick, or when you are just recovering from illness. At such times your Qì is unbalanced, and if you practice Qìgōng then, you may interfere with the body's natural efforts to achieve a new Qì balance. It is therefore very important to be aware of what is going on with your body and emotions when you practice Qìgōng.

This imbalance will sometimes happen when your Qìgōng training emphasizes one side more than the other. It is always best to develop the Qì evenly. When Qì is developed in a balanced way, your Yì will also be balanced and strong. This will increase the efficiency of your training significantly.

Headache and Eye Ache

For a beginner, the most common cause of headache during Qìgōng practice is failure to keep your breathing smooth. For example, you may hold your breath without even noticing it. This causes your body to be tense, which stagnates the Qì and blood flow and reduces the oxygen supply to the head, causing a headache. There are times when you will want to hold your breath in Qìgōng practice, for example during certain martial practices like Iron Shirt training. However, as a Qìgōng beginner, you should not practice holding your breath.

Eye ache is a common phenomenon during still meditation. There are two main reasons for eye ache. Sometimes, to help a student keep his mind within his body, a Qìgōng master will ask him to focus his eyes on the tip of his nose. It is said in Qìgōng society "Yǎnguānbí, Bíguānxīn,"[2] which means "the eyes watch the nose, and the nose watches the heart." In order to keep your mind within your body and to avoid being distracted by what is going on around you, you should first restrain your vision. Once you have done this, you are able to move your mind to your heart and regulate your emotional mind. However, you should understand that you do this with your mind, not with your physical body. The actual meaning of this sentence is that first you should pay attention to your breathing (i.e., nose or regulating the breathing) and later pay attention to your Xīn (i.e., heart or regulating the mind). It is a common problem that a beginner will actually use his eyes to stare at his nose. This is the major cause of eye ache. When you practice, your eyes may be open or closed, but your mind is focused on your nose (i.e., breathing). It is important to always be relaxed

---

2. 眼觀鼻，鼻觀心。

and comfortable. Any time the eye muscles are not kept relaxed, they will tense up and cause pain.

Another time when the eyes may ache during Qìgōng practice is when you are training to focus the Shén at its residence. You should remember that when you do this you must not use force. Use your mind to lead the Shén to its center constantly but gently. If you use mental force to reach the goal, you will cause not only eye aches but also headaches.

Trembling Body

Body trembling is a very common phenomenon in Qìgōng practice. While this occurs most commonly in the limbs, sometimes you may also experience trembling in part of your torso. This is a spontaneous movement that happens without any intention on your part. There are a number of possible causes. One is when your Qì is redistributing itself. When you have learned how to regulate your body and mind during Qìgōng practice, you will be very relaxed, and Qì will be able to get to certain places more easily than ever before. This extra Qì flow may activate the muscles and cause them to tremble. Sometimes, during still meditation when your body is very calm and relaxed, your upper body will swing forward and backward by itself following your breathing. All of these phenomena during training are good signs. They indicate that you have had some success in regulating your body, breathing, and mind.

Another cause of trembling, however, is over-training. When your muscles are over-exercised or overloaded for a period of time, your mind will gradually lose control of them. This will cause trembling, and frequently also cramping. This kind of trembling happens most often in moving Qìgōng training, especially in martial Qìgōng.

The third cause of body trembling is muscle tension. When the muscles are tensed, the Qì will not be able to move smoothly. If this continues without improving, the Qì will be disturbed and will cause the muscles to tremble or cramp. If this happens, you have not reached even the most fundamental level of body relaxation.

If you are practicing Qìgōng correctly, the body may begin to tremble by itself. You should not use your mind to make this happen intentionally. If you are doing this intentionally, you have lost track of how to regulate your mind.

Warm and Hot Sweat

Warm or hot sweat is normal. When you are practicing Qìgōng you are increasing the Qì circulation, which also raises the energy state of your body. Most of the time, sweating occurs during moving Qìgōng training, although it can also happen during still meditation. Many people think that during still meditation, since you are not moving, you should not sweat. As matter of fact, they are wrong. In still meditation, even though you are not moving externally, you are exercising internally. When the Qì increases to a higher level or higher quantity, it will appear on the surface of your skin and you will begin to sweat.

When you sweat, your pores are open, and you are vulnerable to the cold air. In still meditation, make sure that your body is warm enough so that you do not catch cold. After

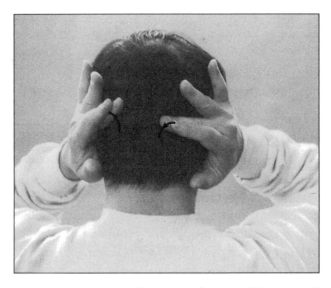

Figure 14-1. Beating the Heavenly Drum (Míngtiāngǔ)

you finish moving Qìgōng training, dry your body immediately and put on extra clothing if necessary. Do not expose your sweaty body to cold wind.

Fright

Fright is one of the worst things that can happen during Qìgōng practice. It generally occurs for two reasons. The first usually happens to beginners during meditation. Sometimes in meditation your mind is very clear but you cannot center it. Your mind may then start to generate a fantasy or illusion. You may feel a cold draft and suddenly think that it is a ghost or evil spirit. Your imagination may come up with just about any kind of idea to disturb you.

If you cannot regulate your mind right away, you may start to believe the illusion and become very scared. The danger lies in the fact that your Yì will no longer be able to lead your Qì, and your Qì circulation will become disturbed. If this happens during very deep meditation, you may cause yourself serious injury. It is therefore very important during meditation that your mind be clear and calm. The emotional mind must be completely controlled.

If you experience this kind of fright, your Yì is too confused to lead your Qì correctly, so you should discontinue practice. There are several ways to help you collect yourself. The first one is to put your palms over your ears and tap your head by snapping your index fingers off the middle fingers (Figure 14-1). This is called "Beating the Heavenly Drum" (Míngtiāngǔ, 鳴天鼓) and is one of the most common way to help your mind to find its center. Alternatively, you may drink some hot tea or coffee, wash your face with warm water, or take a shower.

The second type of fright can happen when you realize that your Qì has been led into the wrong path. For example, suddenly your heart starts beating very fast or your head starts aching seriously. When this happens, your mind is usually disturbed, and you are confused or scared. If this happens, do not stop, calm your mind and move it away from the troublesome spot. The more you keep your mind on the area of concern, the more Qì will flow there and become stagnant. This will worsen the situation instead of help it. Once your mind is calm, use it to lead the Qì to your Lower Dāntián. Sit still for a few minutes and gradually bring your mind back to your surroundings. Do not resume practice, but instead wait until the next session.

Difficulty Sleeping

It is very common for Qìgōng beginners to have difficulty sleeping for a while. This is simply because when you practice Qìgōng, your mind is concentrated, clear, and calm, and your spirit is raised and focused. This raised spirit will prevent you from falling sleep. When this happens, you should regulate your mind. A simple way is to pay attention to your breathing, thinking every time you exhale that your body is becoming more and more relaxed. Do not use your Yì to lead your Qì, but just breathe and relax, and soon you will fall sleep.

Coughing

Beginners sometimes have trouble with coughing during practice. There are several possible reasons. The most common reason is that the breathing is not being regulated smoothly. You may be breathing too fast or holding your breath. If this is the case, use your Yì to regulate the breathing until you do not have to regulate it anymore.

The second possible reason is that your body is not regulated correctly. For example, if you press your head backward too much, the front of the throat will be tense, and will cause you to cough.

The third possible reason is that the air is too dry. When you practice, you often increase the flow of air through your throat. Dry air will cause you to cough. However, if you keep the tip of your tongue touching the roof of your mouth, you will generate enough saliva to keep your mouth moist.

Sexual Excitation

It is normal to have sexual feelings and even to become sexually excited during Qìgōng, especially when practicing Nèidān. This is because you are starting to do abdominal breathing again, and this increases Qì circulation in your lower body and stimulates the production of hormones in the testicles and ovaries. While this increases sexual desire, you should remember that you are practicing Qìgōng to increase the production of hormones and use these hormones to raise your Shén. If you cannot regulate your mind, and waste this extra supply of hormones in excessive sexual activity, you are harming your health and perhaps even shortening your life.

Sexual excitation is especially a problem in Marrow/Brain Washing Qìgōng. This training teaches many methods of stimulating hormone production so that the hormones or essence can be converted into Qì to nourish the Shén and brain. People who do not understand the training or who have a weak will may end up wasting what they have gained through their practice.

14-3. SENSATIONS COMMONLY EXPERIENCED IN STILL MEDITATION (JÌNG-ZUÒ YĪBĀN QÌGǍN, 靜坐一般氣感)

In the beginning stage of Qìgōng practice you learn how to regulate your body, breathing, and mind. Then when you start to practice Qìgōng, especially sitting meditation, you can enter into a deep level of meditation where the Qì readjusts and balances itself, reaching every little place in your body. When this happens, you may experience many kinds of feelings or even have visions in your mind. Many of these feelings cannot be experienced when you are not in meditation. The Chinese call these sensations "Jǐngqì" (景氣), which means "Qì scenery" or "Qì view," because they are generated by the Qì. We will now discuss some of the common sensations you might experience. Do not expect that you will experience all of these sensations, or that everyone will experience them. It all depends on the individual, the time of day, and even the environment in which you are sitting.

The "Eight Touches" (Physical and Sensory Phenomena)

The "Bāchù" (eight touches, 八觸) are sensations which are often felt during Qìgōng practice, such as sensations of heat, someone touching you, or heaviness. In Chinese they are called Chùgǎn (touch and feel, 觸感) or Dòngchù (moving touch, 動觸). Some practitioners list these eight phenomena as: 1. Moving (Dòng, 動); 2. Itching (Yǎng, 癢); 3. Cool (Líang, 涼); 4. Warm (Nuǎn, 暖); 5. Light (Qīng, 輕); 6. Heavy (Zhòng, 重); 7. Harsh (Sè, 澀); and 8. Slippery (Huá, 滑). Other practitioners list a different eight: 1. Shake (Diào, 掉); 2. Ripple (Yī, 猗); 3. Cold (Lěng, 冷); 4. Hot (Rè, 熱); 5. Float (Fú, 浮); 6. Sink (Shěn, 沈); 7. Hard (Jiān, 堅); and 8. Soft (Ruǎn, 軟).

You should understand that all of these sensations are common and normal in Qìgōng practice. Even Qìgōng beginners will sometimes feel them. If you experience something, analyze it to determine the source or cause. If it is a natural phenomenon and the result of the redistribution of Qì, let it happen and don't worry about it. Conversely, if any of the above phenomena occur for other reasons, correct the circumstances that are causing them. For example, if you feel cold because the room temperature is too low, either put on more clothing or turn up the thermostat.

Do not expect these phenomena, do not look for them, and do not be worried about them. Simply follow nature and let it happen. Take it easy and continue your practice. Keep your mind clear and calm, and do not be disturbed or distracted by anything that happens.

Sensations of Movement or Vibration

This is a different sensation from what we mentioned above where one part of the body spontaneously starts to move or tremble. This sensation happens in still meditation in the Dāntián area. When you train your sitting meditation for a while, you might first experience a feeling of warmth in your lower abdomen. After a couple of weeks you may find that the area around your Dāntián starts to vibrate by itself. This means that the Qì is full at the Dāntián and it is time for you to use your Yì to lead the Qì through the Small Circulation. Normally, this is the first sensation which people beginning sitting meditation experience. It gives you the confidence that you are practicing correctly and that you are making progress.

Sensations Inside the Abdomen

Once you feel the warmth and vibration in your Dāntián, the abundant Qì will spread out through your abdomen. The motion of your abdomen as you breathe increases this Qì circulation in your intestines. Sometimes this causes sounds in the intestines, and the release of gas. After this happens for a while, you will feel warmth and other sensations in your abdomen, and you will feel the Qì flowing smoothly and strongly. Sometimes this may make you sweat. After you have practiced for a while, these sensations will disappear as all the channels in the abdomen open up and the Qì is able to move without any stagnation.

The Sensation of Lightness

After you have completed your Small Circulation, and the Qì is circulating smoothly inside your body, you may experience that when you enter into a deep state of meditation, your physical body seems to disappear, or your body feels light and airy. This is a very comfortable sensation. However, if you let your mind be distracted by this sensation, it will disappear. You should be aware of what is happening, but don't pay attention to it. Usually, in order to reach this stage, you must have regulated your body into a very deep state of relaxation, where your breathing and heartbeat slow down to the minimum, and your mind is extremely calm and peaceful.

White Scenery (Clouds) in the Empty Room

Sometimes, when you have entered a deep meditative state, you will suddenly feel your physical body disappear and your Qì mix with the surrounding Qì. When this happens, it seems that the entire room is empty, and filled with a white cloud or fog. If you pay attention to this scenery, it will disappear immediately because your mind is not familiar with emptiness, and generates an image of familiar, physical scenery to fill the void.

If you find yourself experiencing this white emptiness, just sense or feel it, do not put your attention on it. This scenery will happen only when your mind is completely regulated into a highly concentrated and relaxed state. The Daoist Wùyīzi (悟一子) said: "(If you) desire to fill the abdomen (with Qì), must first empty the Xīn (regulate the Xīn). (If you) desire to generate the White, (you) must first empty the room."[3] This sentence tells you that in order to train yourself to make the Qì full in your abdomen, you must first have an empty Xīn. That means you must regulate your Xīn until there is no Xīn. Only then will your mind be able to concentrate your Yì in your Lower Dāntián to Start the Fire (build up the Qì). White here means simple, pure, clean, light, like fog, like clouds, and represents the disappearance of the physical body. In order to make your Qì unite with the surrounding

---

3.   悟一子曰：〝欲實其腹，先虛其心，欲生其白，先虛其室。〞

Qì, you must first let go of and ignore all of the objects in your mind's "room," including your physical body.

Six Other Sensations

When you reach a higher level of Qìgōng meditation, there are six other common sensations which you may experience. These are: 1. Dāntián is hot as if it were on fire; 2. The (internal) kidneys feel like they are boiling in water; 3. The eyes are emitting a beam of light; 4. Winds are being generated behind the ears; 5. An eagle is shouting behind your head; 6. Your body is energized and your nose trembles. These six phenomena are called the Six Verifications (Liùjǐng, 六景) by Daoist Wǔ, Shǒu-Yáng (伍守陽), because they verify that you are following the correct approach in your meditation.

Six Transportations

When you have reached the level of regulating your Shén, your Shén will be high and its Líng (靈) supernatural power will be able to reach farther than any ordinary person's. Your mind will then be able to communicate with the six natural powers:

1. **Seeing the Present.** Your mind is so clear that it can analyze and understand events or incidents clearly and thoroughly. This happens because, when you have learned to regulate your mind, you are able to see things or events from a neutral point of view, without being confused by your Xīn. Since most people cannot do this, you can see more clearly than most people.

2. **Understanding the Past and Seeing the Future.** Your mind is able to understand the past and predict the future. Since your mind is clear, you will be able to analyze what has happened, understand its causes and see the results. As your experience with objectively analyzing the past accumulates, you will be able to see what will happen in the future, since people remain the same and history always repeats itself.

3. **Viewing the Entire Universe.** When your meditation has reached the highest stage, your spirit is able to feel or sense the entire universe. You will (spiritually) see the mountains, the sky, rivers, oceans, etc. At this stage your Qì and the universe's Qì have united into one and you are able to freely exchange information. This stage is called "unification of the heaven and human" (Tiānrén Héyī, 天人合一).

4. **Hearing the Sounds of the Universe.** Through your spirit you are able to listen to and understand all of the sounds generated by the variations of natural Qì, including the wind, rain, waves, and many other things. You will also be able to hear spirits and communicate with them.

5. **Seeing a Person's Destiny.** After you have experienced all of the changes of the natural Qì field, and accumulated all of the past information related to human beings, you will be able to see a person's mind, personality, and true nature, and this will let you see his destiny. You will even be able to see his spiritual future, whether it involves enjoyment (heaven) or suffering (hell).

6. **Knowing a Person's Thoughts.** Since you have energized your spirit and brain to a highly sensitive state, your brain will be open to a much wider band of wavelengths. You will be able to match wavelengths with other people's minds, and see their thoughts.

Daoist Wǔzhēnrén (伍真人) said: "Return to emptiness to combine with the Dao; after you have reached steadiness and (your spirit is) able to leave (your body), (your spirit is) able to suddenly enter, suddenly leave (your body). Then you are able to communicate with the six or ten (nature powers), and are able to transform into thousands of changes and ten thousand variations; nothing cannot be done."[4] This is the stage of Buddhahood and Enlightenment, where you are able to separate your spirit from your body and unite with nature.

14-4. DEVIATIONS AND CORRECTIONS (PIĀNCHĀ YǓ JIǍOZHÈNG, 偏差與 矯正)

Once you are able to build up the Qì in your body, especially at the Dāntián, if you are not cautious your Qì might deviate from the correct path and bring you into a dangerous situation. This is caused by lack of knowledge, misunderstandings, or wrong training methods. In Qìgōng practice, deviations are called Zǒuhuǒ Rùmó (走火入魔), which means "mislead the Fire and enter the Devil." "Mislead the fire" (Zǒuhuǒ, 走火) means to lead the Qì into the wrong path, and "enter the Devil" (Rùmó, 入魔) means that the mind enters the domain of evil. When this happens during Qìgōng practice, serious problems or injury usually result. In this section, we will discuss the causes of common Qìgōng deviations. Then we will discuss the deviations and how to correct them.

Causes of Deviations
The Qìgōng Style Trained Does Not Fit the Individual or the Circumstances. Many practitioners do not understand that every style of Qìgōng has its own special training methods and objectives. Each Qìgōng set was created by a knowledgeable Qìgōng master to train a specific group of people. For example, Iron Shirt Qìgōng is used to train people whose bodies are already stronger than the average person's. If you are weak and force yourself to train Iron Shirt, you will encounter difficulties and deviations. Therefore, when you choose a Qìgōng style for your training, you must first know your body's condition, the purpose of your training, and if the Qìgōng style chosen will help you to improve your health. Naturally, you must first have a good knowledge of each style. Normally, for a beginner, a knowledgeable master must help you to decide the style to practice. However, with Qìgōng styles which are used to improve one's general health, such as the "Eight Pieces of Brocade" and "Five Animal Sports," you do not have to worry too much about deviations caused by

---

4. 伍真人云：〝還虛合道，出定以後，倏出倏定也可，六通十通皆能，千變萬化，無所不能。〞

choosing the wrong style. Such styles were created for the average person, so you are safe as long as you follow the instructions.

Lack of a Firm Mind or a Knowledgeable Teacher. The most important thing in Qìgōng training is to find a knowledgeable teacher and stay with him. Without a qualified teacher, there is a good chance you may be taught incorrect practices. Once you have found a good teacher, do not lose your patience or confidence and change to another teacher. If you do that, you may change from one training theory to another, which will only increase your confusion. If you train Qìgōng without patience, perseverance, confidence, and a strong will, sooner or later you will find yourself in a situation which is confusing, where deviations can occur.

Anticipating Phenomena. One of the most common causes of deviation in Qìgōng is expectation of phenomena that you have heard or read about. Just because someone else has experienced something doesn't mean that you will experience it also. If you expect something to happen, and especially if you try to make it happen, you are very likely to fall into wrong practices. In no time at all you will be mislead by the wrong sensations or by experiences created solely by your mind.

The Body and Mind are Not Regulated. Many Qìgōng practitioners have encountered serious deviations caused by body tension. For example, after a long day at work, your body is tired and the muscles are still tense. Before practicing Qìgōng, you should calm down your mind, regulate your breathing, and help your body to relax and recover from its fatigue. Any attempt to circulate Qì when you are tired is dangerous.

Deviations are also common when people circulate Qì before their minds are regulated. For example, if you are excited or mad, your Yì is unsteady, and it is dangerous to use it to lead your Qì. If you cannot regulate your mind, you should not practice.

If you practice under either of these circumstances, your Qì can become stagnant or enter the wrong paths. It is very common to experience a headache or various pains in the body. You should remember that regulating your body, breathing, and mind are the basic requirements before you regulate your Qì.

Losing Patience. It is very common for some practitioners to lose their patience during practice and use their Yì aggressively to lead the Qì. This is very dangerous, especially for beginners. When you practice Qìgōng, you must take your time, and be patient and confident. Your understanding and experience will grow with practice. When the time is right, what will happen will happen. For example, many Qìgōng beginners practice circulating Qì in the Small Circulation before they really know what Qì is, and before they can move their abdomens in a relaxed and easy way. This will only cause problems. It is like a child playing with fire before he knows what it is or what it can do.

Mixing Imagination with the Qìgōng Exercises. Qìgōng is a science. It is not a religion or a superstitious belief. Imagination will lead you to the wrong path, and it is a major cause of fear. Imagination is the major cause of "entering the domain of the devil." Most people who have imagination are lacking in scientific knowledge and understanding. They are still confused and wondering what they are doing.

External Interference. Some of the worst deviations are caused by external disturbances during Qìgōng meditation. For example, you are meditating when suddenly you are shocked by a ringing telephone, a loud noise, or a friend talking to you. Such things can cause serious injury, especially when you are circulating Qì in the Small Circulation cycle or are practicing other higher levels of Qìgōng that require great concentration. Therefore, before you practice you should prevent all possible disturbances.

Believing Non-professional Opinions. A common human failing that most of us share is that we tend to believe and trust other people's judgment more than our own. We are especially open to advice from our friends. When you encounter a problem during practice, do not discuss it with anyone who is not experienced with Qìgōng. You can discuss it with your teacher or your fellow students, but it is best not to talk about it with friends who are not practicing Qìgōng. You are likely to be much better qualified to evaluate things than they are.

Not Following the Advice and Rules of the Masters. The last part of this section will discuss twenty-four rules which you should observe while practicing Qìgōng. You must believe in and obey these rules to avoid the most common causes of serious problems in practice.

Though we have pointed out many possible causes of deviation and danger, you should not let this scare you away from practicing Qìgōng. Every scientific study or practice always has some level of risk. For example, you would not ban swimming simply because some people drown, and you shouldn't refuse to drive a car even though many people are killed or injured by them. The proper approach to any of these things is to understand what you are doing, know the source of potential problems, define the training rules, and proceed cautiously.

Most of the deviations we will discuss happen to Qìgōng practitioners who are able to generate a strong Qì flow, yet still do not understand and master the regulation of the body, breathing, and mind. You should understand that once you generate strong Qì in your body, if you do not know how to lead it, it may move into the wrong paths and affect your body's normal Qì circulation. This is harmful and even dangerous. That is why they are called "deviations" rather than "phenomena," which is the term we used earlier in the chapter to refer to experiences which beginners have.

Deviations and Corrections:

Headache. Earlier in the chapter we discussed the headaches which beginners have. Here we will discuss the potentially very serious headaches which happen to people who have developed more Qì.

This headache is generally caused by an excess of Qì and blood, or a lack of oxygen in the brain. The excess of Qì and blood is usually caused by forced concentration, which means the mind is not regulated properly. Even when you are concentrating, both your Yì and body should be relaxed. If you force yourself to concentrate, your mind will lead Qì and blood to

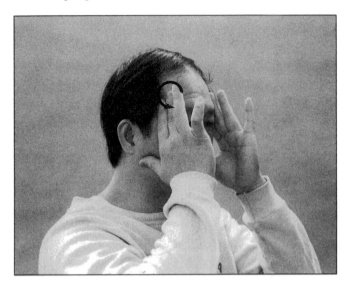

Figure 14-2. Massaging the temples

your head, you will become even more tense, and you will get a headache. It is just like when you can't sleep; it's no good trying to force yourself to sleep. You have to want to fall asleep, but you have to relax and let it happen.

The headache caused by lack of oxygen usually occurs when your breathing is not regulated properly. For example, beginners will frequently try so hard to concentrate their Yì that they unconsciously hold their breath. Holding the breath reduces the oxygen supply to the brain and causes headaches or dizziness. It is therefore very important for the beginner to regulate his breath until it is smooth and natural. That means "regulating the breath without regulating" (Wútiáo Értiáo, 無調而調). Only then should he learn to concentrate his mind on leading the Qì.

If you get a headache while practicing Qìgōng, stop training immediately. Regulate your breathing until it is smooth, and lead your body into a state of deep relaxation. This will help all of the Qì channels in the neck to open, and the Qì and blood which has accumulated in your head will be able to move down to your body. Externally, you may massage both temples (Figure 14-2) and lead the Qì and blood down. You should also massage the Fēngchí (GB-20) (Wind Pond, 風池) cavity (Figure 14-3) on the back of your neck, as well as the muscles there, pushing downward to lead the blood and Qì out of your head. Finally,

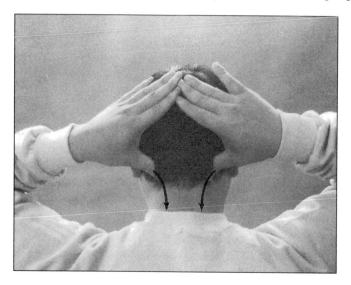

Figure 14-3. Massaging the Fēngchí (GB-20) cavities

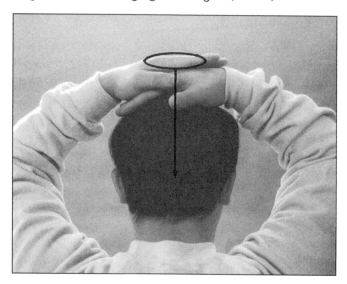

Figure 14-4. Massage the Bǎihuì (Gv-20) cavity down the back

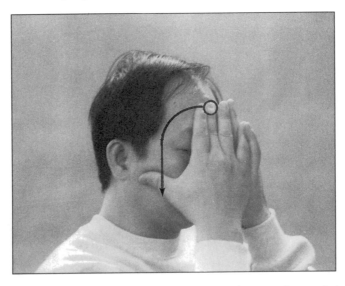

Figure 14-5. Massage from the Upper Dāntián to the temples and downward

put the center of your palm on the Bǎihuì (Gv-20) (Hundred Meetings, 百會) cavity on the crown of your head and lightly circle around for a few times, and then follow the muscles on the back of the neck downward (Figure 14-4).

Stagnant Qì in the Upper Dāntián. When you have stagnant Qì in your Upper Dāntián, it feels like you have a piece of fly paper stuck on your third eye. This usually happens when you have been concentrating there very intensely. Normally, when you concentrate your Shén, your Upper Dāntián area feels comfortably warm. However, if you feel uncomfortable, the Qì is stagnant. When this happens, massage your Upper Dāntián and lead the Qì towards the temples and down the sides of the neck (Figure 14-5). Another way is to massage your Upper Dāntián with your middle finger a few times, then lead the Qì down to the eye bridge, finally spreading the Qì down over your face (Figure 14-6).

Dāntián Feels Expanded and Uncomfortable. Although this is a phenomenon which is more common with beginners, people with some experience may also encounter it. It usually happens when you use too much force to move your abdominal muscles in and out. If you train for a long time, the muscles will be tired and you will not be able to control them. When you train your abdomen to move in and out, it must remain soft and relaxed. If the muscles are tense, the Qì will stagnate there. If you find that your abdomen feels

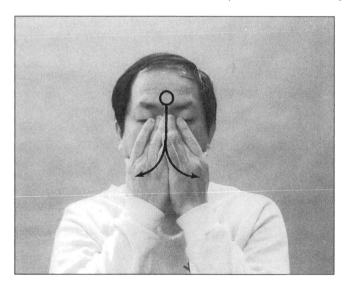

Figure 14-6. Massage from the Upper Dāntián down to the eye bridge and spread over the face

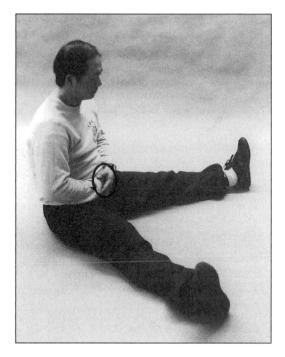

Figure 14-7. Massage from the Lower Dāntián

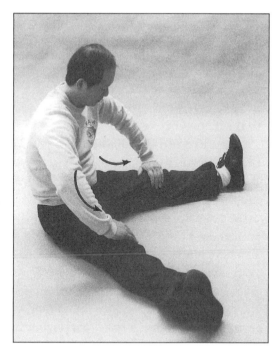

Figure 14-8. From the Lower Dāntián down the thighs

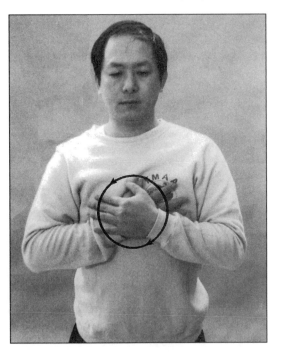

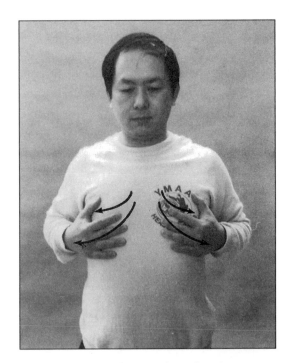

Figure 14-9. Massage the solar plexus (Middle Dāntián)

Figure 14-10. From the solar plexus to the sides

uncomfortable and the Qì is stagnant there, overlap your hands and massage your abdomen in a circular manner a few times (Figure 14-7), then open your hands and brush the Qì down to the thighs (Figure 14-8).

Pressure and Discomfort at the Diaphragm. This uncomfortable feeling usually happens when you use reverse abdominal breathing. It can also happen during normal breathing if you are not regulating your breathing correctly. In reverse abdominal breathing, as you inhale you push the diaphragm down while pulling your abdominal muscles in. This can cause a feeling of pressure and discomfort. Therefore, when you practice, you should start your reverse breathing on a smaller scale, with smaller movements of the abdomen. After you have practiced for a while, you will realize that there is a limit to how far you can move your abdomen without feeling pressure on your diaphragm. However, if you already feel uncomfortable, that means that the Qì is stagnant because of pressure and tension around the diaphragm. You should stop training immediately. Overlap your hands and gently press in on the solar plexus a few times (Figure 14-9), then brush downward and to the sides (Figure 14-10).

Back Pain. Back pain in Qìgōng is usually caused by incorrect posture. This happens especially during sitting meditation. Incorrect posture can cause your Qì circulation to stagnate. It can also increase pressure and tension on the muscles. If you have back pain, stop practice immediately. If you force yourself to continue, you will only disturb your mind and

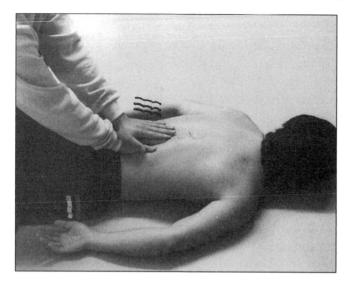

Figure 14-11. Massaging the back

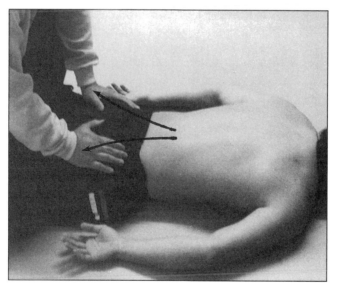

Figure 14-12. Spread the Qì downward to the thighs

make everything worse. If possible, have someone massage the painful area (Figure 14-11), following the spine downward to the hips (Figure 14-12), and spread the Qì to the sides of the body and downward to the legs. If you continue to have back pain when you meditate, you may gently lean against some support. You should not lean directly against a solid wall or anything that can drain your Qì.

Nocturnal Emissions. This happens when you have built up your Qì and do not know how to keep it and circulate it. If you do a lot of Dāntián exercises the Qì will be full there, your sexual organs will be energized, and your body will produce more hormones. This will increase your sexual desire, and cause frequent erections, often without apparent causes such as physical or mental stimulation. If you do not have any sexual activity, internal sexual pressure builds up, and your body will automatically release the pressure through nocturnal emissions about once a month. If you practice Qìgōng and the semen is released automatically more than twice a month, then it is not normal. That means you are not converting the essence into Qì and circulating it properly. In order to convert the essence into Qì and circulate it, when your Qì is full you should coordinate the movement of your Huìyīn cavity and anus with your breathing. This training will be discussed in more detail when we discuss the Small and Grand circulation and the Marrow/Brain Washing Qìgōng in the future volumes.

This problem can also occur when the Qì level in your lower body is lower than normal. When the lower part of your body is deficient due to sickness or excessive walking, there is not enough Qì to keep the muscles functioning normally, and you will occasionally experience nocturnal emissions. This can also happen if you train Qìgōng incorrectly, or if you get involved in Qìgōng before you have completely recovered from an illness. In this case, massage your Lower Dāntián and abdominal area until they are warm after each Qìgōng practice.

The Qì Circulates Strongly by Itself. Sometimes people will build up Qì faster than their Yì can control it. This can be extremely dangerous. It is like driving a car when you don't know how to steer. If you cannot control your Qì, it may go the wrong way and cause serious injury. Many beginning Qìgōng students are enthusiastic and impatient, and try to regulate their Qì before they are able to regulate their body, breathing, and mind. When they feel the Qì move around by itself, especially while training the Small Circulation, they are elated because they think it is a sign that they are making progress. When you find that your Qì is building up and you cannot control it, you should stop practice completely for a period of time. Practice regulating your body, breathing, and mind until you are confident and understand what you are doing. Only then should you start regulating your Qì. The wisest course is to consult with an experienced master. However, many times you will find the Qì moving or distributing itself on a small scale. This usually does not last too long and stops on its own. This is nothing to worry about, and you should simply continue your practice with a calm and peaceful mind.

Do not confuse this experience with what happens when you train certain Qìgōng exercises that build up Qì in a particular area so that it will later circulate strongly by itself. These exercises were designed for that purpose, and the automatic, strong Qì flow is expected.

Qì Entering the Wrong Path. The main reason that Qì enters the wrong path is that your mind is scattered and not regulated. If your Qì is strong and your mind is not regulated, the Qì may go anywhere. It might make your internal organs too Yáng or too Yīn, and you could become ill. Qìgōng without a regulated mind is like a car with a drunken driver—it is extremely dangerous. Always remember: regulate your body, breathing, and mind first before you regulate your Qì. If you are already ill because of Qìgōng practice, stop practice immediately! Relax and get enough rest, and wait until the Qì regains its balance. You usually do not need to see a doctor; if you keep calm and relaxed the Qì will balance itself. When you start again, begin with the most basic regulating exercises first, so that you do not fall into the same problem again.

Stiff Tongue. When the tongue is stiff in Qìgōng practice, it can stagnate the Qì in the Small Circulation. Practice relaxing your tongue as the tip lightly touches the roof of your mouth. Only when you can do this naturally and comfortably should you start practicing the Small Circulation.

14-5. THE TWENTY-FOUR RULES FOR QÌGŌNG PRACTICE (QÌGŌNG LIÀNXÍ ÈRSHÍSÌZÉ, 氣功練習二十四則)

In this section we will list the twenty-four rules which have been passed down by generations of Qìgōng masters. These rules are based on much study and experience, and you should observe them carefully.

1. **Don't Be Stubborn about Plans and Ideas (Yùzhí Wàngniàn, 預執忘念).** This is one of the easiest mistakes for beginners to make. When we take up Qìgōng we are enthusiastic and eager. However, sometimes we don't learn as fast as we would like to, and we become impatient and try to force things. Sometimes we set up a schedule for ourselves: today I want to make my Dāntián warm, tomorrow I want to get through the tailbone cavity, by such and such a day I want to complete the Small Circulation. This is the wrong way to go about it. Qìgōng is not like any ordinary job or task you set for yourself—you cannot make a progress schedule for Qìgōng. This will only make your thinking rigid and stagnate your progress. Everything happens when it is time for it to happen. If you force it, it will not happen naturally.

2. **Don't Place Your Attention in Discrimination (Zhuóyì Fēnbié, 著意分別).** When you practice, do not place your attention on the various phenomena or sensations which are occurring. Be aware of what is happening, but keep your mind centered on wherever it is supposed to be for the exercise you are doing. If you let your mind go to wherever you feel something interesting happening, the Qì will follow your mind and interfere with your body's natural tendency to rebalance itself. Do not expect anything to happen, and don't let your mind wander around looking for the various phenomena. Furthermore, don't start evaluating or judging the phenomena, such as asking "Is my Dāntián warmer today than it was yesterday?" Don't ask yourself "Just where is my Qì now?" When your mind is on your Qì, your Yì is there also, and this stagnant Yì will not lead the Qì. Be aware of what is happening, but don't pay attention to it. When you drive a car, you don't watch yourself steer and work the pedals and shift gears. If you did, you'd drive off the road. You simply

put your mind on where you want to go and let your body automatically drive the car. This is called "regulating without regulating."

3. **Avoid Miscellaneous Thought Remaining on Origins (Zániàn Pānyuán, 雜念 攀緣).** This is a problem of regulating the mind. The emotional mind is strong, and every idea is still strongly connected to its origin. If you cannot cut the ideas off at their source, your mind is not regulated, and you should not try to regulate your Qì. You will also often find that even though you have stopped the flow of random thoughts going through your mind, new ideas are generated during practice. For example, when you discover your Dāntián is warm, your mind immediately recalls where this is mentioned in a book, or how the master described it, and you start to compare your experience with this. Or you may start wondering what the next step is. All of these thoughts will lead you away from peace and calm, and your mind will end up in the Domain of the Devil. Then your mind will be confused, scattered, and very often scared, and you will tire quickly.

4. **Xīn Should Not Follow the External Scenery (Xīnsuí Wàijǐng, 心隨外景).** This is also a problem of regulating the mind (Xīn). When your emotional mind is not controlled, any external distraction will lead it away from your body and to the distraction. You must train yourself so that noises, smells, conversations and such will not disturb your concentration. It is all right to be aware of what is happening, but your mind must remain calmly, peacefully, and steadily on your cultivation.

5. **Regulate Your Sexual Activity (Rùfáng Shījīng, 入房施精).** You should not have sexual relations at least twenty-four hours before or after practicing Qìgōng, especially martial or religious Qìgōng. The essence-Qì conversion training is a very critical part of these practices, and if you practice Qìgōng soon after sex, you will harm your body significantly. Sex depletes your Qì and sperm, and the Qì level in the lower portion of your body is lower than normal. When you practice Qìgōng under these conditions, it is like doing heavy exercise right after sex. Furthermore, when your Qì level is abnormal, your feeling and sensing are also not accurate. Under these conditions, your Yì can be misled and its accuracy affected. You should wait until the Qì level regains its normal balance before you resume Qìgōng practice. Only then will the essence-Qì conversion proceed normally and efficiently.

One of the major purposes of Qìgōng is to increase the essence-Qì conversion and use this Qì to nourish your body. Once a man has built up a supply of Qì, having sex will only pass this Qì on to his partner. As a matter of fact, many Qìgōng masters insist that you should not have sex three days before and four days after practice.

During sexual relations the female usually gains Qì while the male loses Qì during ejaculation. The woman should not practice Qìgōng after sex until her body has digested the Qì she has obtained from the man. There are certain Daoist Qìgōng techniques which teach men how not to lose Qì during sexual activity, and teach women how to receive Qì from the man and digest it. We will leave the discussion of this subject to Qìgōng masters who are qualified and experienced in it.

6. **Don't Be Too Warm or Too Cold (Dàwēn Dàhán, 大溫大寒).** The temperature of the room in which you are training should not be too hot or too cold. You should practice in the most comfortable environment which will not disturb your mind and cultivation.

7. **Be Careful of the Five Weaknesses and Internal Injuries (Wǔláo Ànshāng, 五癆暗傷).** Five weaknesses means the weaknesses of five Yīn organs: the heart, liver, lungs, kidneys, and spleen. When you realize that any of these five organs is weak, you should proceed very gradually and gently with your Qìgōng practice. Qìgōng practice is an internal exercise which is directly related to these five organs. If you do not move gradually and gently, it is like forcing a weak person to run 10 miles right away. This will not build up his strength, instead it will injure him more seriously.

For the same reason, when you have an internal injury your internal Qì distribution and circulation is already disturbed. If you practice Qìgōng your feelings may be misled, and your practice may worsen your problem and interfere with the natural healing process. There are certain Qìgōng exercises which are designed to cure internal injuries, but to use them properly you need to have a very good understanding of the Qì situation of your body.

8. **Avoid Facing the Wind When Sweating (Zuòhàn Dāngfēng, 坐汗當風).** Don't practice in the wind, especially facing the wind. When you practice Qìgōng you are exercising either internally, or both internally and externally. It is normal to sweat, and since you are relaxed, your pores are wide open. If you expose your body to cold wind, you will catch cold.

9. **Don't Wear Tight Clothes and Belt (Jǐnyī Shùdài, 緊衣束帶).** Always wear loose clothes during practice because this will help you to feel comfortable. Keep your belt loose, too. The abdomen is the key area in Qìgōng practice, and you must be careful not to limit the movement of this area because it will interfere with your practice.

10. **Don't Eat Too Much Greasy and Sweet Food (Tāotiè Féigān, 饕餮肥甘).** You should regulate your eating habits while you are practicing Qìgōng. Greasy or sweet food will increase your Fire Qì, making your mind scattered, and your Shén will stray away from its residence. You should eat more fruits and vegetables, and keep away from alcohol and tobacco.

11. **Don't Hang Your Feet Off the Bed (Báchuáng Xuánjiǎo, 跋床懸腳).** In ancient times the most common place in Qìgōng practice was sitting on your bed. Since most beds were high, if you sat on the edge of the bed your feet would hang off the side of the bed above the floor. When you practice Qìgōng your feet should touch the floor. If they do not, all of the weight of your body will press down on the lower part of your thighs and reduce the Qì and blood circulation. Furthermore, when you

practice you should not put your feet up on the table, because this position will also stagnate the Qì and blood circulation.

12. **Don't Practice with a Full Bladder (Jiǔrěn Xiǎobiàn, 久忍小便).** You should go to the toilet before you start your practice. If you need to go during practice, stop your practice and do so. Holding it in disturbs your concentration.

13. **Don't Scratch an Itch (Sāozhuā Yǎngchù, 搔抓癢處).** If you itch because of some external reason, such as an insect walking on you or biting you, do not be alarmed and keep your mind calm. Use your Yì to lead the Qì back to its residence, the Dāntián. Breathe a couple of times and gradually bring your consciousness back to your surroundings. Then you may scratch or think of how to stop the itching. However, if the itching is caused by Qì redistribution in the Qìgōng practice, remain calm and do not move your mind there. Simply ignore it and let it happen. Once it has reached a new balance, the itching will stop. If you scratch this kind of itch it means that your mind has been disturbed, and also that you are using your hands to interfere with the natural rebalancing of your body's Qì.

14. **Avoid Being Suddenly Disturbed or Startled (Cùhū Jīngjì, 猝呼驚悸).** You should avoid being suddenly disturbed or startled. However, if it does happen, calm down your mind. You must absolutely prevent yourself from losing your temper. What has happened has happened, and getting mad cannot change anything. What you should do is prevent it from happening again. Most important of all, though, is learning how to regulate your mind when you are disturbed.

15. **Don't Take Delight in the Scenery (Duìjǐng Huānxǐ, 對景歡喜).** It is very common during practice to suddenly notice something that is going on inside of you. Perhaps you feel Qì moving more clearly than ever before, or you start to sense your bone marrow, and you feel elated and excited. You have just fallen into a very common trap. Your concentration is broken, and your mind is divided. This is dangerous and harmful. You have to learn how to be aware of what is going on inside you without getting excited.

16. **Don't Wear Sweaty Clothes (Jiǔzhuó Hànyī, 久著汗衣).** This happens mostly in moving Qìgōng practice, especially in martial Qìgōng training. When your clothes are wet from sweat you will feel uncomfortable and your concentration will be affected. It is better to change into dry clothes and then resume practice.

17. **Don't Sit When Húngry or Full (Jībǎo Shàngzuò, 飢飽上坐).** You should not practice Qìgōng when you are Húngry or when your stomach is full. When you are Húngry it is hard to concentrate, and when you are full your practice will affect your digestion.

18. **Heaven and Earth Strange Disaster (Tiāndì Zāiguài, 天地災怪).** It is believed that your body's Qì is directly affected by changes in the weather. It is therefore not advisable to practice Qìgōng when there is a sudden weather change, because your practice will interfere with your body's natural readjustment to the new

environment. You will also be unable to feel and sense your Qì flow as you do normally. You must always try to remain emotionally neutral whenever you do Qìgōng; even if you are disturbed by a natural disaster like an earthquake, you must remain calm so that your Qì stays under control.

19. **Listen Sometimes to True Words (Zhēnyán Ǒutīng, 真言偶聽).** You need to have confidence when you practice Qìgōng. You should not listen to advice from people who do not have experience in Qìgōng and who are not familiar with the condition of your body. Some people listen to their classmates explain how they reached a certain level or how they cured a certain problem, and then blindly try to use the same method themselves. You need to understand that everyone has a different body, everyone's health is slightly different, and everyone learns differently. When the time comes for you to learn something new, you will understand what you need. Play it cool and easy, and always have confidence in your training.

20. **Don't Lean and Fall Asleep (Hūnchén Qīngyī, 昏沉傾欹).** You should not continue your Qìgōng training when you are sleepy. Using an unclear mind to lead Qì is dangerous. Also, when you are sleepy your body will not be regulated and will tend to lean or droop, and your bad posture may interfere with the proper Qì circulation. When you are sleepy it is best to take a rest until you are able to regain your spirit.

21. **Don't Meditate When You Have Lost Your Temper or Are Too Excited (Dànù or Dàlè Rùzuò, 大怒、大樂入坐).** You should not meditate when you are too excited due to anger or happiness. Since your mind is scattered, meditation will bring you more harm than peace.

22. **Don't Keep Spitting (Tǔtán Wúdù, 吐痰無度).** It is normal to generate a lot of saliva while practicing Qìgōng. The saliva should be swallowed to moisten your throat. Don't spit out the saliva because this is a waste, and it will also disturb your concentration.

23. **Don't Doubt and Become Lazy (Shēngyí Xièdài, 生疑懈怠).** When you first start Qìgōng, you must have confidence in what you are doing, and not start doubting its validity, or questioning whether you are doing it right. If you start doubting right at the beginning you will become lazy, and you will start questioning whether you really want to continue. In this case, you will not have any success and your practice will never last.

24. **Do Not Ask for Speedy Success (Bùqiú Sùxiào, 不求速效).** This is to remind you that Qìgōng practice is time consuming and progress is slow. You must have patience, a strong will, and confidence to reach your goal. Taking it easy and being natural are the most important rules.

PART THREE

The Qì Channels and Vessels

CHAPTER 15

General Concepts

15-1. INTRODUCTION (JIÈSHÀO, 介紹)

In this chapter we will explain a number of concepts and terms which are used in discussing Qì. You will find that many of the terms have already been discussed in previous chapters. We believe however, that it will be helpful to refresh your memory, as well as introduce new terms, to help you understand later discussions. Chapter 16 will review the twelve Qì channels and their relationship to health and Qìgōng, and Chapter 17 will discuss the eight extraordinary vessels.

Qì

Qì is the energy which circulates within the body. As we noted in chapter 3, your entire body is like a factory and your organs are like many machines operating inside this factory. Your brain is like management, directing the entire operation. In order to keep the factory functioning properly, you need a power supply. The power supply is connected to each machine with many wires and cables. Each machine must receive the appropriate level of power; too much power will damage the machine and shorten its life, and too little power will not enable the machine to function properly. You can see that without a proper power supply in the factory, production will be off, and if the power supply stops, the entire factory is dead. It is the same with your body. When your body does not have a normal energy (Qì) supply, the organs will not function properly, and you will become sick; and if the Qì circulation stops, you will die.

You should realize that your entire body is alive, including every blood cell, every nerve tissue, and every muscle fiber. All of these physical, fundamental structures of the body need Qì to maintain their existence and their ability to function. The system which distributes Qì throughout your body is much like the wiring system in a factory, connecting the power source to the machines.

From the viewpoint of function, Chinese medical science classifies Qì in the following ways:

1. **Organ Qì.** This Qì is responsible for the functioning of the organs.
2. **Channel Qì.** This Qì is responsible for the transportation and moving functions of the channels.
3. **Nourishing Qì.** The main responsibilities of this Qì are transforming and creating blood. Nourishing Qì also moves with the blood and helps the blood to nourish the tissues of the body.
4. **Guardian Qì.** (also commonly translated as Protective Qì). This Qì circulates outside the channels and the organs. Guardian Qì's responsibilities are to warm the organs, to travel between the skin and the flesh to regulate the opening and closing of the pores, and to protect and moisten the skin, hair, and nails. This Qì is able to provide the body with a defense capability against external negative influences such as cold weather.
5. **Ancestral Qì.** This Qì gathers (resides) in the chest with its center at the Shānzhōng cavity (Co-17) (膻中). Ancestral Qì is able to travel up to the throat and down to the abdomen. It is responsible for breathing and speaking, regulating the heart beat, and, when cultivated through meditation, Ancestral Qì can strengthen the body.

Blood

The Western concept of blood is only part of the Chinese conception of blood. Although blood is seen as a red fluid, in Chinese medical science it is also regarded as a force which is involved with the sensitivity of the sense organs and the inner vitality of the body. Since the main responsibility of blood is to carry nourishment to every part of the body, it clearly is closely related to Nourishing Qì.

Qì and Blood

In Chinese medicine, Qì is considered Yáng and blood is considered Yīn. Qì is said to be the "commander" of blood because blood relies on Qì for its generation out of food and air, and for its power to move through and remain in the blood vessels. It is also said that blood is the "mother" of Qì because the strength of Qì depends upon the nutrition and moisture carried in blood. Therefore, Qì and blood are believed to complement each other.

Organs (Viscera)

The concept of the Organs in Chinese medicine differs significantly from that of Western medicine. In Chinese medicine the Organs are systems of functions, and not mere physical objects. Generally, this means that within the description of the Organs, almost all of the body's functions can be defined and explained.

In Chinese medical science, the Organs are divided into two main groups: the Yīn (Inner) and Yáng (Outer) Organs. There are six Yīn organs and six Yáng Organs. Five of the Yīn organs (excluding the Pericardium) are called "Zàng" (臟), which means viscera. These

	WOOD 木	FIRE 火	EARTH 土	METAL 金	WATER 水
Direction	East	South	Center	West	North
Season	Spring	Summer	Long Summer	Autumn	Winter
Climactic Condition	Wind	Summer Heat	Dampness	Dryness	Cold
Process	Birth	Growth	Transformation	Harvest	Storage
Color	Green	Red	Yellow	White	Black
Taste	Sour	Bitter	Sweet	Pungent	Salty
Smell	Goatish	Burning	Fragrant	Rank	Rotten
Yin Organ	Liver	Heart	Spleen	Lungs	Kidneys
Yáng Organ	Gall Bladder	Small Intestine	Stomach	Large Intestine	Bladder
Opening	Eyes	Tongue	Mouth	Nose	Ears
Tissue	Sinews	Blood Vessels	Flesh	Skin/Hair	Bones
Emotion	Anger	Happiness	Pensiveness	Sadness	Fear
Human Sound	Shout	Laughter	Song	Weeping	Groan

Table 15-1. Table of correspondence associated with the Five Phases

five (Liver, Heart, Spleen, Lungs, and Kidneys) are considered the core of the entire system. Usually, when a discussion involves the channels and all the Organs, the Pericardium is added; otherwise it is treated as an adjunct of the Heart. According to Chinese medicine, the Yīn Organs "store and do not drain." That means that their functions are directed toward sustaining homeostasis, both physically and mentally.

The six Yáng Organs are called "Fǔ" (腑), which means 'bowels', and include the Gall Bladder, Small Intestine, Large Intestine, Stomach, Bladder, and Triple Burner. According to Chinese medicine, these Yáng Organs "drain and do not store." This refers to their responsibility in the transformation and the disposal of food and waste. All the Yáng Organs receive food or a by-product of food, and then pass it along.

In Table 15-1, you will notice that each Yáng Organ is associated with a Yīn Organ by a special Yīn/Yáng relationship (or Inner/Outer relationship). Pairs of related Yīn and Yáng Organs belong to the same Phase, and their Qì channels are sequential to each other in Qì circulation. They are so closely linked that a disease in one will usually affect the other.

Yīn and Yáng

We have discussed the concept of Yīn and Yáng in chapter 7. Yīn and Yáng are not contradictory. Nor is one considered "good," and the other "bad." To obtain health, a harmony is sought between them and any imbalance is avoided. Remember, Yīn and Yáng are relative, not absolute.

Five Phases (or Five Elements) (Wǔxíng, 五行)

The Five Phases are Wood, Fire, Earth, Metal, and Water. They are also commonly translated as the "Five Elements." In Chinese, "Xíng" means "to walk or to move"; probably more

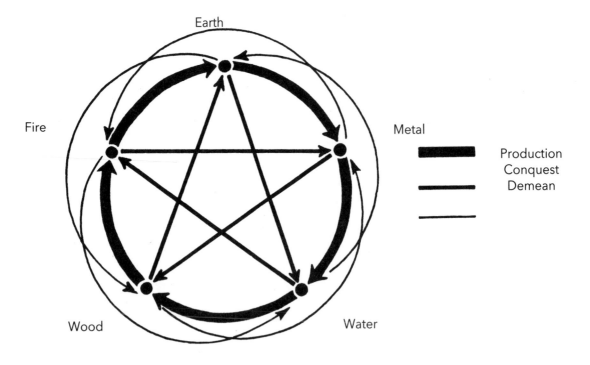

Figure 15-1. The relationships between the Five Phases

pertinent, it means a process. The Five Phases are thought of as the five properties inherent in all things. Each phase symbolizes a category of related functions and qualities. For example, Wood is linked with active functions that are in phase with growth or with increasing. Fire expresses that the functions have reached a maximum state and are ready to decline. Metal represents that the functions are declining. Water symbolizes that the functions have declined and are ready to grow. And finally, Earth is associated with balance or neutrality. Therefore, Earth is the center point of the five phases.

The relationships between the five phases are shown in Figure 15-1.

Qì Channels and Vessels

"Jīng" (經) is commonly translated "meridians" or "primary Qì channels." Your body has twelve channels, which Chinese medicine considers to be like rivers of Qì. Each channel, although referred to in the singular, is actually a pair of mirror-image channels, one on either side of the body. One end of each of these twelve channels is associated with one of the twelve organs, while the other end is connected to a toe or finger (six channels are connected to the fingers and the other six are connected to the toes).

There are eight "Qìmài" (氣脈) or "Qì vessels" in your body. They are often compared to reservoirs because they store Qì for your system. They can also be compared to batteries and capacitors in an electrical system. Batteries store and then release electrical current, and capacitors regulate the electrical current in the same way that the vessels regulate the Qì in your channels and organs.

There are other Qì channels called "Luò" (絡) or "Qì branches." There are millions of Luò spreading out from the channels to distribute Qì to every cell in the body. The Luò carry Qì from the channels outward to nourish the skin, hair, eyes, nails, etc., and also inward to the bone marrow to maintain the production of blood cells. Luò also connect the organs, enabling them to communicate and cooperate with each other.

The next term you must know is "Xuè" (穴), which is translated as "cavity." Your body has more than seven hundred of these cavities, through which acupuncturists access the Qì channels with needles or other methods.

In order for you to be healthy, the Qì must flow smoothly and continuously in the channels. However, sometimes there are blockages, and the flow becomes stagnant. Blockages can be caused by eating poor quality food, by injuries, or by the physical degeneration that occurs as you age. Another problem is when the Qì is not flowing at the proper level. Acupuncturists have several ways of treating these problems, including the insertion of needles in certain cavities to adjust the flow of Qì.

CHAPTER 16

The Twelve Primary Qì Channels

16-1. Introduction (Jièshào, 介紹)

In this chapter we will briefly review the twelve primary Qì channels. As a Qìgōng practitioner you need to know how the Qì in each channel and related organ can be affected by the seasons, the weather, emotions, and food. Table 15-1 offers you a guideline to these relationships.

You should also know the organ's Yīn and Yáng. As seen in the last chapter, there are six Yáng organs and six Yīn organs. Each Yáng organ is associated with a Yīn organ by a special Yīn/Yáng relationship. Pairs of Yīn and Yáng organs belong to the same phase in the Five Phases, their channels are sequential to each other in the circulation of Qì, their functions are closely related, and disease in one usually affects the other. In Chinese medicine, the channel corresponding to the Yáng organ is often used to treat disorders of its related Yīn organ.

In the limbs, the Yáng channels are on the external side of the limbs while the Yīn channels are on the internal side. Generally speaking, the outsides of the limbs are more Yáng and are more resistant and prepared for an attack, while the internal sides are more Yīn and weaker.

The organs are further subdivided in order to distinguish the different levels of the Yīn/Yáng characteristics. The Yáng organs are divided into Greater Yáng (Tàiyáng, 太陽), Lesser Yáng (Shàoyáng, 少陽), and Yáng Brightness (Yángmíng, 陽明). The Yīn organs are divided into Greater Yīn (Tàiyīn, 太陰), Lesser Yīn (Shàoyīn, 少陰), and Absolute Yīn (Juéyīn, 厥陰). In the following discussion, all of the classifications will be shown in the title, for example: the Lung Channel of Hand—Greater Yīn.

16-2. The Twelve Primary Channels (Shíèrjīng, 十二經)

The Lung Channel of Hand—Greater Yīn (Figure 16-1) 手太陰肺經

1. Course

    Course #1:

    (1). stomach (Zhōngjiāo, Middle Triple Burner) (中焦)—(2). large intestine—(3). diaphragm—(4). lung—(5). throat—(6). upper arm—(7). mid-elbow—(8). forearm—(9). wrist—(10). thenar—(11). pollex (Shàoshāng, L-11, (少商).

    Course #2:

    (12). Above the styloid process at the wrist—(13). Index finger (Shāngyáng, LI-1) (商陽).

2. Related Viscera

    Lung (pertaining organ), large intestine, stomach, and kidney.

3. Cavities

    Zhōngfǔ (L-l) (中府), Yúnmén (L-2) (雲門), Tiānfǔ (L-3) (天府), Xiábái (L-4) (俠白), Chǐzé (L-5) (尺澤), Kǒngzuì (L-6) (孔最), Lièquē (L-7) (列缺), Jīngqú (L-8) (經渠), Tàiyuān (L-9) (太淵), Yújì (L-10) (魚際), and Shàoshāng (L-11, 少商).

4. Discussion

    The Lungs (Yīn) and the Large Intestine (Yáng) are considered paired Organs. From Table 15-1 you can see that they belong to Metal in the Five Phases, the westerly direction, the season of autumn, the dry climactic condition, the color white, the pungent taste, the rank odor, the emotion of sadness, and the sound of weeping. Their opening is the nose, and they govern skin and hair.

    In Qìgōng practice, since the Lungs belong to Metal, they are able to regulate heartburn. The Heart belongs to Fire. Whenever the Heart has excess Qì, deep breathing is able to lead the Heart's fire to the Lungs, and therefore cool the heartburn. When the weather is changing from damp, hot summer into drier and chilly autumn, Lungs are the first organ to sense the change. If your Lungs are not able to readjust themselves to fit the new situation smoothly, you will catch a cold. The lung access the outside world through your nose. The Lungs are responsible for taking Qì from the air, and for the energy (Qì) state of the body.

    Breathing is considered a strategy for leading Qì to the extremities such as skin and hair. When your breathing is regulated properly, you are able to strengthen your body's Guardian Qì and generate an expansive Qì shield to protect your body. You are also able to raise or lower your Qì state through your breathing. For example, when you are angry, deep breathing is able to calm your excited Qì state.

    The Lungs are sensitive to emotional changes, especially when you are sad or angry. They also control that part of the liquid metabolism which distributes liquid to the skin.

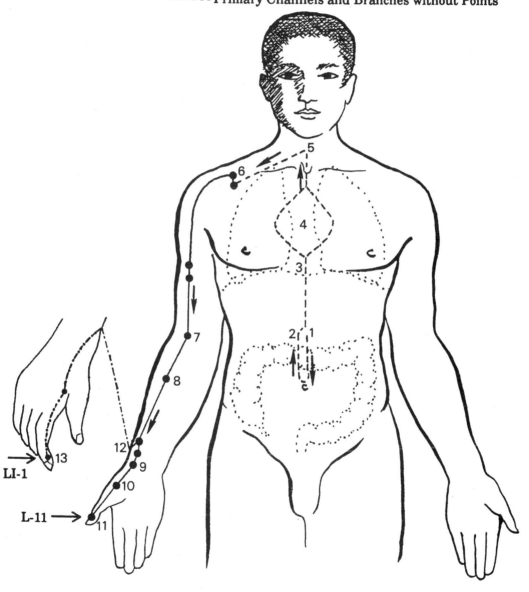

Figure 16-1. The Lung Channel of Hand-Greater Yīn

Because the Lungs are usually the first to be attacked by exogenous diseases, they are called "the Delicate Organ." These diseases can also cause what is called "the Non-Spreading of the Lung Qì." The main symptom of a problem with the Lungs is coughing, which is a form of Rebellious Qì (since the Lung Qì normally flows downward). If coughing is also accompanied by lassitude, shortness of breath, light foamy phlegm, and weakness in the voice, it is called "Deficient Lung Qì." However, if the cough is a dry one, with little phlegm, a parched throat and mouth, and Deficient Yīn symptoms (such as night sweating, low grade fever, red cheeks, etc.), the condition is referred as Deficient Lung Yīn.

The Large Intestine Channel of Hand—Yáng Brightness (Figure 16-2)
手陽明大腸經

1. **Course**

   Course #1:

   (1). Index finger (Shāngyáng, LI-1) (商陽)—(2). Wrist—(3). Elbow—(4). Shoulder joint—(5). Governing Vessel at Dàchuī (Gv-14)(大椎)—(6). Supraclavicular fossa (Quēpén, S-12) (缺盆)—(7). Lung—(8). Diaphragm—(9). Large intestine.

   Course #2:

   (6). Supraclavicular fossa—(10). Neck—(11). Cheek—(12). Lower gum—(13). Rénzhōng (Gv-26) (人中)—(14). Side of the nose (Yíngxiāng, LI-20) (迎香).

2. **Related Viscera**

   Large Intestine (Pertaining Organ), Lung, and Stomach.

3. **Cavities**

   Shāngyáng (LI-1) (商陽), Èrjiān (LI-2) (二間), Sānjiān (LI-3) (三間), Hégǔ (LI-4) (合谷), Yángxī (LI-5) (陽溪), Piānlì (LI-6) (偏曆), Wēnliū (LI-7) (溫溜), Xiàlián (LI-8) (下廉), Shànglián (LI-9) (上廉), Shǒusānlǐ (LI-10) (手三里), Qūchí (LI-11) (曲池), Zhǒuliáo (LI-12) (肘髎), Shǒuwǔlǐ (LI-13) (手五里), Bìnào (LI-14) (臂臑), Jiānyú (LI-15) (肩髃), Jùgǔ (LI-16) (巨骨), Tiāndǐng (LI-17) (天鼎), Fútú (LI-18) (扶突), Héliáo (LI-19) (禾髎), and Yíngxiāng (LI-20) (迎香).

4. **Discussion**

   The Lungs (Yīn) and the Large Intestine (Yáng) are considered paired Organs. From Table 15-1 you can see that they belong to Metal in the Five Phases, the westerly direction, the season of autumn, the dry climactic condition, the color white, the pungent taste, the rank odor, the emotion of sadness, and the sound of weeping. Their opening is the nose, and they govern skin and hair.

   The main function of the Large Intestine is the metabolism of water and the passing of water. It extracts water from the waste material received from the Small Intestine, sends it on to the Urinary Bladder, and excretes the solid material as stool. Many disorders affecting this

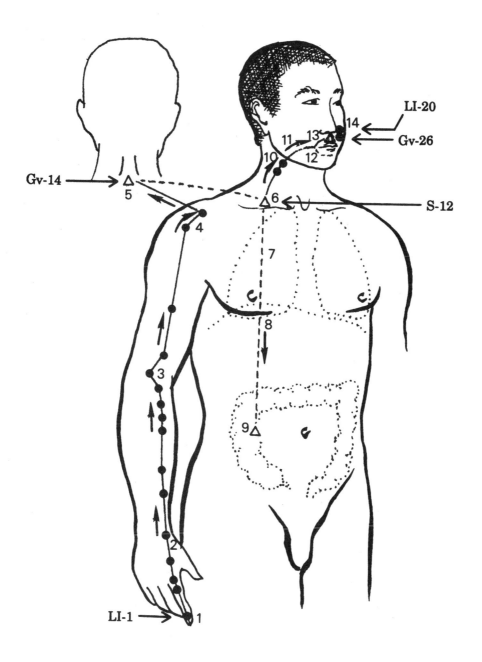

Figure 16-2. The Large Intestine Channel of Hand-Yáng Brightness

Organ are categorized as Spleen and Stomach patterns. Certain abdominal pains are considered manifestations of a blockage of Qì or blood in the Large Intestine.

In Qìgōng, the Dāntián in the lower abdomen is considered the residence of Original Qì. In order to keep this Qì at its residence, this area must be strong and healthy. The Qì circulating around the intestines must not be stagnant. When you practice Qìgōng you must learn how to regulate your breathing to smooth the Qì flow in the Large Intestine and the Lungs. This will allow you to relax the front of your body and regulate the Qì flow in the other organs.

The Stomach Channel of Foot—Yáng Brightness (Figure 16-3) 足陽明胃經

1. **Course**

    Course #1:

    (1). Sides of the nose (Yíngxiāng, LI-20) (迎香)—(2). Root of the nose—(3). Lateral side of the nose—(4). Upper gum—(5). Rénzhōng (Gv-26) (人中)—(6). Chéngjiāng (Co-24) (承漿)—(7). Dàyíng (S-5) (大迎)—(8). Jiáchē (S-6) (頰車)—(9). Ear—(10). Hair line—(11). Shéntíng (Gv-24) (神庭).

    Course #2:

    (7). Dàyíng (S-5) (大迎)—(12). Rényíng (S-9) (人迎)—(13). Throat—(14). Into the chest—(15). Through the diaphragm to Zhōngwǎn (Co-12) (中脘).

    Course #3:

    (16). Infraclavicular fossa—(17). Along the sides of the umbilicus—(18). Qìchōng (S-30) (氣衝)—(19). Bìguān (S-31) (髀關)—(20). Fútù (S-32) (伏兔)—(21). Dúbí (S-35) (犢鼻)—(22). Lateral side of tibia—(23). Dorsal aspect of the foot—(24). Lateral side of the tip of the second toe (Lìduì, S-45) (歷兌).

    Course #4:

    (25). Below the knee—(26). Lateral side of the middle toe.

    Course #5:

    (27). Dorsum of the foot (Chōngyáng, S-42) (衝陽)—(28). Along the medial margin of the hallus and emerges out at its tip (Yǐnbái, Sp-l) (隱白).

2. **Related Viscera**

    Stomach (Pertaining Organ), Spleen, Heart, Small Intestine, and Large Intestine.

3. **Cavities**

    Chéngqì (S-1) (承泣), Sìbái (S-2) (四白), Jùliáo (S-3) (巨髎), Dìcāng (S-4) (地倉), Dàyíng (S-5) (大迎), Jiáchē (S-6) (頰車), Xiàguān (S-7) (下關), Tóuwéi (S-8) (頭維), Rényíng (S-9) (人迎), Shuǐtú (S-10) (水突), Qìshè (S-11) (氣舍), Quēpén (S-12) (缺盆), Qìhù (S-13) (氣戶), Kùfáng (S-14) (庫房), Wūyì (S-15) (屋翳), Yīngchuāng

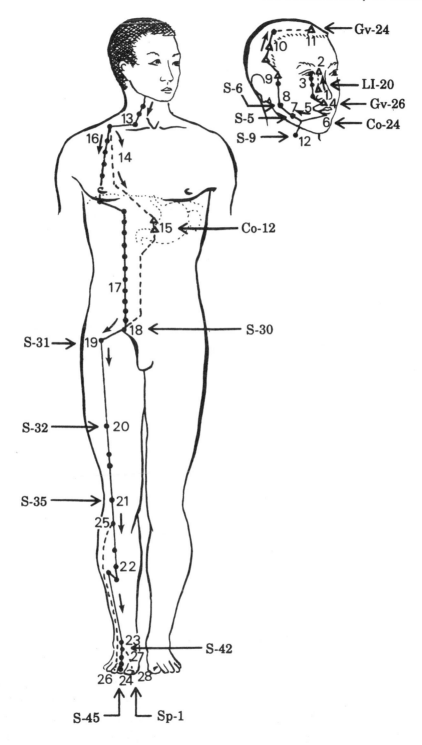

Figure 16-3. The Stomach Channel of Foot-Yáng Brightness

(S-16) (膺窗), Rǔzhōng (S-17) (乳中), Rǔgēn (S-18) (乳根), Bùróng (S-19) (不容), Chéngmǎn (S-20) (承滿), Liángmén (S-21) (梁門), Guānmén (S-22) (關門), Tàiyǐ (S-23) (太乙), Huáròumén (S-24) (滑肉門), Tiānshū (S-25) (天樞), Wàilíng (S-26) (外陵), Dàjù (S-27) (大巨), Shuǐdào (S-28) (水道), Guīlái (S-29) (歸來), Qìchōng (S-30) (氣衝), Bìguān (S-31) (髀關), Femur-Fútù (S-32) (伏兔), Yīnshì (S-33) (陰市), Liángqiū (S-34) (梁丘), Dúbí (S-35) (犢鼻), Zúsānlǐ (S-36) (足三里), Shàngjùxū (S-37) (上巨虛), Tiáokǒu (S-38) (條口), Xiàjùxū (S-39) (下巨虛), Fēnglóng (S-40) (豐隆), Jiěxī (S-41) (解溪), Chōngyáng (S-42) (衝陽), Xiàngǔ (S-43) (陷谷), Nèitíng (S-44) (內庭), Lìduì (S-45) (歷兌).

4. Discussion

The Spleen (Yīn) and the Stomach (Yáng) are paired Organs. They belong to Earth in the Five Phases, the central direction, the season of long summer (the end of summer), the climactic condition of dampness, the color yellow, the emotion of pensiveness, the taste of sweetness, fragrant odor and the sound of singing. Their opening is the mouth and they control the flesh and the limbs.

The Yīn/Yáng relationship between the Spleen and the Stomach is a particularly strong example of the relationship between organs. The Stomach receives food while the Spleen transports nutrients. The Stomach moves things downward while the Spleen moves things upward. The Stomach likes dampness while the Spleen likes dryness.

Though there are some patterns relating to deficiency of the Stomach (many of these originate in the Spleen), most Stomach disorders are caused from Excess. Stomach Fire gives a painful, burning sensation in the Stomach, unusual hunger, bleeding of the gums, constipation, and halitosis.

The Stomach, which is located in the middle Sānjiāo (Middle Triple Burner, 三焦) area, is the first step in converting food into Qì. Food is dissolved in the Stomach before being sent to the intestines for absorbing. The absorbed essence is then converted into Qì and circulated through the entire body.

The Stomach is related to the emotion of pensiveness. When you are upset, the Stomach will not function normally. In Qìgōng, regulating the mind is the first step to maintaining the Stomach in a healthy condition. What food you eat is the second consideration. The proper amount and the proper quality of food will help you to obtain high quality Qì to circulate in your body.

The Spleen Channel of Foot—Greater Yīn (Figure 16-4) 足太陰脾經

1. Course

Course #1:

(1). Medial tip of the big toe (Yīnbái, Sp-l) (隱白)—(2). Anterior border of the medial malleolus—(3). Along the posterior border of the tibia—(4). Medial aspect of

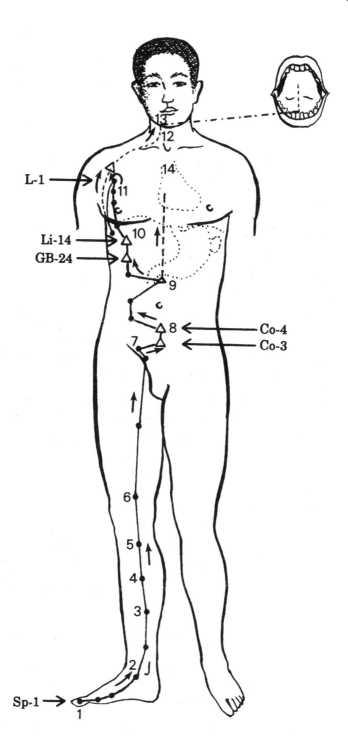

Figure 16-4. The Spleen Channel of Foot-Greater Yīn

the leg—(5). Medial aspect of the *art. genus*—(6). Anterior medial aspect of the thigh—(7). Enter the abdomen—(8). Zhōngjí (Co-3) (中極) and Guānyuán (Co-4) (關元)—(9). Pertains to the Spleen and communicates with the Stomach—(10). Rìyuè (GB-24) (日月) and Qīmén (Li-14) (期門)—(11). Penetrates the diaphragm through Zhōngfǔ (L-1) (中府)—(12). Throat—(13). Root of the tongue.

Course #2:

(9). Stomach—(14). Through the diaphragm and disperses into the Heart.

2. **Related Viscera**

   Spleen (Pertaining Organ), Stomach, Heart, Lung, and Intestines.

3. **Cavities**

   Yǐnbái (Sp-l) (隱白), Dàdū (Sp-2) (大都), Tàibái (Sp-3) (太白), Gōngsūn (Sp-4) (公孫), Shāngqiū (Sp-5) (商丘), Sānyīnjiāo (Sp-6) (三陰交), Lòugǔ (Sp-7) (漏谷), Dìjī (Sp-8) (地機), Yīnlíngquán (Sp-9) (陰陵泉), Xuèhǎi (Sp-10) (血海), Jīmén (Sp-11) (箕門), Chōngmén (Sp-12) (衝門), Fǔshě (Sp-13) (府舍), Fùjié (Sp-14) (腹結), Dàhéng (Sp-15) (大橫), Fùāi (Sp-16) (腹哀), Shídòu (Sp-17) (食竇), Tiānxī (Sp-18) (天溪), Xiōngxiāng (Sp-19) (胸鄉), Zhōuróng (Sp-20) (周榮), Dàbāo (Sp-21) (大包).

4. **Discussion**

   The Spleen (Yīn) and the Stomach (Yáng) are paired Organs. They belong to Earth in the Five Phases, the central direction, the season of long summer (the end of summer), the climactic condition of dampness, the color yellow, the emotion of pensiveness, the taste of sweetness, fragrant odor, and the sound of singing. Their opening is the mouth and they control the flesh and the limbs.

   The Spleen is the main Organ of digestion. Its function is to transport nutrients and regulate the blood (regulate means to keep it within the channels). It is responsible for the transformation of food into nourishment.

   When the Spleen is weak, the body will not be able to use the nourishment available in food. This will cause general lassitude and fatigue, and a pasty complexion. The upper abdomen is considered the province of the Spleen. Deficient Spleen Qì is shown by a sense of malaise or fullness in that area. Because it is required that the transportive function of the Spleen distribute its Qì upward, weakness in the Spleen will usually cause diarrhea. Spleen Qì is also regarded as the Middle Qì, and it is responsible for holding the Viscera in place. Insufficiency of the Middle Qì will presage prolapsed Stomach, Kidneys, etc. In more serious cases, the Spleen Yáng Qì will be deficient, which is manifested in diarrhea, cold limbs, and abdominal pain that can be soothed by the warmth of frequent hot drinks.

   If many of the above symptoms are accompanied by bleeding, especially from the digestive tract or uterus, it is called "Spleen Not Controlling the Blood."

Cold and Dampness Harassing the Spleen is a manifestation type characterized by a pent-up feeling in the chest and a bloated sensation in the abdomen, lassitude, lack of appetite and taste, a feeling of cold in the limbs, a dark yellowish hue to the skin, some edema and diarrhea or watery stool. The Cold and Dampness prevent the Spleen from performing its transforming and transporting functions. This leads to a great disturbance in water metabolism and is one of the origins of Phlegm.

In Qìgōng training, one of the final goals is to regulate the Qì flow to its original (normal) level in the five Yīn Organs. Among them, the Spleen is the last and the hardest organ to regulate. It is believed that if you are able to regulate the Qì in your Spleen to a normal and healthy condition, you will have grasped the key to health and longevity.

The Heart Channel of Hand—Lesser Yīn (Figure 16-5) 手少陰心經

1. Course

   Course #1:

   (1). Heart—(2). Lung—(3). Below the axilla—(4). Upper arm—(5). Antecubital fossa—(6). Between ossa metacarpal IV and V—(7). Tip of the little finger (Shǎochōng, H-9) (少衝).

   Course #2:

   (1). Heart—(8). Diaphragm—(9). Small intestine.

   Course #3:

   (1). Heart—(10). Throat—(11). Tissues surrounding the eye.

2. Related Viscera

   Heart (Pertaining Organ), Small Intestine, Lung, and Kidney.

3. Cavities

   Jíquán (H-l) (極泉), Qīnglíng (H-2) (青靈), Shǎohǎi (H-3) (少海), Língdào (H-4) (靈道), Tōnglǐ (H-5) (通里), Yīnxì (H-6) (陰郄), Shénmén (H-7) (神門), Shǎofǔ (H-8) (少府), Shǎochōng (H-9) (少衝).

4. Discussion

   The Heart and the Small Intestine are paired Organs. The Heart is considered Yīn, and the Small Intestine is considered Yáng, balancing this paired channel. These two organs correspond to Fire in the Five Phases, the southerly direction, the summer season, the climactic condition of heat, the color red, the emotion of happiness, the sound of laughter, the taste of bitterness, the odor of burning. Their point of entry is the tongue, they control the blood vessels and are reflected in the face.

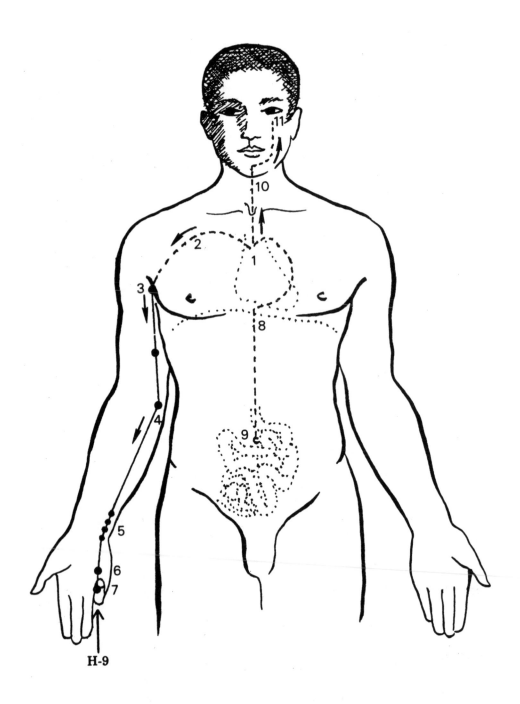

Figure 16-5. The Heart Channel of Hand-Lesser Yīn

Almost all of the problems and disorders of the Heart are associated with weakness. The four major types of Heart weakness are Deficient Heart Qì, Deficient Heart Yáng, Deficient Heart Blood, and Deficient Heart Yīn.

The main functions of the Heart are associated with the spirit and the blood vessels. The Heart governs the blood vessels and is responsible for moving blood through them. It also stores the spirit, and is the Organ usually associated with mental processes. Therefore, some forms of emotional distress, dizziness, palpitations, shortness of breath, and lack of vitality are common to the Heart's diseases. Deficient Heart Qì is symbolized by general lassitude, panting and shallow breathing, and frequent sweating. If the face is swollen to an ashen gray or bluish-green and the limbs are cold, it is called "Deficient Heart Yáng." The symptoms of restlessness, irritability, dizziness, absentmindedness, and insomnia are typical signs of Deficient Heart Blood. In Deficient Heart Yīn cases, developments with a flushed feeling in the palms and face, low grade fever, and night sweating will occur.

The symptom of Heart Excess arises from an excess of Heart Fire. This is manifested by fever, occasionally accompanied by delirium, a racking pulse, intense restlessness, insomnia or frequent nightmares, a bright red face, a red or blistered and painful tongue, and often a burning sensation during urination. The latter symptom is the result of Heat being transferred from the Heart to the Small Intestine, which interferes with the Small Intestine's role in metabolism and the body's management of water.

In Qìgōng society, it is believed that the mind is associated with the Heart, and that it is also directly related to the spirit. As discussed in the third chapter, the term Heart (Xīn) is usually used to represent the emotional mind or idea. The Middle Dāntián at the solar plexus is considered the residence of the Fire Qì. This Fire is used to nourish the brain and the spirit (Shén) at its residence, the Upper Dāntián or third eye. In Chinese medicine it is said that the Heart is the temple of the spirit because it supplies Fire Qì and can nourish the spirit without limit.

Generally speaking, the Heart is very sensitive during the summertime. The Heart is a Yīn channel, and when the summer Yáng comes it can increase the Heart's Qì level and cause problems. Emotional disturbances, such as excitement from happiness, is considered harmful to the Heart as well, especially during the summertime. Qìgōng emphasizes regulating the Heart in the summer.

The Small Intestine Channel of Hand—Greater Yáng (Figure 16-6) 手太陽小腸經

1. Course

Course #1:

(1). Tip of the digitus minimus (Shǎozé, SI-1) (少澤)—(2). Wrist—(3). Top of elbow—(4). Dorsal surface of the upper arm—(5). Shoulder—(6). Circle around the superior and inferior fossa of the scapula—(7). Meets Dàzhuī (Gv-14) (大椎)—(8). Enters

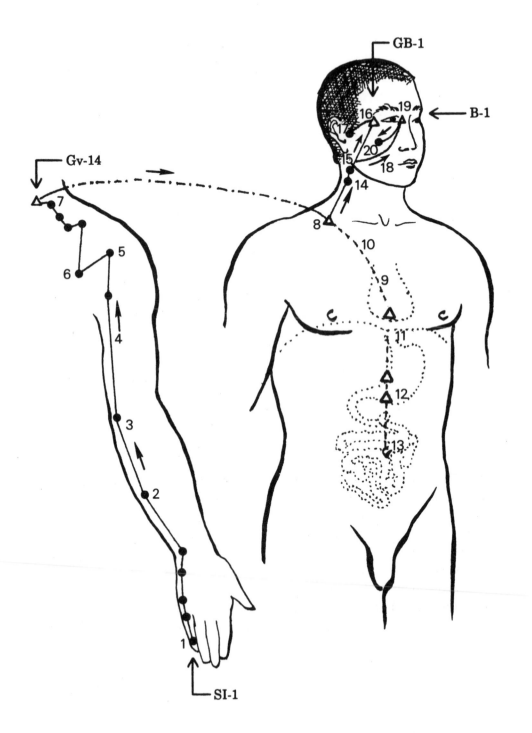

Figure 16-6. The Small Intestine Channel of Hand-Greater Yáng

the supraclavicular fossa—(9). Heart—(10). Passes along the esophagus—(11). Diaphragm—(12). Stomach—(13). Small intestine.

Course #2:

(8). Supraclavicular fossa—(14). Neck—(15). Cheek—(16). Tóngziliào (GB-1) (瞳子髎)—(17). Into the ear.

Course #3:

(18). Cheek—(19). Jīngmíng (B-l) (睛明)—(20). Distributes over zygoma obliquely.

2. **Related Viscera**

Small Intestine (Pertaining Organ), Heart, and Stomach.

3. **Cavities**

Shǎozé (SI-1) (少澤), Qiángǔ (SI-2) (前谷), Hòuxī (SI-3) (後溪), Hand-Wàngǔ (SI-4) (腕骨), Yánggǔ (SI-5) (陽谷), Yǎnglǎo (SI-6) (養老), Zhīzhèn (SI-7) (支正), Xiǎohǎi (SI-8) (小海), Jiānzhēn (SI-9) (肩貞), Nàoshū (SI-10) (臑俞), Tiānzōng (SI-11) (天宗), Bǐngfēng (SI-12) (秉風), Qūyuán (SI-13) (曲垣), Jiānwàishū (SI-14) (肩外俞), Jiānzhōngshū (SI-15) (肩中俞), Tiānchuāng (SI-16) (天窗), Tiānróng (SI-17) (天容), Quánliào (SI-18) (顴髎), Tīnggōng (SI-19) (聽宮).

4. **Discussion**

The Heart and the Small Intestine are paired Organs. The Heart is considered Yīn, and the Small Intestine is considered Yǎng, balancing this paired channel. These two organs correspond to Fire in the Five Phases, the southerly direction, the summer season, the climactic condition of heat, the color red, the emotion of happiness, the sound of laughter, the taste bitterness, the odor of burning. Their point of entry is the tongue. They control the blood vessels and are reflected in the face.

The major function of the Small Intestine is to separate waste material from the nutritious elements in food. The nutritious elements are then distributed throughout the body and the waste is sent on to the Large Intestine.

The Small and Large Intestines are located in the Lower Dāntián. In order to store the Original Qì converted from Original Essence, the abdomen must be healthy and the Qì circulation in the area of the Intestines must be smooth and natural. The best way to reach this goal is through abdominal breathing exercises. One such exercise is to lead the Original Qì upward following the Heart and Small Intestine Qì Channels to cool down the Heart Fire.

The Urinary Bladder Channel of Foot—Greater Yáng (Figure 16-7) 足太陽膀胱經

1. **Course**

   Course #1:

   (l). Canthus medial—(2). Shéntíng (Gv-24) (神庭)—(3). Bǎihuì (Gv-20) (百會).

   Course #2:

   (3). Bǎihuì (Gv-20) (百會)—(4). Fúbái (GB-10) (浮白), Head-Qiàoyīn (GB-11) (頭竅陰), and Wángǔ (Head-Wángǔ, GB-12) (完骨), etc.

   Course #3:

   (3). Bǎihuì (Gv-20) (百會)—(5). Nǎohù (Gv-17) (腦戶)—(6). Neck—(7). Dàzhuī (Gv-14) (大椎) and Táodào (Gv-l3) (陶道)—(8). Lumbar region—(9). Kidney—(10). Urinary bladder.

   Course #4:

   (8). Lumbar region—(11). Crosses the buttock—(12). Popliteal fossa.

   Course #5:

   (6). Neck—(13). Medial side of the scapula—(14). Lumbar region (15). Lateral side of the thigh—(16). Popliteal fossa—(17). M. gastrocnemius—(18). Púshēn (B-61) (僕參)—(19). The lateral side of the tip of the small toe (Zhìyīn, B-67) (至陰).

2. **Related Viscera**

   Urinary Bladder (Pertaining Organ), Kidney, Brain, and Heart.

3. **Cavities**

   Jīngmíng (B-l) (睛明), Zǎnzhú (B-2) (攢竹), Méichōng (B-3) (眉衝), Qūchà (B-4) (曲差), Wǔchù (B-5) (五處), Chéngguāng (B-6) (承光), Tōngtiān (B-7) (通天), Luòquè (B-8) (絡卻), Yùzhěn (B-9) (玉枕), Tiānzhù (B-10) (天柱), Dàzhù (B-11) (大杼), Fēngmén (B-12) (風門), Fèishū (B-13) (肺俞), Juéyīnshū (B-14) (厥陰俞), Xīnshū (B-15) (心俞), Dūshū (B-16) (督俞), Géshū (B-17) (膈俞), Gānshū (B-18) (肝俞), Dǎnshū (B-19) (膽俞), Píshū (B-20) (脾俞), Wèishū (B-21) (胃俞), Sānjiāoshū (B-22) (三焦俞), Shènshū (B-23) (腎俞), Qìhǎishū (B-24) (氣海俞), Dàchángshū (B-25) (大腸俞), Guānyuánshū (B-26) (關元俞), Xiǎochángshū (B-27) (小腸俞), Pángguāngshū (B-28) (膀胱俞), Zhōnglǚshū (B-29) (中膂俞), Báihuánshū (B-30) (白環俞), Shàngliào (B-31) (上髎), Cìliào (B-32) (次髎), Zhōngliào (B-33) (中髎), Xiàliào (B-34) (下髎), Huìyáng (B-35) (會陽), Fùfēn (B-36) (附分), Pòhù (B-37) (魄戶), Gāohuāngshū (B-38) (膏肓俞), Shéntáng (B-39) (神堂), Yīxī (B-40) (譩譆), Géguān (B-41) (膈關), Húnmén (B-42) (魂門), Yánggāng (B-43) (陽綱), Yìshè (B-44) (意舍), Wèicāng (B-45) (胃倉), Huāngmén (B-46) (肓門), Zhìshì (B-47) (志室), Bāohuāng (B-48) (胞肓), Zhìbiān (B-49) (秩邊), Chéngfú

(B-50) (承扶), Yīnmén (B-51) (殷門), Fúxì (B-52) (浮郄), Wěiyáng (B-53) (委陽), Wěizhōng (B-54) (委中), Héyáng (B-55) (合陽), Chéngjīn (B-56) (承筋), Chéngshān (B-57) (承山), Fēiyáng (B-58) (飛揚), Fūyáng (B-59) (跗陽), Kūnlún (B-60) (崑崙), Púshēn (B-61) (僕參), Shēnmài (B-62) (申脈), Jīnmén (B-63) (金門), Jīnggǔ (B-64) (京骨), Shùgǔ (B-65) (束骨), Foot-Tōnggǔ (B-66) (足通骨), and Zhìyīn (B-67) (至陰).

4. Discussion

The Kidneys (Yīn) and the Urinary Bladder (Yáng) are paired Organs. They correspond to Water in the Five Phases, the winter season, the cold climactic condition, the northerly direction, the color black, the emotion of fear, the taste of salt, a rotten smell, and the sound of groaning. Their sensory organ is the ear. Their opening is the urethra. They control the bones, marrow, and brain, and their health is reflected in the hair of the head.

The main function of the Urinary Bladder is to transform fluids into urine and excrete it from the body.

In Qìgōng, the Urinary Bladder has never enjoyed serious attention. However, its pairing partner the Kidney is one of the most important organs—one with which all Qìgōng practitioners are concerned and train most often. The reason for this is simply that the Kidneys are the residence of the Original Essence.

The Kidney Channel of Foot—Lesser Yīn (Figure 16-8) 足少陰腎經

1. Course

   Course #1:

   (1). Small toe—(2). Inferior aspect of the navicular tuberosity (Rángǔ, K-2) (然谷)—(3). Behind the malleolus medialis—(4). Spreads to the heel—(5). M. gastrocnemius—(6). Medial side of the popliteal fossa—(7). Posterior aspect of the thigh—(8). Enters kidney—(9). Communicates with the urinary bladder—(10). Guānyuán (Co-4) (關元) and Zhōngjí (Co-3) (中極).

   Course #2:

   (9). Kidney—(11). Liver and diaphragm—(12). Enters the lung—(13). Along the throat—(14). Root of the tongue.

   Course #3:

   (12). Lung—(15). Heart and spreads to the chest.

2. Related Viscera

   Kidney (Pertaining Organ), Urinary Bladder, Liver, Lung, Heart, and other organs.

3. **Cavities**

    Yǒngquán (K-l) (湧泉), Rángǔ (K-2) (然谷), Tàixī (K-3) (太溪), Dàzhōng (K-4) (大鐘), Shuǐquán (K-5) (水泉), Zhàohǎi (K-6) (照海), Fùliū (K-7) (復溜), Jiāoxìn (K-8) (交信), Zhúbīn (K-9) (築賓), Yīngǔ (K-I0) (陰谷), Hénggǔ (K-11) (横骨), Dàhè (K-12) (大赫), Qìxuè (K-13) (氣穴), Sìmǎn (K-14) (四滿), Abdomen-Zhōngzhù (K-15) (中注), Huāngshū (K-16) (肓俞), Shāngqū (K-17) (商曲), Shíguān (K-18) (石關), Yīndū (K-19) (陰都), Abdomen-Tōnggǔ (K-20) (腹通谷), Yōumén (K-21) (幽門), Bùláng (K-22) (步廊), Shénfēng (K-23) (神封), Língxū (K-24) (靈墟), Shéncáng (K-25) (神藏), Yùzhōng (K-26) (彧中), and Shūfǔ (K-27) (俞府).

4. **Discussion**

    The Kidneys (Yīn) and the Urinary Bladder (Yáng) are paired Organs. They correspond to Water in the Five Phases, the winter season, the cold climactic condition, the northerly direction, the color black, the emotion of fear, the taste of salt, a rotten smell, and the sound of groaning. Their sensory organ is the ear. Their opening is the urethra. They control the bones, marrow, and brain, and their health is reflected in the hair of the head.

    The Kidneys store Original Essence (Yuánjīng, 元精) and are therefore responsible for growth, development, and reproductive functions. They play the primary role in water metabolism and control the body's liquids, and also hold the body's most fundamental Yīn and Yáng.

    Because the Kidneys are the repositories of the basal Yīn and Yáng of the body, any disorder, if sufficiently chronic, will involve the Kidneys. More significantly, a disease of the Kidneys will usually lead to problems in other Organs. Methods of strengthening the Kidneys are therefore used by both medical and Qìgōng societies to increase or maintain vitality and health. The symptoms of Deficient Kidney Yáng or Yīn are typical symptoms of the disorder, and will appear to a certain extent as Deficient Yáng or Yīn patterns in any Organ.

    It is easy to understand and memorize the symptoms of Deficient Kidney Yīn if one learns the correspondences of the Kidneys and remembers that Yīn represents the constructive, nourishing, and fluid aspects of the body. Usually, the lower back is weak and sore, there is ringing in the ears and loss of hearing acuity, the face is ashen or dark, especially under the eyes. It is common to feel dizziness and thirst, and to experience night sweats and low grade fevers. In addition, men have little semen and tend toward premature ejaculation, while women have little or no menstruation.

    Deficient Kidney Yáng symptoms are significantly associated with loss of energy or warmth. Similar to Deficient Kidney Yīn, there is commonly ringing in the ears, dizziness, and soreness in the lower back. However, the soreness is characterized by a feeling of coldness, lassitude, and fatigue. Weakness in the legs can be noticed. In men, there is a tendency toward impotence, and in both sexes, clear and voluminous urine or incontinence.

    Usually, Deficient Kidney Yīn generates similar disorders in the Heart and Liver, while Deficient Kidney Yáng disturbs the functions of the Spleen and Lungs. The progression

2.

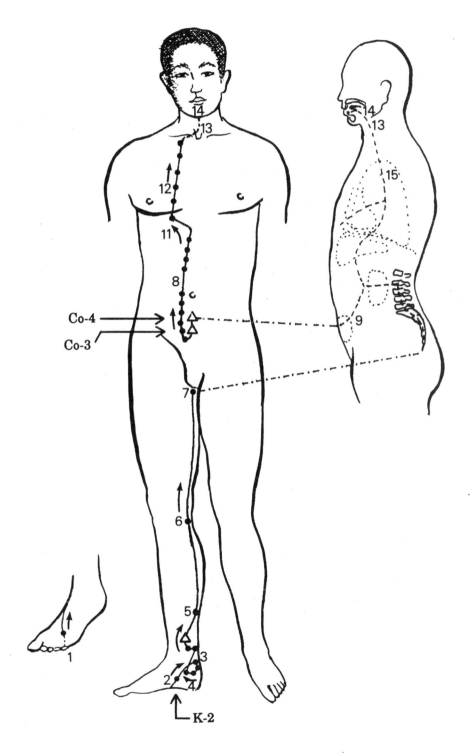

Figure 16-8. The Kidney Channel of Foot-Lesser Yīn

could be in the opposite direction. When this pattern is associated with the Lungs, it is called "Kidney Not Receiving Qì," a type of wheezing characterized by difficult breathing, mainly during inhalation. In addition to the Deficient Kidney Yáng symptoms, this condition is also manifested by a faint voice, coughing, puffiness in the face, and spontaneous sweating.

The Kidneys perform an important role in the metabolism of water. If these functions are disrupted, the condition of Deficient Kidneys will lead to Spreading Water.

In Qìgōng practice, essence (Jīng) is considered the most original source of human vitality. Qì is converted from essence, and this Qì supplies the entire body and nourishes the brain and spirit. It is believed by both Chinese medical and Qìgōng societies that the Kidneys are the residence of Original Essence. In order to protect your inherent essence, you must strengthen your Kidneys. Only when your Kidneys are strong will you be able to keep your essence at its residence. Therefore, keeping the Kidneys healthy has become one of the most important subjects in Qìgōng.

Maintaining the Kidneys in a healthy state includes protecting the physical kidneys from degeneration, and maintaining a smooth and correct level of Qì flow. In order to reach this goal, the diet must be considered. For example, too much salt is harmful to the Kidneys. Eating too much eggplant will weaken the Kidneys. In addition, the condition of the body is also important. Such things as over-working without proper rest will increase tension on the Kidneys and make the Qì flow stagnant. In winter, the Kidneys will have more tension than in summer. Due to this, the Qì flow is more stagnant in the wintertime than in the summertime. Therefore, back pain problems increase in the winter.

In order to protect the Kidneys, Qìgōng practitioners have studied the relationship of the Kidneys to nature, food, and even to emotional states. They have developed massage techniques and specific exercises to increase Qì circulation in the Kidneys during the winter. Since the health of the Kidneys is related to the emotions as well, learning how to regulate the mind in order to regulate the Qì has become one of the major training methods in Qìgōng.

The Pericardium Channel of Hand—Absolute Yīn (Figure 16-9) 手厥陰心包絡經

1. **Course**

   Course #1:
   (1). Pericardium—(2). Below the armpit—(3). Axilla—(4). Forearm—(5). Wrist—(6). Palm—(7). Tip of middle finger (Zhōngchōng, P-9) (中衝).

   Course #2:
   (1). Pericardium—(8). Diaphragm—(9). Connects Triple Burner (Sānjiāo, 三焦).

   Course #3:
   (6). Palm (Láogōng, P-8) (勞宮)—(10). Tip of ring finger (Guānchōng, TB-1) (關衝).

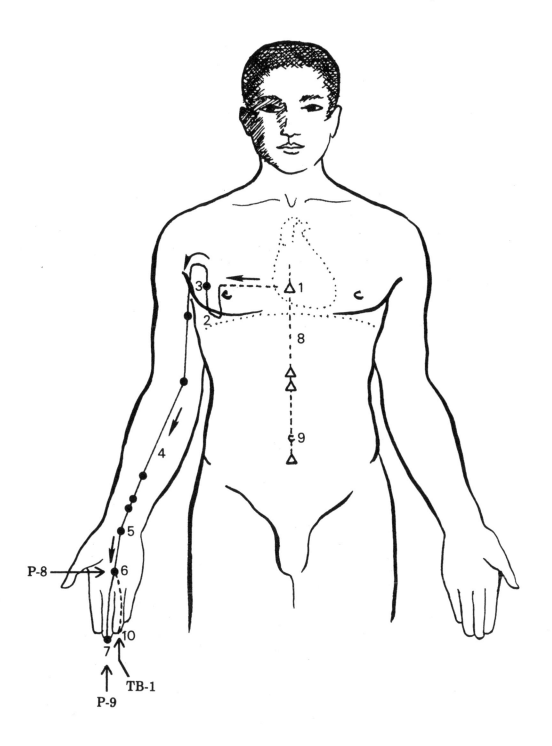

Figure 16-9. The Pericardium Channel of Hand-Absolute Yīn

Related Viscera

Pericardium (Pertaining Organ) and Triple Burner (Sānjiāo, 三焦).

3. **Cavities**

Tiānchí (P-1) (天池), Tiānquán (P-2) (天泉), Qūzé (P-3) (曲澤), Xìmén (P-4) (郄門), Jiānshǐ (P-5) (間使), Nèiguān (P-6) (內關), Dàlíng (P-7) (大陵), Láogōng (P-8) (勞宮), and Zhōngchōng (P-9) (中衝).

4. **Discussion**

The Pericardium (Yīn) and the Triple Burner (Yáng) are paired Organs. They are said to correspond to the "Ministerial Fire," as opposed to the "Sovereign Fire" of the Heart and Small Intestine. Though the Pericardium has no separate physiological functions, it is generally mentioned with regard to the delirium induced by high fevers.

The regulation of Qì in the Pericardium is considered a very important subject in Qìgōng. It is believed that the Heart, the most vital organ in your body, must have a proper level of Qì circulation in order to function normally. The Qì level of the Heart can be raised easily to an abnormal state by illness, emotional disturbance, exercise, or injury. The function of the Pericardium is to dissipate the excess Qì from the Heart and direct it to the Láogōng cavity (P-8) (勞宮), located in the center of the palm. From Láogōng, the excess Qì will be released naturally and hence, regulate the Heart's Qì level. The Láogōng cavity is used in Qìgōng massage to reduce the body's temperature during a fever. You can see that the purpose of the Pericardium is to regulate the Qì in the Heart through the Láogōng cavity.

You should understand that in Qìgōng it is believed that there are five centers (called "gates") where the Qì of the body is able to communicate with the surrounding environment, and, consequently, regulate the Qì level in your body. Two of these five centers are the Láogōng cavities, and two others are Yǒngquán (K-1) (湧泉), used to regulate the Qì in the Kidneys. The fifth one is your face. The face is connected and related to many of your organs. Whenever any of your organ Qì is not normal, it shows on your face.

The Triple Burner Channel of Hand—Lesser Yáng (Figure 16-10) 手少陽三焦經

1. **Course**

Course #1:

(1). Tip of the ring finger (Guānchōng, TB-1) (關衝)—(2). Between the ossa metacarpal IV and V—(3). Wrist—(4). Dorsal side of the forearm—(5). Passing the olecranon—(6). Lateral aspect of the upper arm—(7). Shoulder—(8). Jiānjǐng (GB-21) (肩井)—(9). Enters the supraclavicular fossa—(10). Branches out in the chest, communicating with the pericardium—(11). Diaphragm—(12). Links successively the upper, middle, and lower portions of the body cavity.

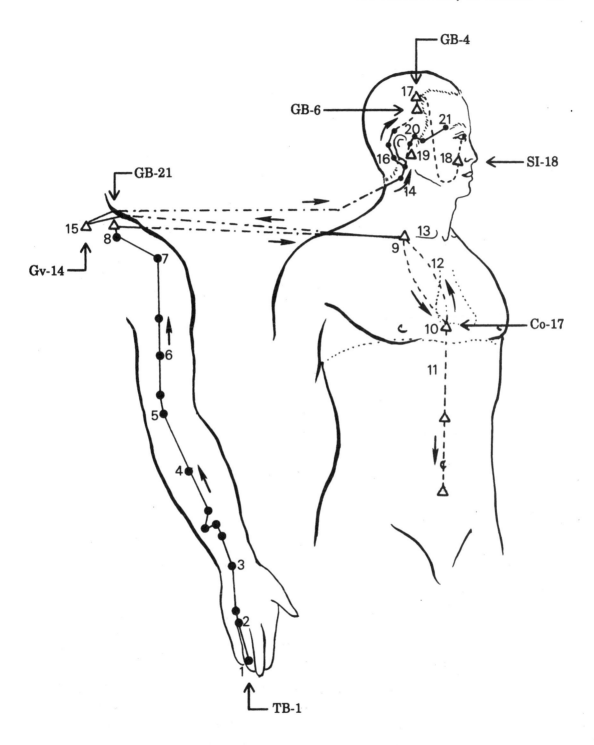

Figure 16-10. The Triple Burner Channel of Hand-Lesser Yáng

Course #2:

(10). Shānzhōng (Co-17) (膻中)—(13). Supraclavicular fossa—(14). Neck—(15). Dazhui (Gv-14) (大椎)—(16). Posterior border of the ear—(17). Xuánxī (GB-6) (懸釐) and Hànyàn (GB-4) (頷厭)—(18). Quánliáo (SI-18) (顴髎).

Course #3:

(19). Retro-auricular region where it enters the ear—(20). Emerges in front of the ear—(21). Lateral canthus.

2. Related Viscera

It pertains to the upper, middle and lower portions of the body cavity (Sānjiāo, 三焦) and communicates with the Pericardium.

3. Cavities

Guānchōng (TB-1) (關衝), Yèmén (TB-2) (液門), Hand-Zhōngzhǔ (TB-3) (中渚), Yángchí (TB-4) (陽池), Wàiguān (TB-5) (外關), Zhīgōu (TB-6) (支溝), Huìzōng (TB-7) (會宗), Sānyángluò (TB-8) (三陽絡), Sìdú (TB-9) (四瀆), Tiānjǐng (TB-10) (天井), Qīnglěngyuān (TB-11) (清冷淵), Xiāoluò (TB-12) (消濼), Nàohuì (TB-13) (臑會), Jiānliáo (TB-14) (肩髎), Tiānliáo (TB-15) (天髎), Tiānyǒu (TB-16) (天牖), Yìfēng (TB-17) (翳風), Chìmài (TB-18) (瘈脈), Lúxī (TB-19) (顱息), Jiǎosūn (TB-20) (角孫), Ěrmén (TB-21) (耳門), Ear-Héliào (TB-22) (耳和髎), and Sīzhúkōng (TB-23) (絲竹空).

4. Discussion

At least as far back as the 3rd century CE, in the *Classic on Disorders* (Nànjīng, 難經) the Triple Burner was regarded as "having a name but no form." In the *Inner Classic* (Nèijīng, 內經), the Triple Burner was considered an Organ that coordinated all the functions of water metabolism. In other traditional documents, the Burners were considered three regions of the body that were used to group the Organs. The Upper Burner includes the chest, neck, and head as well as the functions of the Heart and Lungs. The Middle Burner is the region between the chest and the navel, and includes the functions of the Stomach, Liver, and Spleen. The Lower Burner spans the lower abdomen, and the functions of the Kidneys and Urinary Bladder. Therefore, the Upper Burner has been compared to a mist which spreads the blood and Qì, the Middle Burner is like a foam which churns up food in the process of digestion, and the Lower Burner resembles a swamp where all the impure substances are excreted.

Regulating the Qì to a normally "smooth-flow" state is one of the main Qìgōng training methods for maintaining health. It is normally done through Wàidān exercises, and it is believed that the Qì must flow around internal organs smoothly in order for them to maintain their normal functions. This means that in order to keep Qì flow smooth and the organs healthy, you must first learn how to regulate and relax muscles that are holding and related to a given organ. External movements also exercise internal muscles. One of the most common external exercises is regulating the Triple Burner by lifting your hands up above your head and then moving them down slowly. These up and down arm movements extend and relax the internal muscles and therefore increase Qì flow.

The Gall Bladder Channel of Foot—Lesser Yáng (Figure 16-11) 足少陽膽經

1. **Course**

   Course #1:

   (1). Outer canthus of the eye (Tóngzǐliào, GB-1) (瞳子髎)—(2). Nose-Heliao (TB-22) (耳和髎)—(3). Jiǎosūn (TB-20) (角孫)—(4). Dàzhuī (Gv-14) (大椎)—(5). Enters the supraclavicular fossa.

   Course #2:

   (6). Retro-auricular region, passes through Yìfēng (TB-17) (翳風)—(7). Tīnggōng (SI-19) (聽宮) and Xiàguān (S-7) (下關).

   Course #3:

   (1). Outer canthus of the eye—(8). Dàyíng (S-5) (大迎)—(9). Infraorbital region—(10). Jiáchē (S-6) (頰車)—(11). Supraclavicular fossa—(12). Into the chest—(13). Tiānchí (P-l) (天池)—(14). Communicates with the Liver—(15). Pertains to the gall bladder—(16). Inside of the hypochondrium—(17). Around the pubes—(18). Hip (Huántiào, GB-30) (環跳).

   Course #4:

   (19). Supraclavicular fossa—(20). Axilla—(21). Lateral aspect of the chest—(22). Through the hypochondrium—(23). Zhāngmén (Li-13) (章門)—(24). Along the lateral aspect of thigh—(25). Knee—(26). Anterior aspect of the fibula—(27). Anterior aspect of the malleolus—(28). Lateral side of the tip of the fourth toe or foot-Qiàoyīn (GB-44) (足竅陰).

   Course #5:

   (29). Dorsum of the foot (Línqì, GB-41) (臨泣)—(30). Big toe (Dàdūn, Li-l) (大敦).

2. **Related Viscera**

   Gall Bladder (Pertaining Organ), Liver, and Heart.

3. **Cavities**

   Tóngzǐliào (GB-1) (瞳子髎), Tīnghuì (GB-2) (聽會), Shàngguān (GB-3) (上關), Hànyàn (GB-4) (頷厭), Xuánlú (GB-5) (懸顱), Xuánxī (GB-6) (懸釐), Qūbìn (GB-7) (曲鬢), Shuàigǔ (GB-8) (率谷), Tiānchōng (GB-9) (天衝), Fúbái (GB-10) (浮白), Head-Qiàoyīn (GB-11) (頭竅陰), Head-Wángǔ (GB-12) (完骨), Běnshén (GB-13) (本神), Yángbái (GB-14) (陽白), Head-Línqì (GB-15) (頭臨泣), Mùchuāng

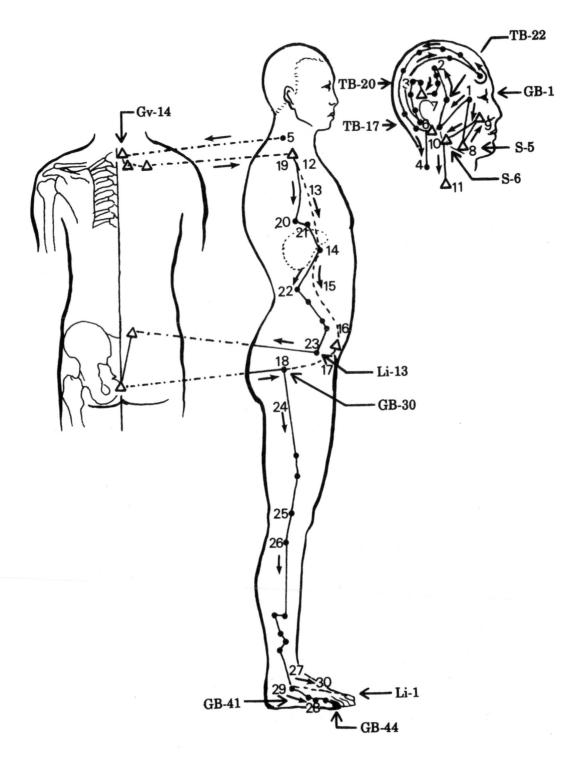

Figure 16-11. The Gall Bladder Channel of Foot-Lesser Yáng

(GB-16) (目窗), Zhèngyíng (GB-17) (正營), Chénglíng (GB-18) (承靈), Nǎokōng (GB-19) (腦空), Fēngchí (GB-20) (風池), Jiānjǐng (GB-21) (肩井), Yuānyè (GB-22) (淵腋), Zhéjīn (GB-23) (輒筋), Rìyuè (GB-24) (日月), Jīngmén (GB-25) (京門), Dàimài (GB-26) (帶脈), Wǔshū (GB-27) (五樞), Wéidào (GB-28) (維道), Femur-Jūliào (GB-29) (居髎), Huántiào (GB-30) (環跳), Fēngshì (GB-31) (風市), Femur-Zhōngdú (GB-32) (中瀆), Xīyángguān (GB-33) (膝陽關), Yánglíngquán (GB-34) (陽陵泉), Yángjiāo (GB-35) (陽交), Wàiqiū (GB-36) (外丘), Guāngmíng (GB-37) (光明), Yángfǔ (GB-38) (陽輔), Xuánzhōng (GB-39) (懸鐘), Qiūxū (GB-40) (丘墟), Foot-Línqì (GB-41) (足臨泣), Dìwǔhuì (GB-42) (地五會), Xiáxī (GB-43) (俠溪), Foot-Qiàoyīn (GB-44) (足竅陰).

4. **Discussion**

The Liver (Yīn) and the Gall Bladder (Yáng) are paired Organs. They correspond to Wood in the Five Phases, the direction east, the spring season, the climactic wind, the color green, the emotion of anger, the taste of sour, the odor goatish, and the sound of shouting. Their point of entry is the eyes. They control the sinews (muscles and joints), and their health is reflected in the fingernails and toenails.

The main function of the Gall Bladder is storing and excreting the gall produced by the Liver. Together with the Heart, the Gall Bladder is responsible for decision-making.

The main disease related to the Gall Bladder is a disorder affecting the flow of gall, usually caused by Dampness and Heat. This is commonly manifested by pain in the region of the Liver, an oppressive sensation of fullness in the abdomen, and yellowish eyes, skin, urine, and tongue.

The Gall Bladder has never enjoyed serious attention during Qìgōng training. Its paired partner the Liver however, has received much more attention.

The Liver Channel of Foot—Absolute Yīn (Figure 16-12) 足厥陰肝經

1. **Course**

Course #1:

(1). Behind the nail of the big toe—(2). Malleolus medialis —(3). Sānyīnjiāo (Sp-6) (三陰交)—(4). Side of shin—(5). Side of knee—(6). Medial aspect of the thigh—(7). Chōngmén (Sp-12) (衝門) and Fǔshè (Sp-13) (府舍)—(8). Pubic region—(9). Lower abdomen—(10). Qūgǔ (Co-2) (曲骨), Zhōngjí (Co-3) (中極), and Guānyuán (Co-4) (關元)—(11). Liver—(12). Lower chest—(13). Neck posterior—(14). Upper palate—(15). Tissues of the eye—(16). Forehead—(17). Vertex.

Course #2:

(15). Eye—(18). Cheek—(19). Curves around the inner surface of the lips.

Course #3:

(20). Liver—(21). Through diaphragm—(22). Lung.

2. Related Viscera

Liver (Pertaining Organ), Gall Bladder, Lung, Stomach, and brain.

3. Cavities

Dàdūn (L-l) (大敦), Xíngjiān (L-2) (行間), Tàichōng (L-3) (太衝), Zhōngfēng (L-4) (中封), Lígōu (L-5) (蠡溝), Tibia-Zhōngdū (L-6) (中都), Xīguān (L-7) (膝關), Qūquán (L-8) (曲泉), Yīnbāo (L-9) (陰包), Femur-Wǔlǐ (L-10) (足五里), Yīnlián (L-11) (陰廉), Jímài (L-12) (急脈), Zhāngmén (L-13) (章門), and Qīmén (L-14) (期門).

4. Discussion

The Liver (Yīn) and the Gall Bladder (Yáng) are considered paired Organs. They correspond to Wood in the Five Phases, the direction east, the spring season, the climactic of wind, the color of green, the emotion of anger, the taste of sour, the odor goatish, and the sound of shouting. Their point of entry is the eyes. They control the sinews (muscles and joints), and their health is reflected in the finger and toe nails.

The main task of the Liver is spreading and regulating Qì throughout the entire body. Its unique character is flowing and free. Therefore, depression or frustration can disturb the functioning of the Liver. In addition, the Liver is also responsible for storing blood when the body is at rest. This characteristic, together with its control over the lower abdomen, makes it the most critical Organ in regards to women's menstrual cycle and sexuality.

Depression or long-term frustration can stagnate the Liver's spreading function and result in continuing depression, a bad temper, and a painful, swollen feeling in the chest and sides. If this condition worsens, it may cause disharmony between the Liver and the Stomach and/or Spleen. This disorder is symbolized by the "rebellion" of Qì in the latter Organs, whereby Qì moves in the opposite direction than is normal. For example, the Stomach Qì normally descends, so rebellious Qì means hiccoughing, vomiting, etc. In the case of the Spleen, the Qì ordinarily moves upward, so rebellious Qì in this Organ means diarrhea.

Depression of the Liver Qì is the main cause of many women's disorders, including menstrual irregularities, swollen and painful breasts, etc.

One of the most important responsibilities of the Liver is the storage of blood with intended emphasis upon nourishing and moistening. Whenever the Liver blood is deficient, the Liver will not be able to handle the function of moistening. This is generally shown as dry and painful eyes with blurred or weak vision, lack of suppleness or pain in moving the joints, dry skin, dizziness, and infrequent or spotty menstruation. If the Deficient Liver Yīn has become serious, the conditions Rising Liver Fire or Hyper Liver Yáng Ascending occur. These occurrences are evidenced in ill-temper, restlessness, headache, vertigo, red face and eyes, and a parched mouth. If the Liver Yīn is so deficient that it is incapable of securing the

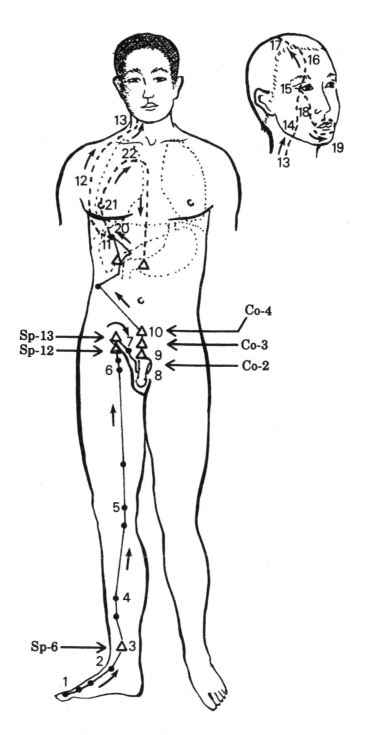

Figure 16-12. The Liver Channel of Foot-Absolute Yīn

Liver Yáng, many of the symptoms appear as disorders of the head. Weakness in the lower joints may also be manifested.

The Liver is one of the five Yīn Organs whose Qì level the Qìgōng practitioner wants to regulate. Since the Liver and the Gall Bladder are directly connected, when the Liver's Qì is regulated, the Qì circulating in the Gall Bladder will also be regulated. Many methods have been developed for regulating the Liver Qì. Wàidān Qìgōng works through the limbs. For example, when the arms are moved up and down, the internal muscles surrounding the Liver will be moved and the Qì around the Liver will be circulated smoothly. In Nèidān Qìgōng, it is believed that the Liver is closely related to your mind. It is also believed that when your mind is regulated, the Qì circulation in the Liver will be normal and therefore the Liver will function properly.

16-3. IMPORTANT POINTS (ZHÒNGDIĂN, 重點)

1. The Spleen, Liver, and Heart are the Organs with the most direct relationship with the blood. The Spleen filters the blood (modifying the blood's structure), the Liver stores the blood, and the Heart moves it. Any problem associated with the blood will involve at least one of these Organs.

2. The Liver and the Kidneys are closely related. Their channels cross in many places. The Liver stores blood; the Kidneys store essence. These substances, both of which are Yīn, have a considerable influence on the reproductive functions.

3. The Heart (Upper Burner, Fire) and the Kidneys (Lower Burner, Water) keep each other in check and are dependent upon one another. The spirit of the Heart and the essence of the Kidneys cooperate in establishing and maintaining human consciousness.

4. The Spleen's digestive function is associated with the distributive functions of the Liver. Disharmony between these two results in various digestive troubles. The transportive and digestive functions of the Spleen (also called "the Middle Qì") depend upon the strength of the Kidney Yáng.

5. Although the Lungs govern Qì, Qì from the Lungs must mix with essence from the Kidneys before Original Qì can be produced. The Lungs govern Qì, the Liver spreads Qì, and the Kidneys provide its basis.

CHAPTER 17

The Eight Extraordinary Qì Vessels

17-1. INTRODUCTION (JIÈSHÀO, 介紹)

The eight extraordinary Qì vessels and the twelve primary Qì channels (meridians) comprise the main part of the channel system. Most of the eight vessels branch out from the twelve primary channels and share the function of circulating Qì throughout the body. These vessels form a web of complex interconnections with the channels. At the same time, each has its own functional characteristics and clinic utility independent of the channels.

Traditional Chinese medicine emphasizes the twelve primary organ-related channels and only two of the eight vessels (the Governing and the Conception Vessels). The other six vessels are not used very often simply because they are not understood as well as the other channels, and there is still a lot of research being conducted on them. Although they were discovered two thousand years ago, little has been written about them. There is a lot of research on the extraordinary vessels being conducted today, especially in Japan, but the results of one researcher often contradict the results that another has achieved.

In this section we would like to compile and summarize the important points from the limited number of available documents. Since references from original Chinese sources are very scarce, and references from Western textbooks are tentative, esoteric, or in disagreement with one another, I have used my own judgment in selecting ideas and details.

What are the Eight Vessels?

The eight vessels are called "Qíjīng Bāmài" (奇經八脈). "Qí" means "odd, strange, or mysterious." "Jīng" means "meridian or channels." "Bā" means "eight" and "Mài" means "vessels." Qíjīng Bāmài is then translated as "Odd Meridians and Eight Vessels" or "extraordinary meridian (EM)." Odd has a meaning of strange in Chinese. It is used simply because these eight vessels are not well understood yet. Many Chinese doctors explain that they are called "Odd" simply because there are four vessels that are not paired. Since these eight vessels also serve the function of homeostasis, sometimes they are called "Homeostatic Meridians." French acupuncturists call them "Miraculous Meridians" because they were able to create therapeutic effects when all other techniques had failed. In addition, because each of these channels exerts a strong effect upon psychic functioning and individuality, the command points are among the most important psychological points in the body. For this reason, they are occasionally called the "Eight Psychic Channels."

These vessels are: 1. Governing Vessel (Dūmài, 督脈); 2. Conception Vessel (Rènmài, 任脈); 3. Thrusting Vessel (Chōngmài, 衝脈); 4. Girdle (or Belt) Vessel (Dàimài, 帶脈); 5. Yáng Heel Vessel (Yángqiāomài, 陽蹻脈); 6. Yīn Heel Vessel (Yīnqiāomài, 陰蹻脈); 7. Yáng Linking Vessel (Yángwéimài, 陽維脈); and 8. Yīn Linking Vessel (Yīnwéimài, 陰維脈).

History

The first brief mention of some of these eight vessels is found in the second part of the Nèijīng chapter of the book *Huángdì Nèijīng Sùwèn* (*The Yellow Emperor's Classic*, 黃帝內經素問) (Hàn dynasty, circa 100–300 BCE, 漢). Also, some of the vessels were mentioned in Biǎnquè's classic *Nànjīng* (*Classic on Disorders*, 難經) (Qín and Hàn dynasty, 221 BCE to 220 CE, 秦、漢). It was not until the 16th century that all eight vessels were deeply studied by Lǐ, Shí-Zhēn (1518-1593 CE, 李時珍) and revealed in his book *Qíjīng Bāmài* Kǎo (*Deep Study of the Extraordinary Eight Vessels*, 奇經八脈考). From then until only recently, very few documents have been published on this subject. Although there is more research being published, as yet, there is still no single document which is able to define this subject systematically and in depth.

General Functions of the Eight Vessels

Serving as Qì Reservoirs. Because the eight vessels are so different from each other, it is difficult to generalize their characteristics and functions. However, one of the most common characteristics of the eight vessels was specified by Biǎnquè (扁鵲) in his Nànjīng. He reported that the twelve organ-related Qì channels constitute rivers, and the eight extraordinary vessels constitute reservoirs. The reservoirs, especially the Conception and Governing Vessels, absorb excess Qì from the main channels, and then return it when they are deficient.

You should understand however, that because of the limited number of traditional documents, as well as the lack of modern, scientific methods of Qì research, it is difficult to determine the precise behavior and characteristics of these eight vessels. The main difficulty probably lies in the fact that they can be taken at different levels, because they perform different functions and contain every kind of Qì such as Yíngqì (營氣), Wèiqì (衛氣), Jīngqì (精氣), and even blood.

When the twelve primary channels are deficient in Qì, the eight vessels will supply it. This store of Qì can easily be tapped with acupuncture needles through those cavities which connect the eight vessels with the twelve channels. The connection cavities behave like the gate of a reservoir, which can be used to adjust the strength of the Qì flow in the rivers and the level of Qì in the reservoir. Sometimes, when it is necessary, the reservoir will release Qì by itself. For example, when a person has had a shock, either physically or mentally, the Qì in some of the main channels will be deficient. This will cause particular organs to be stressed, and Qì will accumulate rapidly around these organs. When this happens, the reservoir must release Qì to increase the deficient circulation and prevent further damage.

Guarding Specific Areas Against "Evil Qì." The Qì which protects the body from outside intruders is called Wèiqì (Guardian Qì, 衛氣). Among the eight vessels, the Thrusting Vessel, the Governing Vessel, and the Conception Vessel play major roles in guarding the abdomen, thorax, and the back.

Regulating the Changes of Life Cycles. According to chapter 1 of *"Sùwèn"* (素問), the Thrusting Vessel and the Conception Vessel also regulate the changes of the life cycles which occur at seven-year intervals for women and 8 year intervals for men.

Circulating Jīngqì to the Entire Body, Particularly the Five "Ancestral Organs." One of the most important functions of the eight vessels is to deliver Jīngqì (Essence Qì, which has been converted from Original Essence and sexual essence) to the entire body, including the skin and hair. They must also deliver Jīngqì to the five ancestral organs: the brain and spinal cord, the liver and gall bladder system, the bone marrow, the uterus, and the blood system.

17-2. THE EIGHT EXTRAORDINARY VESSELS (BĀMÀI, 八脈)

The Governing Vessel (Dūmài, 督脈) (Figure 17-1)

1. Course

Course #1:

(1). Perineum—(2). Along the middle of the spine—(3). Fēngfǔ (Gv-16) (風府)—(4). Enters the brain—(5). Vertex—(6). Midline of the forehead across the bridge of the nose—(7). Upper lip.

Course #2:

(8). Pelvic region—(9). Descends to the genitals and perineum—(10). Tip of the coccyx—(11). Gluteal region (intersects the Kidney and Urinary Bladder Channels)—(12). Returns to the spinal column and then joins with the kidneys.

Course #3:

(13). Inner canthus of the eye—(14). Two (bilateral) branches, ascend across the forehead—(15). Converge at the vertex (enters the brain)—(16). Emerges at the lower end of the nape of the neck—(17). Divides into two branches which descend along opposite sides of the spine to the waist—(18). Kidneys.

Course #4:

(19). Lower abdomen—(20). Across the navel—(21). Passes through the heart—(22). Enters the trachea—(23). Crosses the cheek and encircles the mouth—(24). Terminates at a point below the middle of the eye.

***This vessel intersects Fengmen (B-12) (風門) and Huìyīn (Co-l) (會陰).

2. **Cavities**

Chángqiáng (Gv-l) (長強), Yāoshū (Gv-2) (腰俞), Yāoyángguān (Gv-3) (腰陽關), Mìngmén (Gv-4) (命門), Xuánshū (Gv-5) (懸樞), Jízhōng (Gv-6) (脊中), Zhōngshū (Gv-7) (中樞), Jīnsuō (Gv-8) (筋縮), Zhìyáng (Gv-9) (至陽), Língtái (Gv-10) (靈台), Shéndào (Gv-11) (神道), Shēnzhù (Gv-12) (身柱), Táodào (Gv-13) (陶道), Dàzhuī (Gv-14) (大椎), Yǎmén (Gv-15) (啞門), Fēngfǔ (Gv-16) (風府), Nǎohù (Gv-17) (腦戶), Qiángjiān (Gv-18) (強間), Hòudǐng (Gv-19) (後頂), Bǎihuì (Gv-20) (百會), Qiándǐng (Gv-21) (前頂), Xìnhuì (Gv-22) (囟會), Shàngxīng (Gv-23) (上星), Shéntíng (Gv-24) (神庭), Sùliào (Gv-25) (素髎), Rénzhōng or Shuǐgōu (Gv-26) (人中、水溝), Duìduān (Gv-27) (兌端), and Kěnjiāo (Gv-28) (齦交).

3. **Discussion**

The Governing Vessel is the confluence of all the Yáng channels, over which it is said to "govern." Because it controls all the Yáng channels, it is called the "Sea of Yáng Meridians." This is apparent from its pathway because it flows on the midline of the back, a Yáng area, and in the center of all Yáng channels (except the Stomach Channel which flows in the front). The Governing Vessel governs all the Yáng channels, which means that it can be used to increase the Yáng energy of the body.

Since the Governing Vessel is the "Sea of Yáng Meridians" and it controls or governs the back, the area richest in Guardian Qì (Wèiqì, 衛氣), it is also responsible for the circulation of the body's Guardian Qì to guard against external evil intruders. The circulation of Guardian Qì starts from Fēngfǔ (Gv-16) (風府), and moves down the Governing Vessel to Huìyīn (Co-1) (會陰). It is said that it takes twenty-one days for the Guardian Qì to flow from Fēngfǔ to Huìyīn, and nine days from Huìyīn to the throat, making it a monthly cycle.

According to Chinese medical science, Guardian Qì is Yáng Qì and therefore represents the "Fire" of the body. Its quick and ubiquitous circulation keeps the fire going in the body and controls the loss of body heat. Guardian Qì is also inextricably linked with the fluids that flow outside the channels, in the skin and flesh. Consequently, through the breathing (under control of the Lungs), Guardian Qì is responsible for the opening and the closing of the pores, and also controls the sweat.

The Governing Vessel is also responsible for nourishing the five ancestral organs, which include the brain and spinal cord. This is one of the ways in which the Kidneys "control" the brain, as is said in Chinese medicine.

Because of their importance to health, the Governing Vessel and the Conception Vessel are considered the two most important Qì channels to be trained in Qìgōng, especially in Nèidān (內丹). Training related to these two vessels includes: 1. How to fill them with Qì so that you have enough to regulate the twelve channels; 2. How to open up stagnant areas in these two vessels so that the Qì flows smoothly and strongly; 3. How to effectively direct the Qì to nourish the brain and raise up the Shén; 4. How to effectively govern the Qì in the

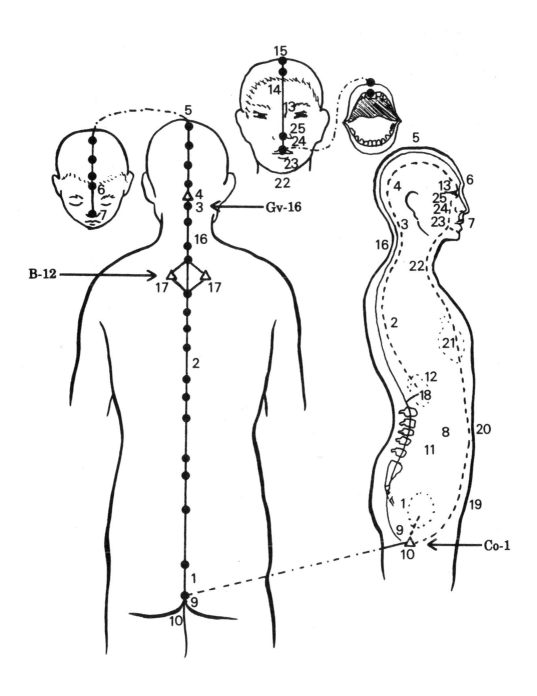

Figure 17-1. The Governing Vessel (Dūmài)

twelve channels, and nourish the organs; 5. How to use your raised Shén to lead the Guardian Qì to the skin and strengthen the Guardian Qì shield covering your body

In Nèidān Qìgōng training, when you have filled up the Qì in these two vessels and can effectively circulate the Qì in them, you have achieved the "Small Circulation." In order to do this, you must know how to convert the essence stored in the Kidneys into Qì, circulate this Qì in the Governing and Conception Vessels, and finally lead this Qì to the head to nourish the brain and Shén (spirit). If you are interested in "Small Circulation," please refer to the book: *Qìgōng Meditation—Small Circulation*, by YMAA Publication Center.

The Conception Vessel (Rènmài, 任脈) (Figure 17-2)

1. Course

   Course #1:

   (1). Lower abdomen below Qūgǔ (Co-2) (曲骨)—(2). Ascends along the midline of the abdomen and chest—(3). Crosses the throat and jaw—(4). Winds around the mouth—(5). Terminates in the region of the eye.

   Course #2:

   (6). Pelvic cavity—(7). Enters the spine and ascends along the back.

   ***This vessel intersects Chéngqì (S-1) (承泣) and Kěnjiāo (Gv-28) (齦交).

2. Cavities

   Huìyīn (Co-l) (會陰), Qūgǔ (Co-2) (曲骨), Zhōngjí (Co-3) (中極), Guānyuán (Co-4) (關元), Shímén (Co-5) (石門), Qìhǎi (Co-6) (氣海), Abdomen-Yīnjiāo (Co-7) (陰交), Shénquè (Co-8) (神闕), Shuǐfèn (Co-9) (水分), Xiàwǎn (Co-10) (下脘), Jiànlǐ (Co-11) (建里), Zhōngwǎn (Co-12) (中脘), Shàngwǎn (Co-13) (上脘), Jùquè (Co-14) (巨闕), Jiūwěi (Co-15) (鳩尾), Zhōngtíng (Co-16) (中庭), Shānzhōng (Co-17) (膻中), Yùtáng (Co-18) (玉堂), Chest-Zǐgōng (Co-19) (紫宮), Huágài (Co-20) (華蓋), Xuánjī (Co-21) (璇璣), Tiāntú (Co-22) (天突), Liánquán (Co-23) (廉泉), and Chéngjiāng (Co-24) (承漿).

3. Discussion

   "Rèn" (任) in Chinese means "direction, responsibility." Rènmài, the "Conception Vessel," has a major role in Qì circulation, directing and being responsible for all of the Yīn channels (plus the Stomach Channel). The Conception Vessel is connected to the Thrusting and Yīn Linking Vessels, and is able to increase the Yīn energy of the body.

   This vessel nourishes the uterus (one of the five ancestral organs) and the whole genital system. It is said in the *Nèijīng* (內經) that the Conception and Thrusting Vessels contain both blood and essence (Jīng), and both flow up to the face and around the mouth. They

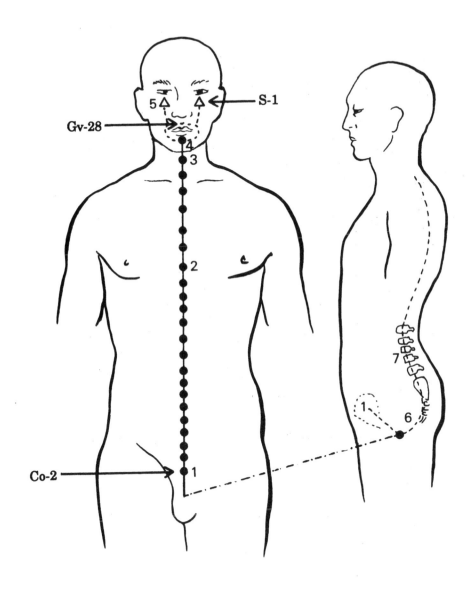

Figure 17-2. The Conception Vessel (Rènmài)

contain more blood than essence in men, and thus promote the growth of the beard and body hair. Because women lose blood with their menstruation, they contain proportionately less blood and hence, no beard or body hair.

It was described in the *Sùwèn* (素問) that both the Conception and Thrusting Vessels control the life cycles every seven years for women and every eight years for men. It is the changes taking place in these vessels at those intervals that promote the major alterations in our lives.

In addition, the Conception Vessel also controls the distribution and "dispersion" of Guardian Qì all over the abdomen and thorax via numerous small Qì branches (Luò, 絡). This vessel also plays an important role in the distribution of body fluids in the abdomen.

In Qìgōng society, this vessel and the Governing Vessel are considered the most important among the Qì channels and vessels, and must be trained first. It is believed that there is usually no significant Qì stagnation in the Conception Vessel. However, it is important to increase the amount of Qì you are able to store, which also increases your ability to regulate the Yīn channels.

The Thrusting Vessel (Chōngmài, 衝脈) (Figure 17-3)

1. Course

   Course #1:

   (1). Lower abdomen—(2). Emerges along the Path of Qì—(3). Tracks the course of the Kidney Channel—(4). Ascends through the abdomen—(5). Skirts the navel—(6). Disperses in the chest.

   Course #2:

   (6). Chest—(7). Ascends across the throat—(8). Face—(9). Nasal cavity.

   Course #3:

   (1). Lower abdomen—(10). Below the Kidney—(11). Emerges along the Path of Qì—(12). Descends along the medial aspect of the thigh—(13). Popliteal fossa—(14). Medial margin of the tibia and the posterior aspect of the medial malleolus—(15). Bottom of the foot.

   Course #4:

   (16). Tibia—(17). Toward the lateral margin of the bone—(18). Enters the heel—(19). Crosses the tarsal bones of the foot—(20). Big toe.

   Course #5:

   (21). Pelvic cavity—(22). Enter the spine and circulates through the back.

***This vessel intersects Huìyīn (Co-l) (會陰), Yīnjiāo (Co-7) (陰交), Qìchōng (S-30) (氣

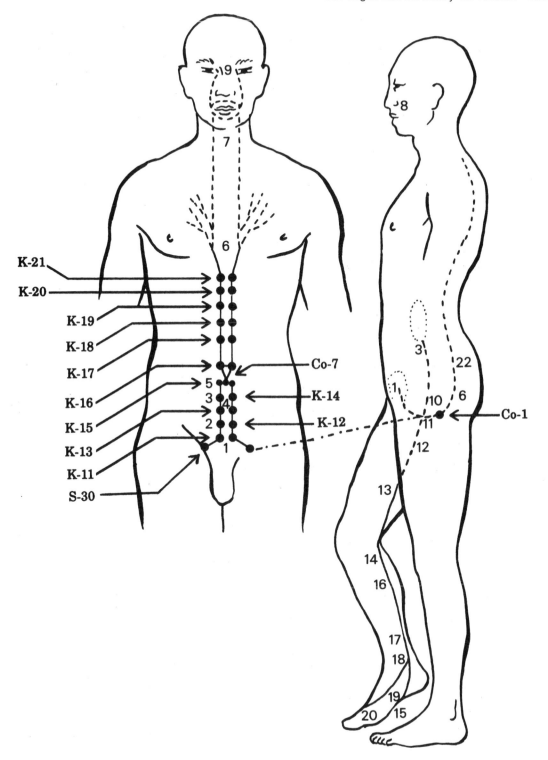

Figure 17-3. The Thrusting Vessel (Chōngmài)

衝), Hénggǔ (K-11) (橫骨), Dàhè (K-12) (大赫), Qìxuè (K-13) (氣穴), Sìmǎn (K-14) (四滿), Abdomen-Zhōngzhù (K-15) (中注), Huāngshū (K-16) (肓俞), Shāngqū (K-17) (商曲), Shíguān (K-18) (石關), Yīndū (K-19) (陰都), Abdomen-Tōnggǔ (K-20) (腹通谷), and Yōumén (K-21) (幽門).

2. Discussion

One of the major purposes of the Thrusting Vessel is to connect, to communicate, and to mutually support the Conception Vessel. Because of this mutual Qì support, both can effectively regulate the Qì in the Kidney Channel. The Kidneys are the residence of Original Qì and are considered one of the most vital Yīn organs.

The Thrusting Vessel is considered one of the most important and decisive vessels in successful Qìgōng training, especially in Marrow/Brain Washing. There are many reason for this. The first reason is that this vessel intersects two cavities on the Conception Vessel: Huìyīn (Co-1) (會陰) and Yīnjiāo (Co-7) (陰交). Huìyīn means "meeting with Yīn" and is the cavity where the Yáng and Yīn Qì is transferred. Yīnjiāo means "Yīn junction" and is the cavity where the Original Qì (Water Qì, or Yīn Qì) interfaces with the Fire Qì created from food and air. The Thrusting Vessel also connects with eleven cavities on the Kidney Channel. The Kidney is considered the residence of Original Essence (Yuánjīng, 元精), which is converted into Original Qì (Yuánqì, 元氣).

The second reason for the importance of the Thrusting Vessel in Qìgōng training is that this vessel is connected directly to the spinal cord and reaches up to the brain. The major goal of Marrow/Brain Washing Qìgōng is to lead the Qì into the spinal cord and then further on to the head, nourishing the brain and spirit (Shén).

And finally, the third reason is found in actual Qìgōng practice. There are three common training paths: Fire, Wind, and Water. In Fire path Qìgōng, the emphasis is on the Fire or Yáng Qì circulating in the Governing Vessel and therefore strengthening the muscles and organs. The Fire path is the main Qì training in Muscle/Tendon Changing (Yìjīnjīng, 易筋經) Qìgōng. However, the Fire path can also cause the body to become too Yáng, and therefore speed up the process of degeneration. In order to adjust the Fire to a proper level, Marrow/Brain Washing (Xǐsuǐjīng, 洗髓經) Qìgōng is also trained. This uses the Water Path, in which Qì separates from the route of the Fire Path at the Huìyīn cavity (Co-1) (會陰), enters the spinal cord, and finally reaches up to the head. The Water Path teaches how to use Original Qì to cool down the body, and then to use this Qì to nourish the brain and train the spirit. Learning to adjust the Fire and Water Qì circulation in the body is called Kǎn-Lí (坎-離), which means Water-Fire. You can see from this that the Thrusting Vessel plays a very important role in Qìgōng training.

The Girdle Vessel (Dàimài, 帶脈) (Figure 17-4)

1. Course

  (1). Below the hypochondrium at the level of the 2nd lumbar vertebra—(2). Turns downward and encircles the body at the waist like a girdle.

***This vessel intersects Dàimài (GB-26) (帶脈), Wǔshū (GB-27) (五樞), and Wéidào (GB-28) (維道).

2. **Discussion**

The major purpose of the Girdle Vessel is to regulate the Qì of the Gall Bladder. It is also responsible for the Qì's horizontal balance. If you have lost this balance, you will have lost your center and balance both mentally and physically.

From the point of view of Qìgōng, the Girdle Vessel is also responsible for the strength of the waist area. When Qì is full and circulating smoothly, back pain will be avoided. In addition, because the Kidneys are located nearby, this vessel is also responsible for Qì circulation around the Kidneys, maintaining the Kidneys' health. Most important of all for the Girdle Vessel is the fact that the Lower Dāntián is located in its area. In order to lead Original Qì from the Kidneys to the Lower Dāntián, the waist area must be healthy and relaxed. This means that the Qì flow in the waist area must be smooth. The training of the Girdle Vessel is discussed in the book: *The Essence of Shàolín White Crane*, available from YMAA Publication Center.

The Yáng Heel Vessel (Yángqiāomài, 陽蹻脈) (Figure 17-5)

1. **Course**

(1). Below the lateral malleolus at Shēnmài (B-62) (申脈)—(2). Ascends along the lateral aspect of the leg—(3). Posterior aspect of the hypochondrium—(4). Lateral side of the shoulder—(5). Traverses the neck—(6). Passes beside the mouth—(7). Inner canthus (joins the Yīn Heel Vessel and the Urinary Bladder Channel)—(8). Ascends across the forehead—(9). Winds behind the ear to Fēngchí (GB-20) (風池)—(10). Enters the brain at Fēngfǔ (Gv-16) (風府).

***This vessel intersects Shēnmài (B-62) (申脈), Púshēn (B-61) (僕參), Fūyáng (B-59) (跗陽), Jīngmíng (B-1) (睛明), Jūliào (GB-29) (居髎), Fēngchí (GB-20) (風池), Nàoshū (SI-10) (臑俞), Jùgǔ (LI-16) (巨骨), Jiānyú (LI-15) (肩髃), Dìcāng (S-4) (地倉), Jùliào (S-3) (巨髎), Chéngqì (S-l) (承泣), and Fēngfǔ (Gv-16) (風府).

2. **Discussion**

While the preceding four vessels (Governing, Conception, Thrusting, and Girdle) are located in the trunk, this and the next three are located in the trunk and legs. (In addition, each of these four vessels is paired.) For millions of years, man has been walking on his legs, which do much more strenuous work than the arms. I believe that because of this, as evolution proceeded, the legs gradually developed these vessels for Qì storage and supply. If this is true, it may be that as time goes on and man uses his legs less and less, in a few million years these vessels will gradually disappear.

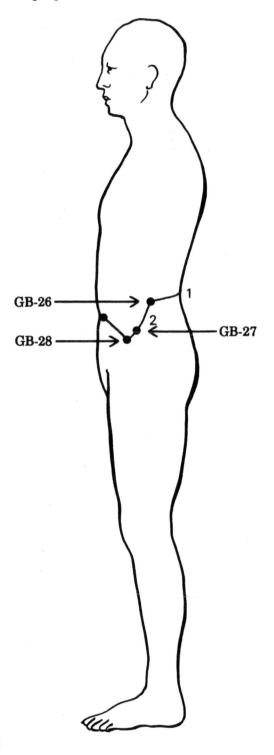

Figure 17-4. The Girdle Vessel (Dàimài)

You can see from the way that the Yáng Heel Vessel intersect with other Qì channels that it regulates the Yáng channels, such as the Urinary Bladder, the Gall Bladder, the Small Intestine, and the Large Intestine. The Yáng Heel Vessel is also connected with the Governing Vessel. The Qì filling this vessel is supplied mainly through exercising the legs, which converts the food essence or fat stored in the legs. This Qì is then led upward to nourish the Yáng channels. It is believed in Qìgōng that, since this vessel is also connected with your brain, certain leg exercises can be used to cure headaches. Since a headache is caused by excess Qì in the head, exercising the legs will draw this Qì downward to the leg muscles and relieve the pressure in the head.

Most of the training that relates to this vessel is Wàidān (外丹). Wàidān Qìgōng is considered Yáng, and specializes in training the Yáng channels, while Nèidān (內丹) Qìgōng is considered relatively Yīn and emphasizes the Yīn channel more.

The Yīn Heel Vessel (Yīnqiāomài, 陰蹺脈) (Figure 17-5)

1. **Course**

    (1). Zhàohǎi (K-6) (照海) below the medial malleolus—(2). Extends upward along the medial aspect of the leg—(3). Crossing the perineum and chest entering the supraclavicular fossa—(4). Ascends through the throat and emerges in front of Rényíng (S-9) (人迎)—(5). Traverses the medial aspect of the cheek—(6). Inner canthus (joins the Urinary Bladder Channel and Yáng Heel Vessels)—(7). Ascends over the head and into the brain.

    ***This vessel intersects Zhàohǎi (K-6) (照海), Jiāoxìn (K-8) (交信), and Jīngmín (B-1) (睛明).

2. **Discussion**

The Yīn Heel Vessel is connected with two cavities of the Kidney Channel. Therefore, one of the major sources of Qì for this vessel is the conversion of the Kidney Essence into Qì. It is believed in Qìgōng society that the other major Qì source is the essence of the external Kidneys (testicles). In Marrow/Brain Washing (Xǐsuǐjīng, 洗髓經) Qìgōng, one of the training processes is to stimulate the testicles in order to increase the hormone production and increase the conversion of the essence into Qì. At the same time, you would learn how to lead the Qì in this vessel up to the head to nourish the brain and spirit (Shén). With this nourishment, you would be able to reach Buddhahood or enlightenment. From a health and longevity point of view, the raised spirit will be able to efficiently direct the Qì of the entire body and maintain your health.

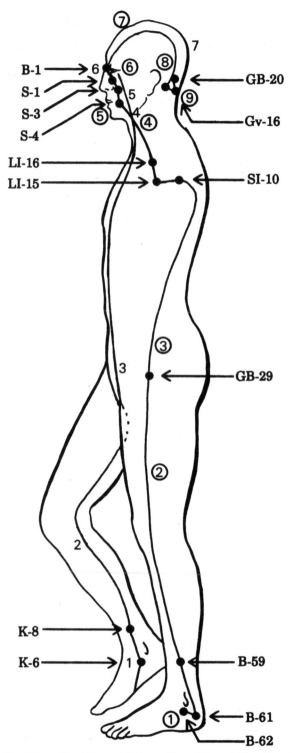

B-1
S-1
S-3
S-4
LI-16
LI-15

GB-20
Gv-16
SI-10

GB-29

K-8
K-6

B-59

B-61
B-62

Figure 17-5. The Yáng Heel Vessel (Yángqiāomài) and The Yīn Heel Vessel (Yīnqiāomài)

The Yáng Linking Vessel (Yángwéimài, 陽維脈) (Figure 17-6)

1. Course

(1). Jīnmén (B-63) (金門) on the heel—(2). Ascends along the lateral aspect of the leg—(3). Lower abdomen—(4). Slants upward across the posterior aspect of the hypochondrium—(5). Across the posterior axillary fold to the shoulder—(6). Ascends the neck and crosses behind the ear—(7). Proceeds to the forehead—(8). Doubles back over the head—(9). Fēngfǔ (Gv-16) (風府).

***This vessel intersects Jīnmén (B-63) (金門), Yángjiāo (GB-35) (陽交), Jiānjǐng (GB-21) (肩井), Fēngchí (GB-20) (風池),

Nǎokōng (GB-19) (腦空), Chénglíng (GB-18) (承靈), Zhèngyíng (GB-17) (正營), Mùchuāng (GB-16) (目窗), Head-Línqì (GB-15) (頭臨泣), Yángbái (GB-14) (陽白), Běnshén (GB-13) (本神), Tiānliào (TB-15) (天髎), Nàoshū (SI-10) (臑俞), Yǎmén (Gv-15) (啞門), Fēngfǔ (Gv-16) (風府), and Tóuwéi (S-8) (頭維).

2. Discussion

The Yáng Linking Vessel regulates the Qì mainly in the Yáng channels: the Urinary Bladder, Gall Bladder, Triple Burner, Small Intestine, and Stomach Channels. It is also connected with the Governing Vessel at Yǎmén (Gv-15) (啞門) and Fēngfǔ (Gv-16) (風府). This vessel and the Yáng Heel Vessel have not been emphasized much in Qìgōng, except in Iron Shirt training where these two and the Governing Vessel are trained.

The Yīn Linking Vessel (Yīnwéimài, 陰維脈) (Figure 17-6)

1. Course

(1). Lower leg at Zhúbīn (K-9) (築賓)—(2). Ascending along the medial aspect of the leg—(3). Enters the lower abdomen—(4). Upward across the chest—(5). Throat (meets Tiāntú (Co-22) (天突) and Liánquán (Co-23) (廉泉).

***This vessel intersects Zhúbīn (K-9) (築賓), Chōngmén (Sp-12) (衝門), Fǔshě (Sp-13) (府舍), Dàhéng (Sp-15) (大橫), Fùāi (Sp-16) (腹哀), Qīmén (Li-14) (期門), Tiāntú (Co-22) (天突), and Liánquán (Co-23) (廉泉).

2. Discussion

The Yīn Linking Vessel has connections with the Kidney, Spleen, and Liver Yīn channels. The Yīn Linking Vessel also communicates with the Conception Vessel at two cavities. This vessel is not trained much in Qìgōng.

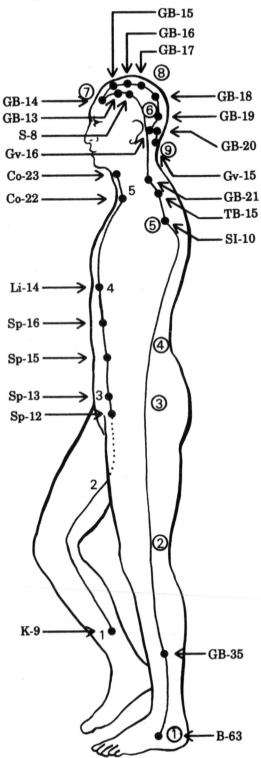

GB-15
GB-16
GB-17
⑧
GB-14
GB-13
S-8
Gv-16
Co-23
Co-22
⑦
⑥
GB-18
GB-19
GB-20
⑨
Gv-15
GB-21
TB-15
⑤
SI-10
5
Li-14 — 4
Sp-16
Sp-15
④
Sp-13 — 3
Sp-12
③
2
②
K-9 — 1
GB-35
① — B-63

Figure 17-6. The Yáng Linking Vessel (Yángwéimài) and the Yīn Linking Vessel (Yīnwéimài)

PART FOUR

Conclusion

CHAPTER 18

One Hundred and One Questions

Because many of the Qìgōng practices have been kept secret in the past, many theories and methods have been passed down randomly. Only in the last twenty years have most of these secrets been revealed to the general public. Finally, interested practitioners have the opportunity to learn the secrets of other styles. Even so, because of the long years of secrecy, many of the documents that are available to us remain incomplete or unconfirmed. To compile all of these documents and finalize a systematic summary of theoretical explanations is very difficult. During the course of my study and research, many questions and answers have arisen. Some answers seem accurate but need further verification through modern technology. Some of the questions are beyond any test which can be done with modern scientific equipment.

In addition, you should understand that since most Qìgōng was created in an ancient time, and with different cultural foundations than our society, many new situations must be considered and studied. For example, human beings never had the opportunity to travel from one side of the world to the other in twelve hours until very recently. What happens to the Qì circulation in a human body after such a trip? How is the Qì circulation affected by the inverted schedule of a night shift worker? How does the gasoline exhaust produced by automobiles affect the Qì circulation? How do nuclear experiments affect the natural Qì balance? How do radio waves influence the body's Qì circulation?

Many other questions have been generated as we recognize the affect of the Earth's magnetic field on our bodies' energy. When you meditate on the North Pole it will be different from meditating on the South Pole. Since most traditional Qìgōng and meditating methods were developed in the Northern Hemisphere of the earth, can the people living in the Southern Hemisphere use the same theory and methods to obtain the same results, or must we modify the methods and theory?

These questions keep appearing in my mind. Some questions may be due to my limited understanding of Qìgōng training, while others are generated from advances in modern science. I believe that during the course of my continuing research, over the rest of my life, many of these questions will be answered. I also hope that I will obtain some of the answers from other experienced Qìgōng masters. Many of the questions need to be tested or proven through experimentation involving modern equipment. These questions will be answered when a thorough scientific study is conducted. Some of the questions may remain mysteries, since I firmly believe that nobody is able to reach the level of Qìgōng practice attained by earlier masters.

The following are some of the questions I have had. I hope that you will keep these questions or any question you might have in your mind during the course of your study, so that one day you will come to realize that you know much more than anybody else.

About Essence

1. How is Original Essence stored in the Kidneys? Chinese medicine and Qìgōng society tell us that a person's Original Essence is stored in the Kidneys. How is it stored?

2. Why is Original Essence stored in the Kidneys instead of other organs? We need a theoretical explanation and experimental proof for this.

3. If Original Essence is stored in the Kidneys, then what about those people who have only one Kidney? Will the person with only one Kidney die earlier? Will the Original Essence stored in the single Kidney be enough for life? Will the Original Essence-Qì conversion be reduced?

4. How can we tell a person whose Original Essence is strong from someone whose is weak? Normally, it was judged from the spirit of vitality and the state of health of a person, but there is no standard for this. Is there any scientific way of judging this?

5. Can we see Original Essence? Is it material? Is it the source of hormones? Can we see it in a dead body?

6. Is Original Essence the genes or hormones? Judging from descriptions in many sources, I am led to believe that the genes and hormones might be what the ancient Chinese called "Original Essence," or at least be closely related.

7. Can the quantity of the Original Essence be increased and the quality improved through modern technology?

About Qì and Bioenergy

1. Is the traditional concept of human Qì the same as bioelectromagnetic energy, or is it a mixture of a number of types of energy? Many Qìgōng practitioners are not completely convinced that Human Qì is merely a bioelectromagnetic energy circulating in the body. Many Qìgōng phenomena cannot be explained satisfactorily by bioelectromagnetic science. For example, how can a Qìgōng master hold a burning coal in his hand without being burned?

2. How do we standardize the measurement of Qì level? A unit system is necessary. Many different types of equipment have been designed to measure the Qì level in terms of heat (infrared), temperature rise, and electricity. Since Human Qì has not been defined, there is no specific equipment which we are convinced is the most accurate method for measuring Qì. However, if it is proven that Qì is human

electromagnetic energy, then we will be able to use an electric unit system to define the level of Qì.

3. Since the general definition of Qì is universal energy, how do we relate all kinds of different energy into one, if it is possible? To me, there is no absolute way to relate them. You cannot use the unit system which is used for measuring heat to measure electricity. Therefore, it may be more feasible to add an extra word in front of Qì to distinguish them, for example "heat Qì" or "electric Qì."

4. When Qì is transferred from one person to another, what, other than heat and bioelectricity, is transferred? I have often wondered how one person can be more effective in transferring his Qì than another person. There must be some extra power which is transferred to the patient emotionally to help the patient himself build up an EMF and cure himself internally. What is this power—brain wave, emotional touch, or self-confidence buildup?

5. Why was the character for the Chinese word Qì changed? Was this change caused by confusion due to similar pronunciation? Many times it is found that ancient words are confused with other words because their pronunciation is similar. Since most Chinese people could neither write nor read, this idea seems plausible. If it was so, how could those Qìgōng experts or medical doctors let it happen? Or was it changed purposely in order to distinguish Human Qì (Chinese word meaning "no fire") from other natural energies? I cannot find any document which explains this difference satisfactorily.

6. Why has the character for "air" supplanted the ancient word for Qì (which meant "no fire")? The character meaning "air" is commonly used by the Chinese as a general term for different kinds of energy. This has confused me from the beginning of my Qìgōng practice. One of the most plausible explanations is the following: Air or oxygen (called Kōngqì) does not change its form when it is taken into the body and delivered to the cells to be converted through biochemical reaction into carbon dioxide. On the other hand, the food essence must be converted into a form of bioenergy before it can be absorbed by the body. Is it why the "air" Qì is used to represent energy?

7. What is the scientific explanation for the halo around the head, or the glow around the body, of a meditator? Though I try to explain these phenomena as air de-ionization generated by the body's electrical charge, an experiment needs to be conducted to determine whether this is true.

8. How can Qì be used to bounce someone away with only a touch? We have heard in the Chinese martial arts that a very good Qìgōng master is able to bounce (or shock) an enemy away with a simple touch. When someone touches a high voltage wire, his body reacts instinctively to protect him, and bounces him away. The wire does not exert any physical power. Is this what happens with the Qìgōng master? Does

he pass electricity into the other person's heart so that his body bounces him away instinctively?

9. How exactly does Qì nourish the blood, nerves, and cells?

10. If Qì is bioelectricity, how can we use modern technology to increase bioelectric circulation in the body and reach the same goals as the Qìgōng practices which allow us to obtain health, longevity and spiritual enlightenment? It was not possible to generate electrical and magnetic fields in ancient times; however, it is very easy to create them today. We should be able to find a way to use external electrical or magnetic fields to increase the circulation, correct the level of Qì, and keep the marrow clean. Naturally, caution is always the first consideration. We do not know yet how this modern technology will affect us. It may produce adverse reactions. How can a field which is created through external processes duplicate the mental calmness necessary for enlightenment? Even if the circulation can be opened, will not attachment to the world inhibit clarity of focus? Won't there then be the danger of people who are exceptionally powerful physically who do not have the discipline to control their power? It will be necessary to do research on a very wide scale.

11. How do clouds and fog affect the Qì circulation in the body? We know that low clouds are able to generate an electric field which affects the human energy field. Does fog do this as well? When you are in fog, do the charges surround you uniformly? Can this affect your Qì circulation?

About Spirit (Shén)

1. When does the spirit start in a baby? How do we know if a baby has spirit or not, and how do we determine when it first has spirit? Does it have spirit before birth, or only after it is separated from its mother?

2. How is spirit generated in a newly born baby? Where does spirit originate? Does it start when a baby starts to think? Does it exist only in humans?

3. What are the differences between the spirit and the soul? Since there is no exact translation from Chinese into English, I will need the exact difference and definition of these words.

4. Can the spirit and soul exist even if there is no physical life form? It is believed in the Chinese religions that the spirit and soul can exist even after death. Are spirit and soul an energy form? Are they part of the non-human natural energy, or are they the residues of human energy?

5. How do we define spirit (Shén) and mind? The relationship between the Shén and the mind is very confusing. Is Shén generated from mind? If Shén must be generated from mind, then can Shén exist after physical death? If Shén can exist after death, does this Shén have a mind and can it think independently? How do they relate to brain waves? Can Shén be measured?

6. How do we generate a "spiritual baby Shén" in Qìgōng training? In Qìgōng, in order to reach the final goal of enlightenment you must train yourself until you have given birth to a baby Shén. Only when this baby has grown to be independent will your spirit not die, but live forever. Is this true? Scientifically, how can this happen? Can we use modern science to explain this, or is it still beyond what today's science can grasp? If we believe that a highly cultivated mind is able to speed up the process of evolution, then this mind may be able to reach many other things which are still beyond human understanding. The science we understand is still in the infant stage. Remember, we cannot use today's science to gauge the potential of science.

7. Does a newborn child need an already-existing spirit? Some religions say that a newborn baby does in order to form a complete human. If so, where does this spirit come from? From the people who died before? If a newborn baby needs this pre-existing spirit, then how does the population keep increasing? Where do the new spirits originate? Do they come from the sun, or universal energy? Could spirits from other planets immigrate to the earth and be born into human bodies?

8. Is there another dimension which we cannot usually see, but, when the time is right, we are able to touch? There are many accounts of very sick or dying people being able to see or sense the same kind of new world. Is this a spirit world? Is this a new dimension which we cannot see until the time is right? How do we reach this dimension from the scientific standpoint?

9. Does spirit make its own decisions or is it affected by natural Qì? Can a spirit think? How can it help a person who is alive? Through brain wave communication? Or is a spirit only some human energy residue roaming around in the energy world and being affected by surrounding energy forces?

10. Do the spirits of enlightened people who have died continue to exist? If so, can these spirits help the living? Remember if your answer is yes, you have agreed that the spirit and soul can exist even after your death. When you pray, do you actually receive help from God or the spirits of the dead, or are you helping yourself by building your self-confidence?

11. Can a highly concentrated mind make an object move without touching it? What is the theory behind this phenomenon? We have heard of people who are able to move things through thinking. If this is true, then how can brain wave energy become so strong that it can do this? Are miracles done with brain waves?

12. Can the spirit really leave a living body and travel, or is it only that the brain waves sense something and match its frequency so that you can be aware of it? Also, we have heard that when someone is hypnotized, he is able to sense many things which are beyond his capability while he is in a normal state of consciousness. Is this similar to what happens when a person seems to leave his body during meditation?

13. When someone is able to communicate with animals, is this brain wave correspondence? I once saw a woman on a live TV show who seemed to be able to communicate with all kinds of dogs. The information she learned was verified by the owners. If this was real, was it brain wave communication? Do the brains of animals and man function on the same frequency band, or do the bands just partially overlap?

14. Can one person affect another person's thinking through brain wave correspondence?

15. CÀnmódern technology create an electromagnetic wave whose wavelength is close to or equivalent to the human brain wave? Our technology seems to have already progressed that far. If this is so, will a brain wave machine be able to generate a wave which will affect your thinking and judgment? This would truly be "brainwashing." Will the wars of the future be wars of brain wave machines?

16. If it is possible to make a brain wave machine, can we determine what frequencies are associated with crime and then somehow block those frequencies? Is it possible to really brainwash criminals? Of course, if such a machine fell into the hands of criminals, they would have a powerful tool for evil. Can we accept the moral responsibility for changing an individual's brain wave?

17. Can a good Qìgōng meditator avoid being controlled and affected by a brain wave machine? Personally, I believe that a Qìgōng practitioner who has reached the stage of regulating his mind effectively would be able to avoid the effects of a brain wave machine. However, how long would he be able to do this?

18. What is the width of the brain wave band? What existing materials can shield them out? Metal is usually a good insulator against radio waves, but can it also keep out brain waves? If not, is there any material which can be used to shield against brain waves?

19. What is the relationship between spirit (Shén) and brain waves? I personally believe that when your Shén is high, your brain waves will be stronger and, probably, more focused. Is this true?

About Channels, Vessels, and Cavities

1. In ancient times, how did they find out about and locate Qì channels, vessels, and cavities? There is no record of how those ancient Chinese doctors discovered this. How did they find them with such accuracy? How did they learn how to use them to cure illness?

2. How do plugged up channels interfere with the Qì flow? This is a simple question, but the answer is not easy. It will take the most advanced technology to find out exactly how the Qì channels are plugged up. Is it caused by an accumulation of fat which significantly reduces the tissue's electric conductivity, or simply by some defect in the body's electrically conductive tissues?

3. How do the channels conduct Qì? How many stimuli can make the Qì move? If Qì is a bioelectric energy, then the question is: how many EMF's are there which can make the energy move, and where are they?

4. How do the vessels store qì? If Qì is bioelectric energy, then is a Qì vessel like a battery or a capacitor which is able to store and release energy when necessary?

5. What do the Qì channels and vessels actually look like? So far, no one has been able to show an accurate drawing. However, if they are areas where the electrical conductivity is different than elsewhere, then we should be able to conduct experiments to find out just how the Qì channels and vessels are shaped.

6. How can we design a highly sensitive machine to accurately locate all of these Qì channels and cavities? This would be very helpful for acupuncture practice.

7. Why are there four vessels on the legs and none on the arms? Is it because people use their legs more than their arms? I believe that the vessels in the legs evolved to supply extra Qì to the legs and regulate it more efficiently.

8. Are there any other vessels which have not been discovered? It is possible that there are other, smaller vessels in the body which have not been discovered yet. For example, I believe that there should be vessels in the arms, since people use their arms a lot.

9. What is the actual meaning of opening a channel (commonly called "opening the gate") in Qìgōng practice? What actually happens? Is it that the channel recovers its electrical conductivity? What is the best way to do this?

10. Can we use modern bioelectric technologies to open the channels and increase the smoothness of the Qì circulation?

11. Can we use modern bioelectric technology to fill up the Qì reservoirs? If the vessels are bioelectric capacitors, then we might be able to use external electrical or magnetic methods to refill them. We would then have enough Qì to nourish the whole body, and slow down the aging process significantly.

12. What actually happens when an experienced Qìgōng master helps a student open his channels? Does the master really use his Qì (electricity) and transport it into the student's body to do the job, or does the master only offer some stimulation and confidence to the student, and in fact, does a student open them by himself? Both are possible.

13. Exactly what are cavities? Do all of the cavities have higher electric conductivity or do they differ in capacity? Is increased electrical conductivity the only criteria for locating cavities, or did the ancients have other criteria in addition to this?

14. Why are there cavities? Is the purpose of cavities to circulate Qì to the surface of the skin to nourish it, and to regulate the Qì channels? Are there any other purposes other than these?

15. What does acupuncture actually do to correct the Qì? We need a more complete explanation through modern experimentation and scientific study.

272 The Root of Chinese Qìgōng

About Mutual Qì Nourishment

1. According to Qìgōng documents, two people can practice together to balance their Qì through mutual Qì nourishment. The person with the stronger Qì lowers his Qì volume while the weaker one gains Qì. Two people with weak Qì can help each other build up their Qì. In this kind of mutual Qì nourishment, both persons must be able to coordinate with each other in every aspect—especially in breathing. Emotionally, they must be willing to share with each other. In this kind of practice, must love get involved? If not, how are you able to touch and share Qì with each other? If the answer is "Yes," isn't it against the principle of meditation that the mind should be simple, calm, and peaceful, with no emotional disturbance?

2. When two people practice mutual Qì nourishment, do they actually share Qì, or do they stimulate each other's minds to enhance the brain's EMF and thereby increase their own Qì circulation, or both?

3. From the Qìgōng point of view, love is a natural way of causing mutual Qì nourishment. A person who loves someone can help him recover from illness. Can this be considered a form of Qìgōng?

4. Is sexual activity the ultimate natural way of mutual Qì nourishment? Sex is a natural human desire. Through regular sexual activity, a person is able to obtain mental calmness and peace, and release the pressure generated by emotional disturbance. Can this be considered a form of Qìgōng practice?

5. When the male ejaculates during sex, he loses Qì to the female. How does this happen? Is this why women live longer? If the female has reached a higher level of Qìgōng, can the male receive the Qì instead of losing it?

6. Exactly how is essence and Qì lost during ejaculation? In certain Qìgōng practices, men are taught how to avoid ejaculation. How is Qì transmitted under such circumstances?

7. If sex is considered beneficial for Qìgōng practice, why did all of the Buddhist monks and many of the Daoists hide in the mountains and avoid sexual contact? Is this because they were afraid that sex and love would destroy the calm and peaceful mind they were cultivating?

8. Why did the Daoists develop so many techniques which used sexual activity for Qì nourishment? Could these techniques have been studied by those Daoists whose minds could not be calm? Or did they want, on the one hand to reach enlightenment, and the other hand to enjoy a natural, normal human life?

9. There are no documents that discuss exchanging Qì with animals, such as dogs and cats. Can a person obtain Qì from animals? Theoretically, it should be possible. It has been found that cats have high Qì levels, which enable them to help older men and women maintain their Qì level. Can ways be developed to help older people through this?

About Health and Longevity

1. Can we use external electric or magnetic stimulation to cure sicknesses in the same way that Qìgōng and acupuncture do? Perhaps the process can be duplicated by using external electric or magnetic stimulation to increase or reinstate the normal bioelectric circulation. Qìgōng has cured many kinds of cancer. Can the equivalent be achieved with modern electric and magnetic technologies?

2. Can the immune system be strengthened through electric and magnetic stimulation to cure AIDS and cancer? It is believed that the immune system is related closely to the body's bioenergy system. Can we increase the EMF of the brain and strengthen the bioenergy circulation in the body?

3. Is it dangerous to use electricity and magnetism in acupuncture when we do not understand Qì science completely? So far, there is no conclusive or theoretical report about the use of electricity and magnetism in acupuncture, even though they are being widely used. Is it safe for general practice, or do we need more research?

4. Is practicing Qìgōng to obtain a longer life the correct goal? I believe that if someone really wants to have a much longer life, he must separate himself from human society to avoid emotional disturbance. However, when he does this he loses the meaning of human life. I believe that the correct purpose of the Qìgōng practice is to obtain a healthy physical and mental body while you are still able to experience life. You will extend your life span somewhat because you are healthy, and you will still be able to experience human life.

5. What is the meaning of life? Can Qìgōng help you understand it? Does a long life meÀnmóre to you than a happy life? If you want to have both, what should you do? Qìgōng practice has helped me understand myself, nature, and what I was, am, and will be. It has stopped my wondering and confusion. How about you? Are you expecting the same thing?

6. Can we use modern technology to reach the same goal as marrow washing training and obtain a longer life without giving up our emotional feelings? I feel certain that once we understand exactly how marrow washing Qìgōng training works, we will be able to use modern technology to quickly reach the same goal.

About Qì and Modern Living

1. Can we use ice to maintain the body's Qì balance during the summer? It was not possible to research this before refrigerators were invented. In the summertime, when the Heart is on fire, can we place a piece of ice on the center of the palm to cool the Heart, or will the ice quench the Heart fire too quickly and cause problems? How about if we use alcohol instead of ice?

2. How does being on the night shift affect a person's Qì circulation? In ancient times, few people worked at night, so there are no documents available today which discuss this. Since the time of day has to be taken into account when giving acupuncture treatments, will being on the night shift affect the treatment?
3. How is Qì circulation affected when you travel several time zones in a short period of time? Does jet lag indicate that the body's Qì is disturbed?

About the Human Magnetic Field

1. Theoretically, there are two magnetic poles formed in the human body by the Earth's magnetic field. Do these two poles reverse when you move from the Northern Hemisphere to the Southern Hemisphere?
2. The Earth's magnetic field starts at the South Magnetic Pole and goes to the North Magnetic Pole. Since the human's south magnetic pole seems to be on the head if one is on the Northern Hemisphere, does this mean that his brain constantly receives energy nourishment? If the human magnetic poles are reversed in the Southern Hemisphere, does this mean that the brains of people there constantly lose nourishment?
3. Does this explain why the most highly developed technology has been created in the Northern Hemisphere?
4. If people in the Southern Hemisphere have their south magnetic poles in the abdomen, do they have more Lower Dāntián energy, and does this help them live longer?
5. When people are sick, can they speed their recovery by flying to the equator, where the effect of the Earth's magnetic field is minimized? I believe that many human sicknesses are caused, or worsened, by disturbances in the body's electromagnetic field. The energy of the Earth can worsen the situation, since your body has lost its natural balance. Can you remove this hindrance to your recovery by moving to the Equator?
6. We are surrounded by energy fields, both natural and man-made. Can we insulate a room against them to help people convalesce? Would this also be a good place to meditate?

Others

1. Are there specific spots on the Earth where the natural energy is especially beneficial for Qìgōng? Many Qìgōng practitioners believe that there are places where Heaven or Earth Qì is able to nourish your Qì and speed up your training. Is this true? Would these areas be good for hospitals?
2. What happens when we are exposed to a strong electric or magnetic field for a long time? How does this affect the body? Can it possibly energize our vital force and improve our health?

3. Since ancient times, Qìgōng practitioners have claimed that there is a Qìgōng practice which can make their bodies light. Is this true? Is this beyond a modern, scientific explanation?

4. Some people can hold a piece of burning charcoal in their hands, or walk barefoot on a bed of glowing coals. How is this done?

5. The Chinese people have been using jade to regulate Qì in their bodies or absorb excess Qì for generations. Has this ever been investigated scientifically?

6. Can we use electrical technology to increase the Qì on the head to prevent hair loss or increase hair growth?

7. Meditators talk about absorbing energy from the Earth through the feet. Is this different from magnetic energy?

8. Can a highly trained Qìgōng practitioner predict the future, or is this simply a matter of judgment, combined with experience and wisdom? It is often said that some Qìgōng masters are able to read your mind and even predict your future. I believe that it is possible to read minds through brain wave correspondence. However, predicting the future requires more than this. Intelligence and wisdom are needed, and a lot of experience. A person's personality is the main cause of success, and it can be read in his face and even in his palms. Is this how the future is read, or is there another way?

9. How does the material your clothing is made of affect your health? Natural materials such as cotton and wool dissipate some of your energy to the surrounding environment. Most man-made materials generate a Qì (or electric) shield which does not allow your Qì to communicate with nature. This affects your body's electromagnetic field and perhaps even disturbs your Qì circulation. This needs to be investigated.

10. How does the weather affect our moods? Moods may be caused by the electric fields generated between low clouds and the ground. These strong, natural, electric fields will affect your body's electromagnetic field, and may cause sickness or emotional disturbance.

11. Is there a way to energize the muscles to a higher level via external electric or magnetic stimulation, or must we rely on traditional practices? If it is possible, would it be fair in competitive sports such as boxing or football? Is the way in which body builders use electrical stimulation of the muscles safe?

12. Is there any danger involved in these experiments? We don't understand the human body very well, and we are such delicate and complicated animals. Naturally, many of the experiments can be performed on other animals first. However, since the inner energy field is closely related to emotions, it is probable that most of the experiments need to be conducted directly on humans.

13. Why do many Daoist Qìgōng practitioners hide themselves in caves for their cultivation? Is it because a cave is able to isolate the individual from external energy disturbances (magnetic fields or ions in the clouds)?

CHAPTER 19

Conclusion

You can see that in order to maintain your health and slow down the aging process, you must keep your twelve Qì rivers running smoothly at the proper Qì level without stagnation. In addition, you must also keep the Qì reservoirs full so that they can properly regulate the Qì flow in the Qì rivers.

Qìgōng was designed to focus on these two targets. It keeps Qì running smoothly in the channels by opening up areas which can cause the flow to stagnate. The first step is learning how to regulate your body into a deep, relaxed state. The next step is regulating your breathing and your mind to lead your mind and spirit into a deep, peaceful, and calm state. Now your organs will not be stressed by emotional disturbances, and can function most efficiently. Only when you have reached the stage at which you can regulate your body, breathing, and mind, will you be able to feel and sense the Qì flow in your body. Only then will you be able to regulate your Qì effectively.

Wàidān (external elixir) Qìgōng is based on this principle. It relies on limb exercises in coordination with mind concentration to build Qì in the limbs, and then lets this Qì flow back into the organs. Wàidān Qìgōng is aimed at the Qì channels.

However, in order to fill up the Qì in the vessels, another method must be used. Nèidān Qìgōng builds up Qì in the Dāntián, which is located in the Qì vessels. First the Conception and Governing Vessels are filled, and then the other six.

These achievements did not satisfy the Qìgōng practitioners. In order to reach a deeper level of Qìgōng training and approach the goals of longevity and enlightenment, two more things are required. One of these is keeping the blood healthy. Blood cells carry nutrition and oxygen to every cell of your body. When the blood is healthy, it will significantly slow the aging process. Since the blood cells are manufactured in the bone marrow, it is essential to keep the marrow clean.

The higher Qìgōng practitioners also seek spiritual independence. In order to attain this goal, the Qì must be led to the head to nourish the brain and spirit, making it possible for the practitioner to reach the stage of enlightenment or Buddhahood.

Hundreds of Qìgōng styles were created based on these requirements. However, the most important ones are the *Muscle/Tendon Changing Classic* and the *Marrow/Brain Washing Classic*. The *Muscle/Tendon Changing Classic* was designed to change the physical body (including the organs) from weak to strong, and to keep the twelve Qì channels running smoothly while filling up the Qì in the two major vessels (Conception and Governing Vessels). When you train Muscle/Tendon Changing Qìgōng, you build the foundation of physical health.

After you have reached an advanced stage of Muscle/Tendon Changing Qìgōng training, for example completing the Small and Grand Circulation, you should start Marrow/Brain Washing Qìgōng. Marrow/Brain Washing Qìgōng fills up the other six vessels, keeps the marrow clean and fresh, and uses the Qì to nourish the brain and spirit. When you have completed this, you will have reached the highest level of Qìgōng training. However, it is not easy to reach this stage. It usually requires that you separate yourself from normal human society, and perhaps live in the mountains like a priest or hermit. It will also require more than 30 years of accurate training.

This volume is meant to serve as a map directing you to the Qìgōng treasure. It will give you the directions and knowledge necessary to start your trek to health and longevity. Beyond showing you the What and How of practice, this book is designed to explain the Why, based on my current understanding. It is my wish that this book stimulate the general Western public to open its collective mind to this new concept. Although I have tried my best, it is not surprising that many questions remain. The science of Qìgōng is so wide and deep in knowledge, and so long in history, that it is not possible for one individual to cover every aspect. I hope that other knowledgeable Qìgōng practitioners and researchers will also share their experience and understanding with the general public.

Although I believe that this book has not covered all aspects of the discussion, I do have confidence that it has given you the key to opening the gate to the mystery. With this book as a directory, you should come to understand the general concepts of Chinese Qìgōng. Once you understand this book, you should start walking. Without walking, the target will never be reached. It is a long and challenging job. You will need a lot of enthusiasm, patience, and strong will to accomplish it. The process will help you to understand yourself and nature much better and more clearly and, therefore, help you live your life in a more meaningful way.

On your way to study and research, I would like to remind you that your thoughts should not be restricted and limited by traditional culture and conventional, conservative morality. Accepting a new culture is not a betrayal of tradition. Daring to remove the masks that everyone has put on since they started to be affected by tradition and the world of conventional reality is not shameful but brave. During this new era in which human beings have enjoyed incredible material progress in a mere 100 years, you must dare to face and accept different cultures. Tradition must be examined. In this new era, different cultures have a chance to interact with each other. It is the responsibility of our generation to create and refine this new mixed culture and pass it to the next generation. This is a difficult challenge for all of us. However, you must understand that the future is in our hands, and we must accept the challenge, becoming the pioneers of this era.

In order to accomplish this job, I would like to give you a few things to keep in mind in the course of your study and research. These are:

1. **Avoid Prejudice.** All culture and tradition which has survived must have its benefits. Perhaps some of them do not fit in our world; however, they deserve our respect. Remember, if you get rid of your past, you have pulled out your root. Naturally, you should not be stubborn and claim that the traditional culture is absolutely right, or claim that an alien culture must be better than the traditional culture. What you should do is keep the good of the traditional and absorb the best of the alien.

2. **Be Objective in Your Judgment.** You should consider every new statement you read from both sides so that you can analyze it objectively. When you evaluate, emotional opinions should be considered, but they should not dominate your judgment.

3. **Be Scientific.** Although there are many occurrences which still cannot be explained by modern science, you should always remember to judge scientifically. New sciences will be developed. Phenomena that could not be tested in ancient times should be examined with modern equipment.

4. **Be Logical and Make Sense.** When you read or study, in your mind you should always ask "Is it logical and does it make sense?" When you keep these questions in mind, you will think and understand instead of believe blindly.

5. **Do not Ignore Prior Experience.** Prior experience that has been passed down is the root of research. You should always be sincere and respectful when you study the past. From the past, you will come to understand the present. By understanding the present, you will be able to create the future. The accumulation of experience is the best teacher. You should respect the past, be cautious about the present, and challenge the future.

China has more than 7,000 thousand years of culture. There have been many brilliant accomplishments, and Qìgōng is only one of them. There has never been such open communication between different cultures as we have today. It is our responsibility to encourage the general public to accept, study, and research other cultures. In this way, the human race will be able to adopt the good parts of each culture and live in a more peaceful and meaningful way.

Chinese Qìgōng is part of traditional Chinese medical science. It has brought the Chinese thousands of years of calm, peaceful, and happy lives. I believe that this brilliant element of Chinese culture will help Westerners, especially in the spiritual part of training. Further publications must be encouraged. Wide scale scholastic and scientific study, research, and tests must be conducted, especially by universities and medical organizations. In this way, we will be able to introduce this new culture to the Western world in a short time.

I predict that the study of Chinese medical science and internal, meditative Qìgōng will attain great results in the next decade. I invite you to join me and become a pioneer in this new field in the Western world.

Acknowledgments—First Edition

Thanks to A. Reza Farman-Farmaian for the photography, David Ripianzi, David Sollars, John Hughes, Jr. and James O'Leary, Jr. for proofing the manuscript and for contributing many valuable suggestions and discussions, to Dr. Guthiel for writing the foreword, to Wén-Chìng Wú for drawings and general help, and to Sierra for drawings and the cover design. Special thanks to Alan Dougall and Eric Hoffman for editing.

Acknowledgments—Second Edition

In this new edition, I would like to express my thanks to Tim Comrie and Měi-Líng Yáng for general help, to Kain M. Sanderson and June-Marie Mahay for proofreading the manuscript, and to Andrew Murray for editing the new edition. Thanks also to Jerry Leake for typesetting, Ilana Rosenberg and David Lepp for the cover design and artwork, and Sarah Noack for her work with the LifeART images. Special thanks to Dr. Irwin H. Rosenberg and Daniel Reid for writing the forewords to this new edition.

Acknowledgments—Third Edition

The publisher wishes to thank Tim Comrie for typesetting, Doran Hunter for copyediting, Axie Breen for illustration enhancements and cover design, and Johnny Houx for proofreading this updated edition.

Appendix: Translation and Glossary of Chinese Terms

Āi 哀 Sorrow.

Ài 愛 Love, kindness.

Ànmó 按摩 Literally, "Press Rub." Together they mean massage.

Āntiān Lèmìng 安天樂命 Means "Peace with heaven and delight in your destiny."

Ānyáng, Hénán province 河南、安陽 The location of an old Chinese capital during the Shāng dynasty (商朝), 1766-1154 BCE It has become an important site for archeological study.

Bāchù 八觸 Eight Touches. The physical and sensory phenomena in Qìgōng practice.

Bāduànjǐn 八段錦 Eight Pieces of Brocade. A Wàidān Qìgōng practice said to have been created by Marshal Yuè, Fēi (岳飛) during the Southern Sòng dynasty (南宋), 1127–1279 CE.

Bāguà (Bā Kuà) 八卦 Literally, "Eight Divinations." Also called "the Eight Trigrams." In Chinese philosophy, the eight basic variations; shown in the *Yìjīng* (易經) as groups of single and broken lines.

Bāguàzhang 八卦掌 Eight Trigrams Palm. One of the internal Qìgōng martial styles, believed to have been created by Dǒng, Hǎi-Chuān (董海川) between 1866 and 1880 CE.

Báihè 白鶴 Means "White Crane." One of the southern martial arts styles of China.

Bǎihuì (Gv-20) 百會 Literally, "Hundred Meetings." An important acupuncture cavity located on the top of the head. The Bǎihuì cavity belongs to the Governing Vessel.

Bāmài 八脈 Referred to as the eight extraordinary vessels. These eight vessels are considered to be Qì reservoirs, which regulate the Qì status in the primary Qì channels.

Bàopǔzi 抱朴子 The name of a well-known Qìgōng and Chinese medical book written by Gé, Hóng (葛洪) during the Jìn dynasty (晋朝) in the 3rd century CE.

Bǎoshēn Mìyào 保身祕要 A Qìgōng and medical book describing moving and stationary Qìgōng practices. It was written by Cáo, Yuán-Bái (曹元白) during the Qīng dynasty (清朝), 1644–1911 CE.

Biǎnquè 扁鵲 A well-known physician who wrote the book, *Nànjīng* (難經) (*Classic on Disorders*) during the Chinese Qín and Hàn dynasties (秦，漢), 221 BCE–220 CE.

Biānshí 砭石 The stone probes used to press acupuncture cavities for healing before metal needles were available.

Bíxí 鼻息 Means "Nose Breathing."

Cǎixiǎoyào 採小藥 Picked up the little herb. Terminology used in Daoist Qìgōng practice.

Cáo, Yuán-Bái 曹元白 A well-known physician and Qìgōng master who wrote a book called *Bǎoshēn Mìyào* (*The Secret Important Document of Body Protection*, 保身祕要) during the Qīng dynasty (清朝), 1644–1911 CE. The book describes moving and stationary Qìgōng practices.

Chán (Rěn) 禪，忍 A Chinese school of Mahayana Buddhism which asserts that enlightenment can be attained through meditation, self-contemplation and intuition, rather than through study of scripture. Chán is called Zěn in Japan.

Cháng 長 Long.

Chángquán 長拳 Means "Long Range Fist." Chángquán includes all northern Chinese long range martial styles. Chángquán has also been used to refer to Tàijíquán.

Chánzōng 禪宗 The Chán school.

Chánzōng Liùzǔ 禪宗六祖 "Six Ancestors of Chán" who include Dámó (達摩), Huìkě (慧可), Sēngcàn (僧璨), Dàoxìn (道信), Hóngrěn (弘忍), and Huìnéng (慧能).

Chánzōng Qīzǔ 禪宗七祖 "Seven Ancestors of Chán" who include Dámó (達摩), Huìkě (慧可), Sēngcàn (僧璨), Dàoxìn (道信), Hóngrěn (弘忍), Huìnéng (慧能), and Shénhuì (神會).

Cháo, Yuán-Fāng 巢元方 A well-known physician and Qìgōng master who lived during the Suí and Táng dynasties (隋、唐), 581–907 CE. Cháo, Yuán-Fāng compiled the *Zhūbìng Yuánhòu Lùn* (*Thesis on the Origins and Symptoms of Various Diseases*, 諸病源候論), which is a veritable encyclopedia of Qìgōng methods, listing 260 different ways of increasing the Qì flow.

Chén 沈 Sink.

Chén, Jì-Rú 陳繼儒 A well-known physician and Qìgōng master who wrote the book *Yǎngshēng Fūyǔ* (養生膚語) (*Brief Introduction to Nourishing the Body*) during the Qīng dynasty (清朝), 1644–1911 CE. The book is about the three treasures: Jīng (essence), Qì (internal energy), and Shén (spirit).

Chēng, Gīn-Gsào 曾金灶 Dr. Yáng, Jwìng-Mǐng's White Crane master.

Chì (Qì) 氣 The energy pervading the universe, including the energy circulating in the human body.

Chì Kūng (Qìgōng) 氣功 Literally the "Gōngfū of Qì," which means the study of Qì.

Chín Ná (Qín Ná) 擒拿 Literally "Grab Control." A component of Chinese martial arts that emphasizes grabbing techniques to control your opponent's joints, in conjunction with attacking certain acupuncture cavities.

Chōngmài 衝脈 Thrusting Vessel. One of the eight extraordinary Qì vessels.

Chùgǎn 觸感 Literally, "Touch Feel." Chùgǎn refers to the unusual feelings or phenomena experienced during Qìgōng practice.

Confucius (Kǒngzǐ) 孔子 A Chinese scholar of the period 551–479 BCE, whose philosophy has significantly influenced Chinese culture.

Cóngnèi Zhújī 從內築基 Means to build the foundation of health and longevity internally. That means to regulate the breathing, mind, and Qì internally.

Cóngwài Jiàngōng 從外健功 Means to build the physical strength externally.

Dàimài 帶脈 Girdle (or Belt) Vessel. One of the eight Qì vessels.

Dámó 達摩 The Indian Buddhist monk credited with creating the Yìjīnjīng (易筋經) and Xǐsuǐjīng (洗髓經) while at the Shàolín monastery. His last name was Sardili and he was also known as Bodhidarma. He was once the prince of a small tribe in southern India.

Dāndǐng Dàogōng 丹鼎道功 The elixir cauldron way of Qìgōng. The Daoists' Qìgōng training.

Dāntián 丹田 Literally, "Field of Elixir." Locations in the body which are able to store and generate Qì (elixir) in the body. The Upper, Middle, and Lower Dāntián are located, respectively, between the eyebrows, at the solar plexus, and a few inches below the navel.

Dāntiánqì 丹田氣 Usually, the Qì that is converted from Original Essence (Yuánjīng, 元精) and is stored in the Lower Dāntián. This Qì is considered "water Qì" and is able to calm the body. Also called Xiāntiānqì (Pre-Heaven Qì, 先天氣).

Dào 道 The "Way"; by implication the "Natural Way."

Dào Dé Jīng 道德經 Morality Classic. Written by Lǎozi (老子).

Dàojiā 道家 The Dao family. Daoism. Created by Lǎozi (老子) during the Zhōu dynasty (周朝), 1122–934 BCE. In the Hàn dynasty (漢朝)(ca. 58 CE), it was mixed with Buddhism to become the Daoist religion (Dàojiào, 道教).

Dàojiào 道教 Daoist religion created by Zhāng, Dào-Líng (張道陵) who combined the traditional Daoist principles with Buddhism during the Chinese Hàn dynasty (漢朝).

Dàoxìn 道信 One of the six ancestors of Chán.

Dàowài Cǎiyào 道外採藥 Means "Herb picking outside of the Dào." A special Daoist Qìgōng training method.

Dàshǒuyìn 大手印 Large hand stamp. A common Tibetan meditation technique in which some of the meditator's fingers press against each other.

Dàzhōutiānn 大周天 Literally, "Grand Cycle Heaven." Usually translated as "Grand Circulation." After a Nèidān Qìgōng practitioner completes Small Circulation (Xiǎozhōutiān, 小周天), he will circulate his Qì through the entire body or exchange the Qì with nature.

Dì 地 The Earth. Earth, Heaven (Tiān, 天) and Man (Rén, 人) are the "Three Natural Powers" (Sāncái, 三才).

Diǎnmài (Dim Mak) 點脈 Mài means "The blood vessel" (Xuěmài, 血脈) or "The Qì channel" (Qìmài, 氣脈). Diǎnmài means "To press the blood vessel or Qì channel."

Diànqì 電氣 Diàn means "electricity" and so Diànqì means "electrical energy" (electricity). In China, a word is often placed before "Qì" to identify the different kinds of energy.

Diǎnxuè 點穴 Diǎn means "To point and exert pressure" and Xuè means "The cavities." Diǎnxuè refers to those Qín Ná (擒拿) techniques which specialize in attacking acupuncture cavities to immobilize or kill an opponent.

Diǎnxuè massages 點穴按摩 One of the Chinese massage techniques in which the acupuncture cavities are stimulated through pressing. Diǎnxuè massage is also called acupressure and is the root of Japanese Shiatsu.

Diào 掉 Shake.

Dìlǐshī 地理師 Dìlǐ means "Geomancy" and Shī means "Teacher." Therefore Dìlǐshī is a teacher or master who analyzes geographic locations according to the formulas in the *Yijīng* (*Book of Changes*, 易經) and the energy distributions in the earth. Also called Fēngshuǐshī.

Dìng 定 To stabilize or to firm.

Dìngshén 定神 To stabilize the spirit. To keep the spirit at one place (usually the Shàng Dāntián located at the third eye). One of the exercises for regulating the Shén (spirit) in Qìgōng.

Dìqì 地氣 The Qì or the energy of the earth.

Dòng 動 Moving.

Dǒng 懂 Understanding.

Dǒng, Hǎi-Chuān 董海川 A well-known Chinese internal martial artist who is credited as the creator of Bāguàzhǎng (八卦掌) in the late Qīng dynasty (清朝), 1644–1911 CE.

Dòngchù 動觸 Literally, "Moving touch." Refers to the unusual, automatic movements or feelings sometimes experienced during Qìgōng practice. Also called Chùgǎn (觸感).

Dōngmiánfǎ 冬眠法 Hibernation technique. A Qìgōng technique that trains the hibernation breathing.

Dūmài 督脈 Usually translated "Governing Vessel." One of the eight extraordinary vessels.

Eastern Hàn dynasty 東漢 A Chinese dynasty from 25–168 CE.

Éméi 峨嵋 Name of a mountain in Sichuan Province (四川省), China.

Éméi Dàpénggōng 峨嵋大鵬功 Dàpéng is a kind of large bird that existed in ancient China. Dàpénggōng is a style of Qìgōng that imitates the movements of this bird. This style was developed at Éméi mountain in China.

Fan 返 Return. Means to return your breathing to its natural way.

Fǎn Fùhūxī 反腹呼吸 Reverse abdominal breathing. One of the Qìgōng breathing methods. Also called Fǎnhūxī (reverse breathing, 反呼吸)or Daoist breathing.

Fǎnhūxī 反呼吸 Reverse breathing. Also commonly called "Daoist Breathing."

Fǎnjīng Bǔnǎo 返精補腦 Daoist Qìgōng terminology that means "To return the Jīng to nourish the brain."

Fǎntóng Hūxī 返童呼吸 Back to childhood breathing. A breathing training technique in Nèidān Qìgōng (內丹氣功) through which the practitioner tries to regain control of the muscles in the lower abdomen. Also called "abdominal breathing" (Fùhūxī, 腹呼吸).

Fǎnxí 返息 Return breathing. Means to return your breathing to its natural way.

Fēngchí (GB-20) 風池 Wind Pond. An acupuncture cavity belonging to the Gall Bladder Qì channel.

Fēnglù 風路 Wind Path. One of the internal Qì circulation paths.

Fěnsuì Xūkōng 粉碎虛空 Crush the Emptiness. The final stage of Daoist Qìgōng enlightenment training.

Fēngshuǐshī 風水師 Literally, "Wind water teacher." Teacher or master of geomancy. Geomancy is the art or science of analyzing the natural energy relationships in a location, especially the interrelationships between "wind" and "water," hence the name. Also called "Dìlǐshī" (地理師).

Fójiā (Fójiào) 佛家 (佛教) Literally, "Buddhism family." Jiào means religion. Therefore, the Buddhist Religion.

Fǔ 腑 The Bowels. The Yáng organs: the Gall Bladder, Small Intestine, Large Intestine, Stomach, Bladder, and Triple Burner.

Fú 浮 Float.

Fúqìfǎ 伏氣法 Yield Qì methods. Techniques used to calm and tame the Qì.

Fùshì Hūxī 腹式呼吸 Literally, "Abdominal way of breathing." As you breathe, you use the muscles in the lower abdominal area to control the diaphragm. It is also called "back to (the) childhood breathing" (Fǎntóng Hūxī, 返童呼吸).

Fūxí 膚息 Skin Breathing. A Qìgōng breathing technique in which the Qì is led to the surface of the skin.

Gǎnjué 感覺 Literally, "To touch and feel." In the second stage of relaxation, you are able to physically feel what is going on inside your body. This occurs before the sensing stage.

Gé, Hóng 葛洪 A famous physician and Qìgōng master who wrote the book Bàopǔzi during the Jìn dynasty (晉) in the 3rd century CE.

Gézhì Yúlùn 格致餘論 The Chinese name of the book *A Further Thesis of Complete Study*, a medical and Qìgōng thesis written by Zhū, Dān-Xī (朱丹溪) during the Sòng, Jīn, and Yuán dynasties (宋、金、元), 960–1368 CE.

Gǒngshǒu 拱手 Arcing arms or hands. A stationary Tàijí Qìgōng training.

Gōngfū (Kūng Fū) 功夫 Means "Energy-Time." Anything that takes time and energy to learn or accomplish is called "Gōngfū."

Guān 觀 Look. Implies to feel and to sense.

Guànqì 貫氣 Guan means "To thread together." Guànqì is a Qìgōng training method in which a practitioner leads Qì from one place to another.

Guānxí 觀息 Guān means "To look." "Look" here means to feel and to sense. Xí is the breathing. Therefore, Guānxí means "To feel and to sense the breathing."

Guānxiǎngfǎ 觀想法 The Behold and Think Method. A Buddhist technique used to regulate the mind.

Guānxīn 觀心 Means to inspect or look at the behavior of Xīn (the emotional mind).

Guǐ 鬼 Ghost. When you die, if your spirit is strong, your soul's energy will not decompose and return to nature. This soul energy is a ghost.

Guǐ Qì 鬼氣 The Qì residue of a dead person. It is believed by the Chinese Buddhists and Daoists that this Qì residue is a so-called ghost.

Guīxí 龜息 Turtle breathing. In Chinese Qìgōng society, it is believed that a turtle is able to live for a long time because it knows how to breath through its skin. Therefore, skin breathing in Qìgōng is called turtle breathing.

Gùjīng 固精 To solidify the essence. A Qìgōng exercise for keeping and firming the essence.

Guóshù 國術 Abbreviation of "Zhōngguó Wǔshù" (中國武術), which means "Chinese Martial Techniques."

Gùshén 固神 Means "To firm and solidify." An exercise for regulating the Shén in which you firm and strengthen the spirit at its residence.

Gùshèn 固腎 Means "To firm and solidify the kidneys." A method to strengthen the kidneys; therefore, to prevent the loss of the Original Essence.

Gǔsuǐ 骨髓 Bone Marrow.

Hā 哈 A Qìgōng sound commonly used to lead an over-abundance of Qì from inside the body out and therefore reduce over-accumulated Qì.

Hàn dynasty 漢朝 A dynasty from Chinese history, 206 BCE–221 CE.

Hán, Chìng-Táng 韓慶堂 A well-known Chinese martial artist, especially in Táiwān in the last forty years. Master Hán is also Dr. Yáng, Jwìng-Mǐng's Long Fist Grand Master.

Hé 和 Harmony or peace.

Hèn 恨 Hate.

Hēng 哼 A Yīn Qìgōng sound that is the opposite of the Hā Yáng sound.

Hóngrěn 弘忍 One of the six ancestors of Chan.

Hòutiānqì 後天氣 Post-Birth Qì. This Qì is converted from the essence of food and air and is classified as "Fire Qì" because it can make your body too Yáng.

Huá 滑 Slippery.

Huǎn 緩 Slow.

Huátuó 華陀 A well-known Chinese physician who lived during the Jìn dynasty (晉) in the 3rd century CE.

Huánjīng Bǔnǎo 還精補腦 Literally, "To return the essence to nourish the brain." A Daoist Qìgōng training process in which Qì that is converted from essence is led to the brain to nourish it.

Huángdì 黃帝 The Yellow Emperor (2690–2590 BCE).

Huángtíng 黃庭 Yellow yard. 1. A yard or hall in which Daoists, who often wore yellow robes, meditate together. 2. In Qìgōng training, a spot in the abdomen where it is believed that you are able to generate an "embryo."

Hǔbùgōng 虎步功 Tiger Step Gōng. A style of Qìgōng training.

Huìkě 慧可 One of the six ancestors of Chán Buddhism.

Huìnéng 慧能 One of the six ancestors of Chán Buddhism.

Huìyīn (Co-1) 會陰 An acupuncture cavity belonging to the Conception Vessel.

Hún 魂 The soul. Commonly used with the word Líng, which means "Spirit." Daoists believe that a human being's Hún and Pò (魄) originate with his Original Qì (Yuánqì, 元氣), and separate from the physical body at death.

Huǒlónggōng 火龍功 Fire Dragon Gōng. A style of Qìgōng training created by Tàiyáng martial stylists (太陽宗).

Huǒlù 火路 Fire Path. One of the paths in Small Circulation meditation.

Huǒqì 火氣 Fire Qì. Qì which tends to make the body positive, or Yáng.

Huǒqì 活氣 Huo means "Alive." Huǒqì is the Qì of a living person or animal.

Jiǎgǔwén 甲骨文 Oracle-Bone Scripture. It is the earliest evidence of the Chinese use of the written word. Found on pieces of turtle shell and animal bone from the Shāng dynasty (商朝), 1766-1154 BCE. Most of the information recorded was of a religious nature.

Jiǎguān 假觀 The False Look. A technique to regulate the mind in Buddhist meditation.

Jiān 堅 Hard and strong.

Jiànxìng Liǎorán 見性了然 Means "To see Nature and understand what it really is."

Jiàohuāgōng 叫化功 Beggar Gōng. A style of Qìgōng training.

Jìguāng 繼光 Huìkě's layman name. Huìkě is one of the six ancestors of Chán Buddhism.

Jìn dynasty 晉 A Chinese dynasty of the 3rd century CE.

Jīn, Shào-Fēng 金紹峰 Dr. Yáng, Jwìng-Mǐng's White Crane grand master.

Jīndān Dàdào 金丹大道 Golden Elixir Large Way. A special Daoist Nèidān Qìgōng training.

Jīng 精 Essence. The most refined part of anything.

Jīng 經 Channels. Sometimes translated as "Meridians." Refers to the twelve organ-related "rivers" that circulate Qì throughout the body.

Jìng 勁 The martial power in Chinese martial arts that derives from muscles that have been energized by Qì to their maximum potential.

Jìng 淨 Clean. Means "regulated." In this book, Jīng means to use natural breathing to regulate your thoughts.

Jìng 靜 Calm and silent.

Jīngliàn 精煉 Means "To refine or purify a liquid to a high quality."

Jīngliàng 精良 Means "Excellent Quality" (literally "Pure and good").

Jīngmén 精門 Essence Doors. They are located on the back of the body.

Jīngmíng 精明 Means "Keen and Clever."

Jǐngqì 景氣 Means "Qì Scenery" or "Qì View."

Jīngqì 精氣 Essence Qì. The Qì that has been converted from Original Essence.

Jīnguì Yàolüè 金匱要略 The name of a Chinese book, Prescriptions from the Golden Chamber, that discusses the use of breathing and acupuncture to maintain good Qì flow. This book was written by Zhāng, Zhòng-Jǐng during the Qín and Hàn dynasties, 221 BCE–220 CE.

Jīngshén 精神 Literally "Essence Shén," which is commonly translated as "spirit of vitality."

Jìngxí 淨息 Clean. Means "regulated." Xí means "breathing." Therefore Jìngxí means to use natural breathing to regulate your thoughts.

Jīngxì 精細 Means "Delicate and painstaking" (literally, "pure and fine").

Jīngzǐ 精子 Literally, "Essence Son." The most refined part of human essence. The sperm.

Jīnzhōngzhào 金鐘罩 Literally, "Golden bell cover." A higher level of Iron Shirt training.

Jùjīng Huìshén 聚精會神 "Gathering your Jīng to meet your Shén." That means "concentration."

Juéyīn 厥陰 Absolute Yīn. Terminology used in acupuncture.

Jūnqiàn 君倩 A Daoist and Chinese doctor who lived during the Jìn dynasty (晉), 265–420 CE. Jūnqiàn is credited as the creator of the Five Animal Sports Qìgōng practice.

Kǎn 坎 One of the Eight Trigrams.

Kāo, Táo 高濤 Dr. Yáng, Jwìng-Mǐng's first Tàijíquán master.

Kōngguān 空觀 The Empty Look. One of the methods of regulating the mind in Qìgōng meditation.

Kōngqì 空氣 Air.

Kūng (Gōng) 功 Means "Energy" or "Hard Work."

Kūng Fū (Gōngfū) 功夫 Literally, "Energy-Time." Any study, learning, or practice that requires patience, energy, and time to complete. Since practicing Chinese martial arts requires a great deal of time and energy, Chinese martial arts are commonly called "Gōngfū."

Kuóshù (Guóshù) 國術 Literally, "National Techniques." Another name for Chinese martial arts. First used by President Chiang, Kai-Shek (蔣介石) in 1926 at the founding of the Nanking Central Guóshù Institute (南京中央國術館).

Lǎma 喇嘛 A TibetÀn mónk. Also used for Tibetan White Crane style.

Lánshì Mìcáng 蘭室祕藏 *Secret Library of the Orchid Room*. The name of a Chinese medical and Qìgōng book written by Lǐ, Guǒ (李果) during the Sòng, Jīn, and Yuán dynasties (宋、金、元), 960–1368 CE.

Láogōng (P-8) 勞宮 Cavity name. On the Pericardium Channel in the center of the palm.

Lǎozi 老子 The creator of Daoism, also called Lǐěr.

Lè 樂 Joy or happiness.

Lěng 冷 Cold.

Lí 離 A phase of the Bāguà (Eight Trigrams). Lí represents fire.

Lǐ, Guǒ 李果 A well-known Chinese physician and Qìgōng master who wrote a book, *Lánshì Mìcáng* (*Secret Library of the Orchid Room*, 蘭室祕藏) during the Sòng, Jīn, and Yuán dynasties (宋、金、元), 960–1368 CE.

Lǐ, Mào-Chīng 李茂清 Dr. Yáng, Jwìng-Mǐng's Long Fist master.

Lǐ, Shí-Zhēn (1518–1593 CE) 李時珍 A well-known Chinese physician and Qìgōng master who wrote a book about the eight Qì vessels, *Qíjīng Bāmài* Kǎo (*Deep Study of the Extraordinary Eight Vessels*, 奇經八脈考) in the 16th century.

Liànjīng Huàqì 煉精化氣 To refine the essence and convert it into Qì. One of the Qìgōng training processes through which you convert essence into Qì.

Lian Qì 煉氣化神 Lian means "To train, to strengthen and to refine." A Daoist training process through which your Qì grows stronger and more abundant.

Liànqì Huàshén 煉氣化神 To refine the Qì to nourish the spirit. Part of the Qìgōng training process in which you learn how to lead Qì to the head to nourish the brain and Shén (spirit).

Liànshén 煉神 To train the spirit. To refine and strengthen the Shén and make it more focused.

Liànshén Fǎnxū 煉神返虛 To refine the Shén into emptiness. Part of the Daoist Qìgōng training process in which you learn how to lead your Shén (spirit) into the emptiness (i.e., free from emotional bondage).

Liànshén Liǎoxìng 煉神了性 To refine the spirit and end human nature. This is the final stage of spiritual Qìgōng training for enlightenment. In this process you learn to keep your emotions neutral and try to be undisturbed by human nature.

Liáng 涼 Cool.

Liáng dynasty 梁朝 A dynasty in Chinese history, 502–557 CE.

Liěr 李耳 Nickname of Lǎozi, the creator of scholarly Daoism.

Líng 靈 The spirit of being, which acts upon others. Líng only exists in high spiritual animals such as humans and monkeys. It represents an emotional comprehension and understanding. When you are alive, it implies your intelligence and wisdom. When you die, it implies the spirit of the ghost. Líng also means "divine" or "supernatural." Líng is often used together with Shén (Língshén, 靈神) to mean "supernatural spirit." It is believed that Qì is the source that nourishes the Líng and is called "Língqì" (靈氣), "meaning "supernatural energy, power, or force."

Língbǎo Bìfǎ 靈寶閉法 Spiritual Treasure to Reach the End Method. A Tibetan Qìgōng training technique.

Língguǐ 靈鬼 Spiritual ghost.

Línghún 靈魂 Spiritual soul.

Língshén 靈神 Supernatural or divine spirit.

Língzhī 靈芝 Língzhī (Fomes Japonica) is a hard, dark brownish fungus which is supposed to possess supernatural powers. In Qìgōng society, sometimes Língzhī means the elixir that enables you to have a long life.

Liùhé Bāfǎ 六合八法 Literally, "Six combinations eight methods." One of the internal martial arts of China, its techniques are combined from Tàijíquán (太極拳), Xíngyìquán (形意拳) and Bāguàzhang (八卦掌). This internal martial art was reportedly created by Chén, Bó (陳博) during the Sòng dynasty (宋朝), 960–1279 CE.

Liùjǐng 六景 Six Qìgōng Verifications. These are: A. Dāntián is hot as if it were on fire; B. The (internal) kidneys feel like they are boiling in water; C. The eyes are emitting a beam of light; D. Winds are being generated behind the ears; E. An eagle is shouting behind your head; F. Your body is energized and your nose trembles.

Luò 絡 The small Qì channels that branch out from the primary Qì channels and are connected to the skin and to the bone marrow.

Mǎbù 馬步 Horse Stance. One of the basic stances in Chinese martial arts.

Mài 脈 Means "Vessel" or "Qì channel."

Mèngzǐ (Mencius) 孟子 (372–289 BCE) A well-known scholar who followed the philosophy of Confucius during the Chinese Zhōu dynasty (周朝), 909–255 BCE.

Mìzàng Shéngōng 密藏神功 Literally, "Secret Style of Spiritual Gōngfū." This means Tibetan Qìgōng and martial arts, originally passed down secretly.

Mìzōng 密宗 Secret Style. Tibetan Qìgōng is commonly called "Mìzōng" simply because it is not known by outsiders.

Mián 綿 Soft.

Mìng 命 Physical life.

Míng dynasty 明朝 A Chinese dynasty from 1368 to 1644 CE.

Mìngmén (Gv-4) 命門 Name of an acupuncture cavity belonging to the Governing Vessel.

Míngtiāngǔ 鳴天鼓 To beat the heavenly drum. A Qìgōng practice for waking up and clearing the mind in which the back of the head is tapped with the fingers.

Nánhuájīng 南華經 A book written by the Daoist philosopher Zhuāngzi (莊子) circa 300 BCE. This book describes the relationship between health and the breath.

Nànjīng 難經 *Classic on Disorders*. A medical book written by the famous physician Biǎnquè (扁鵲) during the Qín and Hàn dynasties (秦、漢), 221 BCE–220 CE. Nànjīng describes the methods of using breathing to increase Qì circulation.

Nǎosuǐ 腦髓 Brain.

Nèidān 內丹 Literally, "Internal elixir." A form of Qìgōng in which Qì (the elixir) is built up in the body and led out to the limbs.

Nèigōng 內功 Literally, "Internal Gōngfū." Chinese martial arts that start with internal training and the cultivation of Qì.

Nèigōng Túshuō 內功圖說 *Illustrated Explanation of Nèigōng*. The name of the Qìgōng book written by Wáng, Zǔ-Yuán (王祖源) during the Qīng dynasty (清朝). This book presents the Twelve Pieces of Brocade and explains the idea of combining both moving and stationary Qìgōng.

Nèijīng 內經 *Inner Classic*. A Chinese medical book written during the reign of the Yellow emperor (黃帝), 2690–2590 BCE.

Nèishèn 內腎 Literally, "internal kidneys." In Chinese medicine and Qìgōng, the real Kidneys; Wàishèn (external kidneys, 外腎) refers to the testicles.

Nèishì Fǎntīng 內視反聽 Means "To see internally and to listen inwardly."

Nèishì Gōngfū 內視功夫 Nèishì means "To look internally," so Nèishì Gōngfū refers to the art of looking inside yourself to read the state of your health and the condition of your Qì.

Niàn 念 Thoughts that stay with you and do not go away.

Níngshén 凝神 To condense or focus on the spirit. In Qìgōng training, after you are able to keep your spirit in one place, you learn how to condense it into a tiny spot and make it stronger.

Nù 怒 Anger.

Nuǎn 暖 Warm.

Píng 平 Peace and harmony.

Pò 魄 Vigorous life force. The Pò is considered to be the inferior or animal soul. It is the animal or sentient life that is an innat part of the body which, at death, returns to the earth with the rest of the body. When someone is in high spirits and gets vigorously involved in some activity it is said he has Pòlì (魄力), which means he has "vigorous strength or power."

Qì 氣 The general definition of Qì is: universal energy, including heat, light, and electromagnetic energy. A narrower definition of Qì refers to the energy circulating in human or animal bodies. A current popular model is that the Qì circulating in the human body is bioelectric in nature.

Qiángshèn 強腎 Strengthen the kidneys.

Qiānjīnfāng 千金方 *Thousand Gold Prescriptions*. A medical book written by the well know physician Sūn, Sī-Miǎo (孫思邈) during the Suí and Táng dynasties (隋、唐), 581–907 CE. This book describes the method of leading Qì, and also describes the use of the Six Sounds.

Qìgōng (Chì Kūng) 氣功 Gōng means Gōngfū (literally "Energy-time.") Therefore, Qìgōng means study, research, and/or practices related to Qì.

Qìgōng Ànmó 氣功按摩 Qìgōng massage.

Qìhǎi (Co-6) 氣海 An acupuncture cavity belonging to the Conception Vessel.

Qìhuàlùn 氣化論 Qì variation thesis. An ancient treatise that discusses the variations of Qì in the universe.

Qǐhuǒ 起火 To start the fire. In Qìgōng practice, when you start to build up Qì at the Lower Dāntián.

Qíjīng Bāmài 奇經八脈 Literally, "Strange (odd) channels eight vessels." Usually referred to as the eight extraordinary vessels or simply as the vessels. Called odd or strange because they are not well understood and some of them do not exist in pairs.

Qíjīng Bāmài Kǎo 奇經八脈考 *Deep Study of the Extraordinary Eight Vessels*. A book written by Lǐ, Shí-Zhēn (李時珍).

Qìmài 氣脈 Qì vessels. The eight vessels involved with transporting, storing, and regulating Qì.

Qín dynasty 秦朝 A Chinese dynasty from 255-206 BCE.

Qín Ná (Chín Ná) 擒拿 Literally "Grab control." A component of Chinese martial arts that emphasizes grabbing techniques to control your opponent's joints, in conjunction with attacking certain acupuncture cavities.

Qīng 輕 Light, as in weight.

Qīng dynasty 清朝 The last of China's dynasties, from 1644–1912 CE.

Qīngxiūpài 清修派 Peaceful Cultivation Division. A division of Daoist Qìgōng training that is similar to Buddhism.

Qínyuán Zhuōmǎ 擒猿捉馬 To seize the ape and catch the horse. A common name for the practice of regulating the mind in Chinese Qìgōng society. The ape represents the emotional mind and the horse represents the calm wisdom mind. In regulating the mind training, you must be able to control your emotional mind and make your wisdom mind steady.

Qīqíng Liùyù 七情六慾 Seven emotions and six desires. The seven emotions are happiness, anger, sorrow, joy, love, hate and desire. The six desires are the six sensory pleasures associated with the eyes, nose, ears, tongue, body and mind.

Qìshì 氣勢 Shì means the way something looks or feels. Therefore, the feeling of Qì as it expresses itself.

Qìxí 氣息 Qì breathing.

Qì-Xuě 氣血 Literally, "Qì blood." According to Chinese medicine, Qì and blood cannot be separated in our bodies and so the two words are commonly used together.

Rè 熱 Hot.

Rén 人 Man or mankind.

Rén 仁 Humanity, kindness or benevolence.

Rěn 忍 Means "To endure." The Japanese name of Chan.

Rènmài 任脈 Conception Vessel. One of the Eight Extraordinary Vessels.

Rénqì 人氣 Human Qì.

Rénshì 人事 Literally, "Human relations." Human events, activities and relationships.

Rèqì 熱氣 Means "warmth" or "heat." Generally, Rèqì is used to represent heat. It implies that a person or animal is still alive because the body is warm.

Ruǎn 軟 Soft.

Rújiā 儒家 Literally, "Confucian family." Scholars following Confucian thoughts; Confucianists.

Rúmén Shìshì 儒門視事 .A book written by Zhāng, Zi-Hé (張子和) during the Sòng, Jīn, and Yuán dynasties (宋、金、元), 960–1368 CE.

Sānbǎo 三寶 Three treasures. Essence (Jīng, 精), energy (Qì, 氣) and spirit (Shén, 神). Also called "Sānyuán" (three origins, 三元).

Sānběn 三本 The Three Foundations.

Sāncái 三才 Three Powers. The Three Powers are Heaven (Tiān, 天), Earth (Dì, 地), and Man (Rén, 人).

Sàngōng 散功 Literally, "Energy dispersion." A state of premature degeneration of the muscles where the Qì cannot effectively energize them. It can be caused by over-training.

Sānguāng 三光 Three lights. In Chinese Qìgōng it is said that the Liver has the Hún (soul, 魂) light, which shows in the eyes; the Lungs have Pò (vigorous life force, 魄) light, which shows in the nose; and the Kidneys have the Jīng (Essence, 精) light, which show in the ears.

Sānhuā Jùdǐng 三花聚頂 Three flowers reach the top. One of the final goals of Qìgōng whereby the three treasures (essence, Qì, and Shén) are led to the top of the body to nourish the brain and spirit center (Upper Dāntián).

Sānjiāo 三焦 Triple burner. In Chinese medicine, the body is divided into three sections: the upper burner (chest), the middle burner (stomach area), and the lower burner (lower abdomen).

Sānyuán 三元 Three origins. Also called "Sānbǎo" (Three treasures, 三寶). Human Essence (Jīng), energy (Qì) and spirit (Shén).

Sè 澀 Harsh.

Sēngcàn 僧璨 One of the six Chán ancestors.

Shàng Dāntián 上丹田 Upper Dāntián. Located at the third eye, it is the residence of the Shén (spirit).

Shāng dynasty 商朝 A Chinese dynasty from 1766–1154 BCE.

Shànghuǒ 上火 Means the body is "on fire." This means the Qì is too sufficient in the body which makes the body on fire (i.e., too positive).

Shàngjiāo 上焦 Upper Burner. One of the Triple Burners in Chinese medicine. The Upper Burner covers the area between the throat and the solar plexus.

Shàolín 少林 Young woods. Name of the Shàolín Temple.

Shàolín Temple 少林寺 A monastery located in Hénán Province (河南省), China. The Shàolín Temple is well known because of its martial arts training.

Shàoyáng 少陽 Lesser Yáng. Terminology used in Chinese acupuncture.

Shàoyīn 少陰 Lesser Yīn. Terminology used in Chinese acupuncture.

Shén 神 Spirit. According to Chinese Qìgōng, the Shén resides at the Upper Dāntián (the third eye).

Shēn 深 Deep.

Shénbù Shǒushè 神不守舍 The spirit is not kept at its residence. This implies not being able to concentrate, or a scattered mind.

Shèngtāi 聖胎 Holy embryo. Another name for the spiritual embryo (Shéntāi, 神胎).

Shénhuì 神會 One of the Seven Ancestors of Chan. Shénhuì was recognized and became as seventh ancestor during the Tang dynasty of Kāiyuán, 713–742 CE.

Shénhún 神魂 Spiritual soul.

Shénmíng 神明 Spiritual divine.

Shénqì Xiànghé 神氣相合 The Shén and the Qì are combined. The final stage of regulating the Shén.

Shènshū (B-23) 腎俞 An acupuncture cavity belonging to the Bladder Qì Channel.

Shénxí 神息 Spirit breathing. The stage of Qìgōng training where the spirit is coordinated with the breathing.

Shénxí Xiāngyī 神息相依 The Shén and breathing mutually rely on each other. A stage in Qìgōng practice.

Shénxiān 神仙 Means "Immortal."

Shēnxīn Pínghéng 身心平衡 Body and heart (mind) balanced. The balance of the physical body and mental body.

Shénzhì 神志 Spiritual will. Shén (spirit) and Zhì (will) together, because they are related.

Shénzhì Bùqīng 神志不清 Means "The spirit and the will (generated from Yì) are not clear." The mind is confused and not steady.

Shíèrjīng 十二經 The Twelve Primary Qì Channels (Meridians) in Chinese medicine.

Shíèrzhuāng 十二庄 Twelve Postures. A style of Qìgōng practice created during the Qīng dynasty (清朝).

Shǐjì 史紀 *Historical Record*. A book written in the Spring and Autumn and Warring States periods (Chūnqiū Zhànguó, 春秋戰國), 770–221 BCE.

Shìjìa 釋家 Literally, "Sakyamuni family." Since Buddhism was created by Sakyamuni, it means Buddhism.

Shíqì 食氣 Food Qì. Qì converted from food.

Shǒushén 守神 To keep the mind at the spirit. A Qìgōng meditation training.

Shǔ 數 Count.

Shuāngxiū 雙修 Dual cultivation. A Qìgōng training method in which Qì is exchanged with a partner in order to balance the Qì in both people.

Shuǐlù 水路 Water Path. A meditation path in which the Qì is led upward through spinal cord to nourish the brain.

Shuǐqì 水氣 Water Qì. Qì created from Original Essence (Yuánjīng, 元精), which is able to calm your body.

Shǔxí 數息 Count the breaths.

Sìdà Jiēkōng 四大皆空 Four large are empty. A stage of Buddhism where all of the four elements (earth, water, fire, and air) are absent from the mind so that one is completely indifferent to worldly temptations.

Sǐqì 死氣 Dead Qì. The Qì remaining in a dead body. Sometimes called "Ghost Qì" (Guǐqì, 鬼氣).

Sòng dynasty 宋朝 A dynasty in Chinese history from 960–1279 CE.

Southern Sòng dynasty 南宋 After the Sòng dynasty was conquered by the Jīn (金) race from Mongolia, the Sòng people moved to the south and established another country, called Southern Sòng, 1127–1279 CE.

Suànmìngshī 算命師 Literally, "Calculate life teacher." A fortune teller who is able to calculate your future and destiny.

Suí 隋 Follow.

Suí dynasty 隋朝 A dynasty in China during the period of 581–618 CE.

Suíxí 隨息 To follow the breathing. A technique for regulating the mind.

Suíxí 髓息 Suí means the marrow or brain. Therefore, Suíxí means the Qìgōng breathing technique which is able to lead the Qì to the bone marrow and brain.

Sūn, Sī-Miǎo 孫思邈 A well-known Chinese physician and Qìgōng master who wrote the book *Qiānjīnfāng* (*Thousand Gold Prescriptions*, 千金方) during the Sui and Tang dynasties, 581–907 CE.

Sùwèn 素問 A medical book. The complete name of the book is *Huángdì Nèijīng Sùwèn* (*The Yellow Emperor's Classic*, 黃帝內經素問). This book was written during the Hàn dynasty, circa 100–300 BCE.

Tài Chí Chuán (Tàijíquán) 太極拳 A Chinese internal martial style based on the theory of Tàijí (Grand Ultimate).

Tàijí 太極 Means "Grand Ultimate." It is this force that generates two poles, Yīn and Yáng.

Tàijíquán (Tài Chí Chuán) 太極拳 A Chinese internal martial style which is based on the theory of Tàijí (Grand Ultimate).

Tàishàng Lǎojūn 太上老君 Old Lord of the Ultimate. The religious title of Lǎozi (老子) by religious Daoists.

Tāixí 胎息 Embryonic breathing. One of the final goals in regulating the breath, Embryo Breathing enables you to generate a "baby Shén" at the Huángtíng (yellow yard, 黃庭).

Tàiyáng 太陽 Greater Yáng. A special terminology used in acupuncture.

Tàiyáng martial stylists 太陽宗 A school of Chinese martial arts that practices Huǒlónggōng (Fire Dragon Gōng, 火龍功) Qìgōng training.

Tàiyīn 太陰 Greater Yīn. A special terminology used in acupuncture.

Tàizǔquán 太祖拳 A style of Chinese external martial arts.

Táng dynasty 唐朝 A dynasty in Chinese history from 618-907 CE.

Táo, Hóng-Jǐng 陶弘景 A well-known physician and Qìgōng master who compiled the book *Yǎngxìng Yánmìng Lù* (*Records of Cultivating Temperament and Extending Life*, 養性延命錄) between 420 to 581 CE.

Tiān 天 Heaven or sky. In ancient China, people believed that Heaven was the most powerful natural energy in this universe.

Tiānqì 天氣 Heaven Qì. It is now commonly used to mean the weather, since weather is governed by Heaven Qì.

Tiānrén Héyī 天人合一 Literally, "Heaven and man unified as one." A high level of Qìgōng practice in which a Qìgōng practitioner, through meditation, is able to communicate his Qì with heaven's Qì.

Tiānshí 天時 Heavenly timing. The repeated natural cycles generated by the heavens such as: seasons, months, days and hours.

Tiáojīng 調精 To regulate the essence.

Tiáoqì 調氣 To regulate the Qì.

Tiáoshēn 調身 To regulate the body.

Tiáoshén 調神 To regulate the spirit.

Tiáoxí 調息 To regulate the breathing.

Tiáoxīn 調心 To regulate the emotional mind.

Tiěbùshān 鐵布衫 Iron shirt. Gōngfū training that toughens the body externally and internally.

Tiěshāzhǎng 鐵砂掌 Literally, "Iron sand palm." A special martial arts conditioning for the palms.

Tīng 聽 Listen.

Tīngxí 聽息 To Listen to the Breathing. A technique for regulating the mind. If you are able to pay attention to your breathing, your mind will not be distracted by surrounding activities.

Tǐxí 體息 Body breathing or skin breathing. In Qìgōng, the exchanging of Qì with the surrounding environment through the skin.

Tǐzhēnzhǐ 體真止 To Comprehend the Real and Stop Method. One of the methods used to regulate the mind in Qìgōng meditation.

Tōngguān 通關 To pass through the gates. In Qìgōng training, the opening of blockages (gates) that hinder the free flow of Qì through the channels.

Tóngrén Yúxuè Zhēnjiǔ Tú 銅人俞穴鍼灸圖 *Illustration of the Brass Man Acupuncture and Moxibustion*. An acupuncture book written by Dr. Wáng, Wéi-Yī (王唯一) during the Sòng dynasty (宋朝).

Tōngsānguān 通三關 Means "To get through the three gates." A special terminology used in Small Circulation.

Tǔnà 吐吶 To utter and to take in. An alternative name of Qìgōng.

Tuīná 推拿 Means "To push and grab." A category of Chinese massages for healing and injury treatment.

Wàidān 外丹 External elixir. External Qìgōng exercises in which a practitioner will build up the Qì in his limbs and then lead it into the center of the body for nourishment.

Wàigōng 外功 External Gōngfū. Gōngfū that emphasizes the physical body training.

Wàishèn 外腎 External Kidneys. The testicles or ovaries.

Wàitái Mìyào 外台祕要 *The Extra Important Secret*. A Chinese medical book written by Wang Tao during the Sui and Tang dynasties, 581–907 CE. This book discusses the use of breathing and herbal therapies for disorders of Qì circulation.

Wāng, Áng 汪昂 A well-known Chinese physician who wrote the book *Yīfāng Jíjiě* (*The Total Introduction to Medical Prescriptions*, 醫方集解) during the Qīng dynasty.

Wáng, Táo 王燾 A well-known Chinese physician and Qìgōng master who wrote the book *Wàitái Mìyào* (*The Extra Important Secret*, 外台祕要) during the Suí and Táng dynasties (隋、唐), 581–907 CE.

Wáng, Wéi-Yī 王唯一 A well-known Chinese physician who wrote the book *Tóngrén Yúxuè Zhēnjiǔ Tú* (*Illustration of the Brass Man Acupuncture and Moxibustion*, 銅人俞穴鍼灸圖) during the Sòng dynasty (宋朝).

Wáng, Zǔ-Yuán 王祖源 A well-known Chinese physician who wrote the book *Nèigōng Túshuō* (*Illustrated Explanation of Nèigōng*, 內功圖說) during the Qīng dynasty (清朝).

Wèi, Bó-Yáng 魏伯陽 A well-known physician who wrote the book *Zhōuyì Cāntóngqì* (A comparative study of the Zhōu dynasty *Book of Changes*, 周易參同契) during the Qín and Hàn dynasties (秦、漢), 221 BCE–220 CE.

Wèiqì 衛氣 Protective Qì or Guardian Qì. The Qì at the surface of the body that generates a shield to protect the body from negative external influences such as colds.

Wǔ, Shǒu-Yáng (1552–1640 CE) 伍守陽 A Chinese Qìgōng master who lived during the late Míng (c) and early Qīng dynasties (清朝).

Wǔdāng Mountain 武當山 Located in Húběi Province (湖北省) in China.

Wújí 無極 Means "no extremity."

Wújí Qìgōng 無極氣功 A style of Tàijí Qìgōng practice.

Wúniàn Zhīniàn 無念之念 Means "The thought of no thought." The final stage of regulating the mind.

Wǔqì Cháoyuán 五氣朝元 Five Qì(s) toward origins. A goal of Qìgōng wherein the Qì of the five Yīn organs (Heart, Lungs, Liver, Kidneys, and Spleen) is kept at the right (original) level. This will keep the organs from being either too Yáng or too Yīn, and will slow the degeneration process.

Wǔqínxì 五禽戲 Five Animal Sports. A set of medical Qìgōng practices created by Jūnqiàn (君倩) during the Jìn dynasty (晉), 265–420 CE.

Wǔshù 武術 Literally, "Martial techniques." A common name for the Chinese martial arts. Many other terms are used, including: Wǔyì (martial arts, 武藝), Wǔgōng (martial Gōngfū, 武功), Guóshù (national techniques, 國術), and Gōngfū (energy-time, 功夫). Because Wǔshù has been modified in mainland China over the past forty years into gymnastic martial performance, many traditional Chinese martial artist have given up this name in order to avoid confusing modern Wǔshù with traditional Wǔshù. Recently, mainland China has attempted to return modern Wǔshù to its traditional training and practice.

Wǔxīn 五心 Five centers. The face, the Láogōng (勞宮) cavities on both palms, and the Yǒngquán (湧泉) cavities on the bottoms of both feet.

Wǔxíng 五行 Five phases. Also called the five elements. Metal, wood, water, fire, and earth, representing the five phases of any process.

Xì 細 Slender.

Xǐ 喜 Happiness and delight.

Xià Dāntián 下丹田 Lower Dāntián. Located in the lower abdomen, it is believed to be the residence of Water Qì (Original Qì; Yuánqì, 元氣).

Xiàjiāo 下焦 Lower Burner. The lower abdomen is called "the Lower Burner."

Xiān 仙 An immortal. A person who has attained enlightenment or Buddhahood, whose spirit can separate from and returned to his physical body at will.

Xiāntāi 仙胎 Holy Embryo.

Xiāntiānqì 先天氣 Pre-Birth Qì or Pre-Heaven Qì. Also called "Dāntiánqì" (丹田氣). The Qì that is converted from Original Essence (Yuánjīng, 元精) and is stored in the Lower Dāntián (下丹田). Considered to be Water Qì (Shuǐqì, 水氣). It is able to calm the body.

Xiào 孝 Filial Piety.

Xiǎozhōutiān 小周天 Literally, "Small heavenly cycle." Also called "Small Circulation." In Qìgōng, when you can use your mind to lead Qì through the Conception and Governing Vessels, you have completed "Xiǎozhōutiān."

Xīn 心 Means "Heart." Xīn means the mind generated from emotional disturbance.

Xìn 信 Trust.

Xìng 性 Human Nature.

Xìngmìng Shuāngxiū 性命雙修 Human nature life dual cultivation. Originally a Buddhist, though now predominantly Daoist approach to Qìgōng emphasizing the cultivation of both spirituality (human nature) and the physical body.

Xíngyìquán (Hsíng Yì Chuán) 形意拳 Literally, "Shape-mind Fist." An internal style of Gōngfū in which the mind or thinking determines the shape or movement of the body. Creation of the style is attributed to Marshal Yuè, Fēi (岳飛).

Xīnniàn 心念 Emotional mind-thought. The thought generated from the emotional mind.

Xīnshén 心神 Literally, "Heart-spirit." This refers to the emotional mind that affects or is affected by Shén.

Xīnshén Bùníng 心神不寧 Means "The (emotional) mind and spirit are not peaceful." A scattered mind.

Xīnxī Xiāngyī 心息相依 Heart (mind) and breathing (are) mutually dependent.

Xīnyì 心意 Literally, "Heart (Xīn, 心) or emotional mind—Yì (wisdom mind)." This denotes the mind generated from both emotion and thought.

Xīnyuán Yìmǎ 心猿意馬 Literally, "Heart monkey Yì horse." Xīn (heart) is used to represent the emotional mind that acts like a monkey, unsteady and disturbing. Yì is the mind that is generated from calm and clear thinking and judgment (i.e., wisdom mind). The Yì is like a horse, calm and powerful.

Xīnzhúxiàn 新竹縣 Birthplace of Dr. Yáng, Jwìng-Mǐng in Táiwān (台灣).

Xǐsuǐjīng 洗髓經 Literally, "Washing Marrow/Brain Classic," usually translated *Marrow/Brain Washing Classic*. A Qìgōng training that specializes in leading Qì to the marrow to cleanse it or to the brain to nourish the spirit for enlightenment. It is believed that Xǐsuǐjīng training is the key to longevity and spiritual enlightenment.

Xiūqì 修氣 Cultivate the Qì. Cultivate implies to protect, maintain and refine. A Buddhist Qìgōng training.

Xiūshēn Sìmìng 修身俟命 Means "Cultivate the body and await destiny."

Xìyuánzhǐ 繫緣止 Tie to the Origin and Stop Method. One of the methods used to regulate the mind.

Xuè 穴 Literally, "Wave or hole." An acupuncture cavity.

Xūwú 虛無 Means "Nothing."

Yáng 陽 In Chinese philosophy, the active, positive, masculine polarity. In Chinese medicine, Yáng means excessive, overactive, overheated. The Yáng (or outer) organs are the Gall Bladder, Small Intestine, Large Intestine, Stomach, Bladder, and Triple Burner.

Yăng 癢 Itching.

Yăngāo Shǒudī 眼高手低 Literally, "The eyes are high and the hands are low." That means expectations are higher than accomplishments.

Yánluówáng 閻羅王 King of Hell. Title of the King in Hell.

Yăngqì 養氣 Means "To cultivate the Qì."

Yăngshén 養神 Yáng means "To raise, nourish, and maintain." Shén means "Spirit." Yăngshén is the main Buddhist approach to regulating the Shén.

Yăngshēng Fūyǔ 養生膚語 *Brief Introduction to Nourishing the Body.* A book written by Chén, Jì-Rú (陳繼儒) during the Qīng dynasty (清朝).

Yăngshēngjué 養生訣 *Life Nourishing Secrets.* A medical book written by Zhāng, Ān-Dào (張安道) during the Sòng, Jīn, and Yuán dynasties (宋、金、元), 960–1368 CE.

Yăngxìng Yánmìnglù 養性延命錄 *Records of Cultivating Temperament and Extending Life.* A Chinese medical book written by Táo, Hóng-Jǐng (陶弘景) in the period of 420 to 581 CE.

Yáng, Jwìng-Mǐng 楊俊敏 Author of this book.

Yáng, Tim Chùn-Chiéh 楊俊杰 Author's brother.

Yángmíng 陽明 Yáng Brightness. A special terminology used in acupuncture.

Yángqiāomài 陽蹺脈 Yáng Heel Vessel. One of the eight Qì vessels.

Yángwéimài 陽維脈 Yáng Linking Vessel. One of the eight vessels.

Yì 意 Mind. Specifically, the mind generated by clear thinking and judgment, and which is able to make you calm, peaceful, and wise.

Yì 義 Justice or righteousness.

Yī 猗 Ripple.

Yīfāng Jíjiě 醫方集解 *The Total Introduction to Medical Prescriptions.* A Chinese medical book written by Wāng, Áng (汪昂) in the Qīng dynasty (清朝).

Yìjīnjīng 易筋經 Literally, "Changing muscle/tendon classic," usually called the *Muscle/Tendon Changing Classic.* Credited to Dámó (達摩) around 550 CE, this work discusses Wàidān Qìgōng training for strengthening the physical body.

Yìjīng 易經 *Book of Changes*. A book of divination written during the Zhōu dynasty (周朝) (1122–255 BCE).

Yǐjīng Huàqì 以精化氣 Means "To convert the Jīng (essence) into Qì."

Yīn 陰 In Chinese philosophy, the passive, negative, feminine polarity. In Chinese medicine, Yīn means deficient. The Yīn (internal) organs are the Heart, Lungs, Liver, Kidneys, Spleen, and Pericardium.

Yìniàn 意念 Literally, "Wisdom mind-thought." That means the thought generated from wise clear thinking.

Yīnqiāomài 陰蹻脈 The Yīn Heel Vessel. One of the eight vessels.

Yìnggōng 硬功 Hard Gōngfū. Any Chinese martial training which emphasizes physical strength and power.

Yíngqì 營氣 Managing Qì. The Qì that manages the functioning of the organs and the body.

Yīnwéimài 陰維脈 Yīn Linking Vessel. One of the eight vessels.

Yīnxū 殷墟 An archeological site of the late Shāng dynasty (商朝) burial ground.

Yǐqì Huàshén 以氣化神 Means "To nourish the Shén (spirit) with Qì."

Yǐshén Yùqì 以神馭氣 Use the Shén (spirit) to govern the Qì. A Qìgōng technique. Since the Shén is the headquarters for the Qì, it is the most effective way to control it.

Yìshì 意識 Literally, "Yì recognize." To use the Yì (wisdom mind) to sense and understand a situation. In order to do this, your Yì must search for information, evaluate it, and then reach a final decision. Yìshì is similar to "sense" in English; however, Yì Shì is more active and aggressive.

Yìshǒu Dāntián 意守丹田 Keep your Yì on your Lower Dāntián. In Qìgōng training, you keep your mind at the Lower Dāntián in order to build up Qì. When you are circulating your Qì, you always lead your Qì back to your Lower Dāntián before you stop.

Yǐxīn Huìyì 以心會意 Means "Modulate the Xīn (emotional mind) to match the Yì (wisdom mind)."

Yǐyì Huìshēn 以意會身 Means "Use your Yì to meet the body."

Yǐyì Yǐnqì 以意引氣 Use your Yì (wisdom mind) to lead your Qì. A Qìgōng technique. Qì cannot be pushed, but it can be led. This is best done with the Yì.

Yìzhì 意志 Will. Yì is commonly used together with will.

Yǒngquán (K-1) 湧泉 Bubbling Well. Name of an acupuncture cavity belonging to the Kidney Primary Qì Channel.

Yōu 悠 Long, far, meditative, continuous, slow, and soft.

Yù 慾 Desire.

Yuán dynasty 元代 A Chinese dynasty from 1206–1367 CE.

Yuánjīng 元精 Original Essence. The fundamental, original substance you inherited from your parents. It is converted into Original Qì.

Yuánqì 元氣 Original Qì. The Qì created from the Original Essence inherited from your parents.

Yuánqiào 元竅 Original key point. Key points to the training.

Yuánshén 元神 Original Shén.

Yuánshǐ Tiānzūn 元始天尊 The Primal Celestial Excellency. A Daoist deity.

Yuè, Fēi 岳飛 A Chinese hero from the Southern Sòng dynasty (宋朝), 1127–1279 CE. He is said to have created Bāduànjǐn (八段錦), Xíngyìquán (形意拳 and Yuè's Yīngzhǎo (岳家鷹爪).

Yùhuáng Dàdì 玉皇大帝 The Supreme Deity. A Daoist title of the heaven emperor who rules heaven and earth.

Yún 勻 Uniform or even.

Zāijiēpài 栽接派 Plant and Graft Division. A division of Daoist Qìgōng training.

Zàng 臟 Viscera. The six Yīn organs. Five of these are considered the core of the entire human system—the Liver, Heart, Spleen, Lungs, and Kidneys. Usually, when a discussion involves the channels and all the organs, the Pericardium is added; otherwise it is treated as an adjunct of the Heart.

Zhāng, Ān-Dào 張安道 A well-known Chinese physician and Qìgōng master who wrote the book, *Yǎngshēngjué* (*Life Nourishing Secrets*, 養生訣), during the Sòng, Jīn, and Yuán dynasties (宋、金、元), 960–1368 CE.

Zhāng, Dào-Líng 張道陵 A Daoist who combined scholarly Daoism with Buddhist philosophies and created Religious Daoism (Dàojiào, 道教) during the Chinese Eastern Hàn dynasty (東漢), 25–221 CE.

Zhāng, Sān-Fēng 張三豐 Zhāng, Sān-Fēng is credited as the creator of Tàijíquán (太極拳) during the Sòng dynasty (宋朝) in China (960–1127 CE).

Zhāng, Zhòng-Jǐng 張仲景 A well-known Chinese physician who wrote the book *Jīnguì Yàolüè* (*Prescriptions from the Golden Chamber*, 金匱要略) during the Qín and Hàn dynasties (秦、漢), 221 BCE–220 CE.

Zhāng, Zi-Hé 張子和 A well-known Chinese physician who wrote the book *Rúmén Shìshì* (*The Confucian Point of View*, 儒門視事), during the Sòng, Jīn, and Yuán dynasties (宋、金、元), 960–1368 CE.

Zhèng Fùhūxī 正腹呼吸 Formal Abdominal Breathing. More commonly called Buddhist Breathing.

Zhèngqì 正氣 Righteous Qì. When a person is righteous, it is said that he has righteous Qì which evil Qì cannot overcome.

Zhēnxí 真息 The real breathing. That means the breathing has been regulated to a deep and profound level.

Zhǐ 止 Stop.

Zhǐguānfǎ 止觀法 Stop and Look Method. One of the methods used to regulate the mind.

Zhǐniàn 止念 Means "To stop the old thought from coming back."

Zhǐniànfǎ 止念法 Methods of Stopping Thought. One of the methods used to regulate the mind.

Zhìxīnzhǐ 制心止 Restrain the Xīn and Stop Method. One of the methods used to regulate the mind.

Zhōng 忠 Loyalty.

Zhòng 重 Heavy.

Zhōng Dāntián 中丹田 Middle Dāntián. Located in the area of the solar plexus, it is the residence of fire Qì.

Zhōngguān 中觀 The Centered Look. A Qìgōng method for regulating the mind.

Zhōngjiāo 中焦 Middle Burner. One of the Triple Burners.

Zhōu dynasty 周朝 A dynasty in China from 1122–934 BCE.

Zhōuyì Cāntóngqì 周易參同契 *A Comparative Study of the Zhōu (Dynasty) Book of Changes.* A medical and Qìgōng book written by Wèi, Bó-Yáng (魏伯陽) during the Qín and Hàn dynasties (秦、漢), 221 BCE–220 CE.

Zhūbìng Yuánhòu Lùn 諸病源候論 *Thesis on the Origins and Symptoms of Various Diseases.* A Chinese medical book written by Cháo, Yuán-Fāng (巢元方) during the Suí and Táng dynasties (隋、唐), 581–907 CE.

Zhū, Dān-Xī 朱丹溪 A well-known Chinese physician who wrote the book *Gézhì Yúlùn* (*A Further Thesis of Complete Study*, 格致餘論), during the Sòng, Jīn, and Yuán dynasties (宋、金、元), 960–1368 CE.

Zhuānqì Zhìróu 專氣致柔 Means "Concentrate on Qì and achieve softness." A famous sentence line from Lǎozi's *Dào Dé Jīng* (道德經).

Zhuāngzhōu 莊周 A contemporary of Mencius who advocated Daoism.

Zhuāngzi 莊子 Zhuāngzhōu. A contemporary of Mencius who advocated Daoism. Zhuāngzi also means "The works of Zhuāngzhōu" (莊周).

Zǐwǔ Liúzhù 子午流注 Zǐ refers to the period around midnight (11:00 pm to 1:00 am), and Wǔ refers to midday (11:00 am to 1:00 pm). Liúzhù means "The flowing tendency." Therefore:

a schedule of the Qì circulation showing which channel has the predominant Qì flow at any particular time, and where the predominant Qì flow is in the Conception and Governing Vessels.

Zǒuhuǒ Rùmó 走火入魔 Walk into the fire and enter into the devil. In Qìgōng training, if you have led your Qì into the wrong path it is called "walking into the fire" (Zǒuhuǒ, 走火), and if your mind has been led into a confused state, it is called "entering into the devil" (Rùmó, 入魔).

Index

About the Author

Yáng, Jwìng-Mǐng, PhD (楊俊敏博士)

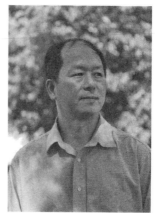

Dr. Yáng, Jwìng-Mǐng was born on August 11, 1946, in Xīnzhúxiàn (新竹縣), Táiwān (台灣), Republic of China (中華民國). He started his Wǔshù (武術) (Gōngfū or Kūng Fū, 功夫) training at the age of fifteen under Shàolín White Crane (Shàolín Báihè, 少林白鶴) Master Chēng, Gīn-Gsào (曾金灶). Master Chēng originally learned Tàizǔquán (太祖拳) from his grandfather when he was a child. When Master Chēng was fifteen years old, he started learning White Crane from Master Jīn, Shào-Fēng (金紹峰) and followed him for twenty-three years until Master Jīn's death.

In thirteen years of study (1961–1974) under Master Chēng, Dr. Yáng became an expert in the White Crane style of Chinese martial arts, which includes both the use of bare hands and various weapons, such as saber, staff, spear, trident, two short rods, and many others. With the same master he also studied White Crane Qìgōng (氣功), Qín Ná or Chín Ná (擒拿), Tuīná (推拿), and Diǎnxué massage (點穴按摩) and herbal treatment.

At sixteen, Dr. Yáng began the study of Yáng Style Tàijíquán (or Tài Chí Chuán, 楊氏太極拳) under Master Kāo, Táo (高濤). He later continued his study of Tàijíquán under Master Lǐ, Mào-Chīng (李茂清). Master Lǐ learned his Tàijíquán from the well-known Master Hán, Chìng-Táng (韓慶堂). From this further practice, Dr. Yáng was able to master the Tàijí bare-hand sequence, pushing hands, the two-man fighting sequence, Tàijí sword, Tàijí saber, and Tàijí Qìgōng.

When Dr. Yáng was eighteen years old, he entered Tamkang College (淡江學院) in Taipei Xiàn to study physics. In college, he began the study of traditional Shàolín Long Fist (Chángquán or Cháng Chuán, 少林長拳) with Master Lǐ, Mào-Chīng at the Tamkang College Guóshù Club (淡江國術社), 1964–1968, and eventually became an assistant instructor under Master Lǐ. In 1971, he completed his MS degree in physics at the National Táiwān University (台灣大學) and then served in the Chinese Air Force from 1971 to 1972. In the service, Dr. Yáng taught physics at the Junior Academy of the Chinese Air Force (空軍幼校) while also teaching Wǔshù (武術). After being honorably discharged in 1972, he returned to Tamkang College to teach physics and resumed study under Master Lǐ, Mào-Chīng. From Master Lǐ, Dr. Yáng learned Northern Style Wǔshù, which includes both bare hand and kicking techniques, and numerous weapons.

In 1974, Dr. Yáng came to the United States to study mechanical engineering at Purdue University. At the request of a few students, Dr. Yáng began to teach Gōngfū, which resulted in the establishment of the Purdue University Chinese Kūng Fū Research Club in the spring of 1975. While at Purdue, Dr. Yáng also taught college-credit courses in Tàijíquán. In May of 1978, he was awarded a PhD in mechanical engineering by Purdue.

In 1980, Dr. Yáng moved to Houston to work for Texas Instruments. While in Houston, he founded Yáng's Shàolín Kūng Fū Academy, which was eventually taken over by his disciple, Mr. Jeffery Bolt, after Dr. Yáng moved to Boston in 1982. Dr. Yáng founded Yáng's Martial Arts Academy in Boston on October 1, 1982.

In January of 1984, he gave up his engineering career to devote more time to research, writing, and teaching. In March of 1986, he purchased property in the Jamaica Plain area of Boston to be used as the headquarters of the new organization, Yáng's Martial Arts Association (YMAA). The organization expanded to become a division of Yáng's Oriental Arts Association, Inc. (YOAA).

In 2008, Dr. Yáng began the nonprofit YMAA California Retreat Center. This training facility in rural California is where selected students enroll in a five to ten-year residency to learn Chinese martial arts.

Dr. Yáng has been involved in traditional Chinese Wǔshù since 1961, studying Shàolín White Crane (Báihè), Shàolín Long Fist (Chángquán), and Tàijíquán under several different masters. He has taught for more than forty-six years: seven years in Táiwān, five years at Purdue University, two years in Houston, twenty-six years in Boston, and more than eight years at the YMAA California Retreat Center. He has taught seminars all around the world, sharing his knowledge of Chinese martial arts and Qìgōng in Argentina, Austria, Barbados, Botswana, Belgium, Bermuda, Brazil, Canada, China, Chile, England, Egypt, France, Germany, Holland, Hungary, Iceland, Iran, Ireland, Italy, Latvia, Mexico, New Zealand, Poland, Portugal, Saudi Arabia, Spain, South Africa, Switzerland, and Venezuela.

Since 1986, YMAA has become an international organization, which currently includes more than fifty schools located in Argentina, Belgium, Canada, Chile, France, Hungary, Ireland, Italy, New Zealand, Poland, Portugal, South Africa, Sweden, the United Kingdom, Venezuela, and the United States.

Many of Dr. Yáng's books and videos have been translated into many languages, including French, Italian, Spanish, Polish, Czech, Bulgarian, Russian, German, and Hungarian.

Books by Dr. Yáng, Jwìng-Mǐng
Analysis of Shàolín Chín Ná, 2nd ed. YMAA Publication Center, 1987, 2004
Ancient Chinese Weapons: A Martial Artist's Guide, 2nd ed. YMAA Publication Center, 1985, 1999
Arthritis Relief: Chinese Qìgōng for Healing & Prevention, 2nd ed. YMAA Publication Center, 1991, 2005

Back Pain Relief: Chinese Qìgōng for Healing and Prevention, 2nd ed. YMAA Publication Center, 1997, 2004

Bāguàzhǎng: Theory and Applications, 2nd ed. YMAA Publication Center, 1994, 2008

Comprehensive Applications of Shàolín Chín Ná: The Practical Defense of Chinese Seizing Arts. YMAA Publication Center, 1995

Essence of Shàolín White Crane: Martial Power and Qìgōng. YMAA Publication Center, 1996

How to Defend Yourself. YMAA Publication Center, 1992

Introduction to Ancient Chinese Weapons. Unique Publications, Inc., 1985

Meridian Qìgōng, YMAA Publication Center, 2016

Northern Shàolín Sword, 2nd ed. YMAA Publication Center, 1985, 2000

Qìgōng for Health and Martial Arts, 2nd ed. YMAA Publication Center, 1995,1998

Qìgōng Massage: Fundamental Techniques for Health and Relaxation, 2nd ed. YMAA Publication Center, 1992, 2005

Qìgōng Meditation: Embryonic Breathing. YMAA Publication Center, 2003

Qìgōng Meditation: Small Circulation, YMAA Publication Center, 2006

Qìgōng—The Secret of Youth: Dá Mó's Muscle/Tendon Changing and Marrow/Brain Washing Qìgōng, 2nd ed. YMAA Publication Center, 1989, 2000

Root of Chinese Qìgōng: Secrets of Qìgōng Training, 2nd ed. YMAA Publication Center, 1989, 1997

Shàolín Chín Ná. Unique Publications, Inc., 1980

Shàolín Long Fist Kūng Fū. Unique Publications, Inc., 1981

Simple Qìgōng Exercises for Health: The Eight Pieces of Brocade, 3rd ed. YMAA Publication Center, 1988, 1997, 2013

Tài Chí Ball Qìgōng: For Health and Martial Arts. YMAA Publication Center, 2010

Tài Chí Chuán Classical Yáng Style: The Complete Long Form and Qìgōng, 2nd ed. YMAA Publication Center, 1999, 2010

Tài Chí Chuán Martial Applications, 2nd ed. YMAA Publication Center, 1986, 1996

Tài Chí Chuán Martial Power, 3rd ed. YMAA Publication Center, 1986, 1996, 2015

Tài Chí Chuán: Classical Yáng Style, 2nd ed. YMAA Publication Center, 1999, 2010

Tài Chí Qìgōng: The Internal Foundation of Tài Chí Chuán, 2nd ed. rev. YMAA Publication Center, 1997, 1990, 2013

Tài Chí Secrets of the Ancient Masters: Selected Readings with Commentary. YMAA Publication Center, 1999

Tài Chí Secrets of the Wǔ and Lǐ Styles: Chinese Classics, Translation, Commentary. YMAA Publication Center, 2001

Tài Chí Secrets of the Wú Style: Chinese Classics, Translation, Commentary. YMAA Publication Center, 2002

Tài Chí Secrets of the Yáng Style: Chinese Classics, Translation, Commentary. YMAA Publication Center, 2001

Tài Chí Sword Classical Yáng Style: The Complete Long Form, Qìgōng, and Applications, 2nd ed. YMAA Publication Center, 1999, 2014

Tàijí Chín Ná: The Seizing Art of Tàijíquan, 2nd ed. YMAA Publication Center, 1995, 2014

Tàijíquan Theory of Dr. Yáng, Jwìng-Mǐng: The Root of Tàijíquan. YMAA Publication Center, 2003

Xíngyìquán: Theory and Applications, 2nd ed. YMAA Publication Center, 1990, 2003

Yáng Style Tài Chí Chuán. Unique Publications, Inc., 1981

Videos by Dr. Yáng, Jwìng-Mǐng
Advanced Practical Chín Ná in Depth, YMAA Publication Center, 2010

Analysis of Shàolín Chín Ná. YMAA Publication Center, 2004

Bāguàzhǎng (Eight Trigrams Palm Kūng Fū). YMAA Publication Center, 2005

Chín Ná in Depth: Courses 1–4. YMAA Publication Center, 2003

Chín Ná in Depth: Courses 5–8. YMAA Publication Center, 2003

Chín Ná in Depth: Courses 9–12. YMAA Publication Center, 2003

Five Animal Sports Qìgōng. YMAA Publication Center, 2008

Knife Defense: Traditional Techniques. YMAA Publication Center, 2011

Meridian Qìgōng. YMAA Publication Center, 2015

Neigong. YMAA Publication Center, 2015

Northern Shàolín Sword. YMAA Publication Center, 2009

Qìgōng Massage. YMAA Publication Center, 2005

Saber Fundamental Training. YMAA Publication Center, 2008

Shàolín Kūng Fū Fundamental Training. YMAA Publication Center, 2004

Shàolín Long Fist Kūng Fū: Basic Sequences. YMAA Publication Center, 2005

Shàolín Saber Basic Sequences. YMAA Publication Center, 2007

Shàolín Staff Basic Sequences. YMAA Publication Center, 2007

Shàolín White Crane Gōng Fū Basic Training: Courses 1 & 2. YMAA Publication Center, 2003

Shàolín White Crane Gōng Fū Basic Training: Courses 3 & 4. YMAA Publication Center, 2008

Shàolín White Crane Hard and Soft Qìgōng. YMAA Publication Center, 2003

Shuāi Jiāo: Kūng Fū Wrestling. YMAA Publication Center, 2010

Simple Qìgōng Exercises for Arthritis Relief. YMAA Publication Center, 2007

Simple Qìgōng Exercises for Back Pain Relief. YMAA Publication Center, 2007

Simple Qìgōng Exercises for Health: The Eight Pieces of Brocade. YMAA Publication Center, 2003

Staff Fundamental Training: Solo Drills and Matching Practice. YMAA Publication Center, 2007

Sword Fundamental Training. YMAA Publication Center, 2009

Tài Chí Ball Qìgōng: Courses 1 & 2. YMAA Publication Center, 2006

Tài Chí Ball Qìgōng: Courses 3 & 4. YMAA Publication Center, 2007

Tài Chí Chuán: Classical Yáng Style. YMAA Publication Center, 2003

Tài Chí Fighting Set: 2-Person Matching Set. YMAA Publication Center, 2006

Tài Chí Pushing Hands: Courses 1 & 2. YMAA Publication Center, 2005

Tài Chí Pushing Hands: Courses 3 & 4. YMAA Publication Center, 2006

Tài Chí Qìgōng. YMAA Publication Center, 2005

Tài Chí Sword, Classical Yáng Style. YMAA Publication Center, 2005

Tài Chí Symbol: Yīn/Yáng Sticking Hands. YMAA Publication Center, 2008

Tàijí 37 Postures Martial Applications. YMAA Publication Center, 2008

Tàijí Chín Ná in Depth. YMAA Publication Center, 2009

Tàijí Saber: Classical Yáng Style. YMAA Publication Center, 2008

Tàijí Wrestling: Advanced Takedown Techniques. YMAA Publication Center, 2008

Understanding Qìgōng, DVD 1: What is Qìgōng? The Human Qì Circulatory System. YMAA Publication Center, 2006

Understanding Qìgōng, DVD 2: Key Points of Qìgōng & Qìgōng Breathing. YMAA Publication Center, 2006

Understanding Qìgōng, DVD 3: Embryonic Breathing. YMAA Publication Center, 2007

Understanding Qìgōng, DVD 4: Four Seasons Qìgōng. YMAA Publication Center, 2007

Understanding Qìgōng, DVD 5: Small Circulation. YMAA Publication Center, 2007

Understanding Qìgōng, DVD 6: Martial Arts Qìgōng Breathing. YMAA Publication Center, 2007

Xíngyìquán: Twelve Animals Kūng Fū and Applications. YMAA Publication Center, 2008

Yáng Tài Chí for Beginners. YMAA Publication Center, 2012

YMAA 25-Year Anniversary. YMAA Publication Center, 2009

BOOKS FROM YMAA

101 REFLECTIONS ON TAI CHI CHUAN
108 INSIGHTS INTO TAI CHI CHUAN
A WOMAN'S QIGONG GUIDE
ADVANCING IN TAE KWON DO
ANALYSIS OF SHAOLIN CHIN NA 2ND ED
ANCIENT CHINESE WEAPONS
ART AND SCIENCE OF STAFF FIGHTING
THE ART AND SCIENCE OF SELF-DEFENSE
ART AND SCIENCE OF STICK FIGHTING
ART OF HOJO UNDO
ARTHRITIS RELIEF, 3D ED.
BACK PAIN RELIEF, 2ND ED.
BAGUAZHANG, 2ND ED.
BRAIN FITNESS
CHIN NA IN GROUND FIGHTING
CHINESE FAST WRESTLING
CHINESE FITNESS
CHINESE TUI NA MASSAGE
COMPLETE MARTIAL ARTIST
COMPREHENSIVE APPLICATIONS OF SHAOLIN CHIN NA
CONFLICT COMMUNICATION
DAO DE JING: A QIGONG INTERPRETATION
DAO IN ACTION
DEFENSIVE TACTICS
DIRTY GROUND
DR. WU'S HEAD MASSAGE
ESSENCE OF SHAOLIN WHITE CRANE
EXPLORING TAI CHI
FACING VIOLENCE
FIGHT LIKE A PHYSICIST
THE FIGHTER'S BODY
FIGHTER'S FACT BOOK 1&2
FIGHTING ARTS
FIGHTING THE PAIN RESISTANT ATTACKER
FIRST DEFENSE
FORCE DECISIONS: A CITIZENS GUIDE
INSIDE TAI CHI
JUDO ADVANTAGE
JUJI GATAME ENCYCLOPEDIA
KARATE SCIENCE
KATA AND THE TRANSMISSION OF KNOWLEDGE
KRAV MAGA COMBATIVES
KRAV MAGA FUNDAMENTAL STRATEGIES
KRAV MAGA PROFESSIONAL TACTICS
KRAV MAGA WEAPON DEFENSES
LITTLE BLACK BOOK OF VIOLENCE
LIUHEBAFA FIVE CHARACTER SECRETS
MARTIAL ARTS OF VIETNAM
MARTIAL ARTS INSTRUCTION
MARTIAL WAY AND ITS VIRTUES
MEDITATIONS ON VIOLENCE
MERIDIAN QIGONG EXERCISES
MINDFUL EXERCISE
MIND INSIDE TAI CHI
MIND INSIDE YANG STYLE TAI CHI CHUAN
NATURAL HEALING WITH QIGONG
NORTHERN SHAOLIN SWORD, 2ND ED.
OKINAWA'S COMPLETE KARATE SYSTEM: ISSHIN RYU
PRINCIPLES OF TRADITIONAL CHINESE MEDICINE
PROTECTOR ETHIC
QIGONG FOR HEALTH & MARTIAL ARTS 2ND ED.
QIGONG FOR TREATING COMMON AILMENTS

QIGONG MASSAGE
QIGONG MEDITATION: EMBRYONIC BREATHING
QIGONG GRAND CIRCULATION
QIGONG MEDITATION: SMALL CIRCULATION
QIGONG, THE SECRET OF YOUTH: DA MO'S CLASSICS
REDEMPTION
ROOT OF CHINESE QIGONG, 2ND ED.
SAMBO ENCYCLOPEDIA
SCALING FORCE
SELF-DEFENSE FOR WOMEN
SHIN GI TAI: KARATE TRAINING
SIMPLE CHINESE MEDICINE
SIMPLE QIGONG EXERCISES FOR HEALTH, 3RD ED.
SIMPLIFIED TAI CHI CHUAN, 2ND ED.
SOLO TRAINING 1&2
SPOTTING DANGER BEFORE IT SPOTS YOU
SPOTTING DANGER BEFORE IT SPOTS YOUR KIDS
SPOTTING DANGER BEFORE IT SPOTS YOUR TEENS
SUMO FOR MIXED MARTIAL ARTS
SUNRISE TAI CHI
SURVIVING ARMED ASSAULTS
TAE KWON DO: THE KOREAN MARTIAL ART
TAEKWONDO BLACK BELT POOMSAE
TAEKWONDO: A PATH TO EXCELLENCE
TAEKWONDO: ANCIENT WISDOM
TAEKWONDO: DEFENSE AGAINST WEAPONS
TAEKWONDO: SPIRIT AND PRACTICE
TAI CHI BALL QIGONG: FOR HEALTH AND MARTIAL ARTS
THE TAI CHI BOOK
TAI CHI CHIN NA, 2ND ED.
TAI CHI CHUAN CLASSICAL YANG STYLE, 2ND ED.
TAI CHI CHUAN MARTIAL POWER, 3RD ED.
TAI CHI CONCEPTS AND EXPERIMENTS
TAI CHI CONNECTIONS
TAI CHI DYNAMICS
TAI CHI FOR DEPRESSION
TAI CHI IN 10 WEEKS
TAI CHI PUSH HANDS
TAI CHI QIGONG, 3RD ED.
TAI CHI SECRETS OF THE ANCIENT MASTERS
TAI CHI SECRETS OF THE WU & LI STYLES
TAI CHI SECRETS OF THE WU STYLE
TAI CHI SECRETS OF THE YANG STYLE
TAI CHI SWORD: CLASSICAL YANG STYLE, 2ND ED.
TAI CHI SWORD FOR BEGINNERS
TAI CHI WALKING
TAIJIQUAN THEORY OF DR. YANG, JWING-MING
FIGHTING ARTS
TRADITIONAL CHINESE HEALTH SECRETS
TRADITIONAL TAEKWONDO
TRAINING FOR SUDDEN VIOLENCE
TRIANGLE HOLD ENCYCLOPEDIA
TRUE WELLNESS SERIES (MIND, HEART, GUT)
WARRIOR'S MANIFESTO
WAY OF KATA
WAY OF SANCHIN KATA
WAY TO BLACK BELT
WESTERN HERBS FOR MARTIAL ARTISTS
WILD GOOSE QIGONG
WINNING FIGHTS
XINGYIQUAN

AND MANY MORE . . .

VIDEOS FROM YMAA

ANALYSIS OF SHAOLIN CHIN NA
BAGUA FOR BEGINNERS 1 & 2
BAGUAZHANG: EMEI BAGUAZHANG
BEGINNER QIGONG FOR WOMEN 1 & 2
BEGINNER TAI CHI FOR HEALTH
CHEN TAI CHI CANNON FIST
CHEN TAI CHI FIRST FORM
CHEN TAI CHI FOR BEGINNERS
CHIN NA IN-DEPTH SERIES
FACING VIOLENCE: 7 THINGS A MARTIAL ARTIST MUST KNOW
FIVE ANIMAL SPORTS
FIVE ELEMENTS ENERGY BALANCE
INFIGHTING
INTRODUCTION TO QI GONG FOR BEGINNERS
JOINT LOCKS
KNIFE DEFENSE
KUNG FU BODY CONDITIONING 1 & 2
KUNG FU FOR KIDS AND TEENS SERIES
LOGIC OF VIOLENCE
MERIDIAN QIGONG
NEIGONG FOR MARTIAL ARTS
NORTHERN SHAOLIN SWORD
QI GONG 30-DAY CHALLENGE
QI GONG FOR ANXIETY
QI GONG FOR ARMS, WRISTS, AND HANDS
QIGONG FOR BEGINNERS: FRAGRANCE
QI GONG FOR BETTER BALANCE
QI GONG FOR BETTER BREATHING
QI GONG FOR CANCER
QI GONG FOR DEPRESSION
QI GONG FOR ENERGY AND VITALITY
QI GONG FOR HEADACHES
QI GONG FOR THE HEALTHY HEART
QI GONG FOR HEALTHY JOINTS
QI GONG FOR HIGH BLOOD PRESSURE
QIGONG FOR LONGEVITY
QI GONG FOR STRONG BONES
QI GONG FOR THE UPPER BACK AND NECK
QIGONG FOR WOMEN WITH DAISY LEE
QIGONG FLOW FOR STRESS & ANXIETY RELIEF
QIGONG MASSAGE
QIGONG MINDFULNESS IN MOTION
QI GONG—THE SEATED WORKOUT
QIGONG: 15 MINUTES TO HEALTH
SABER FUNDAMENTAL TRAINING
SAI TRAINING AND SEQUENCES
SANCHIN KATA: TRADITIONAL TRAINING FOR KARATE POWER
SCALING FORCE
SEARCHING FOR SUPERHUMANS
SHAOLIN KUNG FU FUNDAMENTAL TRAINING 1 & 2
SHAOLIN LONG FIST KUNG FU BEGINNER—INTERMEDIATE—
    ADVANCED SERIES
SHAOLIN SABER: BASIC SEQUENCES
SHAOLIN STAFF: BASIC SEQUENCES
SHAOLIN WHITE CRANE GONG FU BASIC TRAINING SERIES
SHUAI JIAO: KUNG FU WRESTLING
SIMPLE QIGONG EXERCISES FOR HEALTH
SIMPLE QIGONG EXERCISES FOR ARTHRITIS RELIEF
SIMPLE QIGONG EXERCISES FOR BACK PAIN RELIEF
SIMPLIFIED TAI CHI CHUAN: 24 & 48 POSTURES
SIMPLIFIED TAI CHI FOR BEGINNERS 48
SIX HEALING SOUNDS
SUN TAI CHI

SWORD: FUNDAMENTAL TRAINING
TAEKWONDO KORYO POOMSAE
TAI CHI BALL QIGONG SERIES
TAI CHI BALL WORKOUT FOR BEGINNERS
TAI CHI CHUAN CLASSICAL YANG STYLE
TAI CHI FIGHTING SET
TAI CHI FIT: 24 FORM
TAI CHI FIT: ALZHEIMER'S PREVENTION
TAI CHI FIT: CANCER PREVENTION
TAI CHI FIT FOR VETERANS
TAI CHI FIT: FOR WOMEN
TAI CHI FIT: FLOW
TAI CHI FIT: FUSION BAMBOO
TAI CHI FIT: FUSION FIRE
TAI CHI FIT: FUSION IRON
TAI CHI FIT: HEALTHY BACK SEATED WORKOUT
TAI CHI FIT: HEALTHY HEART WORKOUT
TAI CHI FIT IN PARADISE
TAI CHI FIT: OVER 50
TAI CHI FIT OVER 50: BALANCE EXERCISES
TAI CHI FIT OVER 50: SEATED WORKOUT
TAI CHI FIT OVER 60: GENTLE EXERCISES
TAI CHI FIT OVER 60: HEALTHY JOINTS
TAI CHI FIT OVER 60: LIVE LONGER
TAI CHI FIT: STRENGTH
TAI CHI FIT: TO GO
TAI CHI FOR WOMEN
TAI CHI FUSION: FIRE
TAI CHI QIGONG
TAI CHI PUSHING HANDS SERIES
TAI CHI SWORD: CLASSICAL YANG STYLE
TAI CHI SWORD FOR BEGINNERS
TAI CHI SYMBOL: YIN YANG STICKING HANDS
TAIJI & SHAOLIN STAFF: FUNDAMENTAL TRAINING
TAIJI CHIN NA IN-DEPTH
TAIJI 37 POSTURES MARTIAL APPLICATIONS
TAIJI SABER CLASSICAL YANG STYLE
TAIJI WRESTLING
TRAINING FOR SUDDEN VIOLENCE
UNDERSTANDING QIGONG SERIES
WATER STYLE FOR BEGINNERS
WHITE CRANE HARD & SOFT QIGONG
YANG TAI CHI FOR BEGINNERS
YOQI: MICROCOSMIC ORBIT QIGONG
YOQI QIGONG FOR A HAPPY HEART
YOQI:QIGONG FLOW FOR HAPPY MIND
YOQI:QIGONG FLOW FOR INTERNAL ALCHEMY
YOQI QIGONG FOR HAPPY SPLEEN & STOMACH
YOQI QIGONG FOR HAPPY KIDNEYS
YOQI QIGONG FLOW FOR HAPPY LUNGS
YOQI QIGONG FLOW FOR STRESS RELIEF
YOQI: QIGONG FLOW TO BOOST IMMUNE SYSTEM
YOQI SIX HEALING SOUNDS
YOQI: YIN YOGA 1
WU TAI CHI FOR BEGINNERS
WUDANG KUNG FU: FUNDAMENTAL TRAINING
WUDANG SWORD
WUDANG TAIJIQUAN
XINGYIQUAN
YANG TAI CHI FOR BEGINNERS

AND MANY MORE . . .

more products available from . . .

YMAA Publication Center, Inc. 楊氏東方文化出版中心

1-800-669-8892 • info@ymaa.com • www.ymaa.com

YMAA
PUBLICATION CENTER